D1524523

Hearing for the Speech-Language Pathologist and Health Care Professional

Butterworth-Heinemann Series in Communication Disorders

Charlena M. Seymour, Ph.D. Series Editor

Battle, D.E. *Communication Disorders in Muticultural Populations* (1993)

Billeaud, F.P. *Communication Disorders in Infants and Toddlers: Assessment and Intervention* (1993)

Huntley, R.A. & Helfer, K.S. *Communication in Later Life* (1995)

Kricos, P.B. & Lesner, S.A. *Hearing Care for the Older Adult: Audiologic Rehabilitation* (1995)

Maxon, A.B. & Brackett, D. *The Hearing-Impaired Child: Infancy Through High School Years* (1992)

Wall, L.G. *Hearing for the Speech-Language Pathologist and Health Care Professional* (1995)

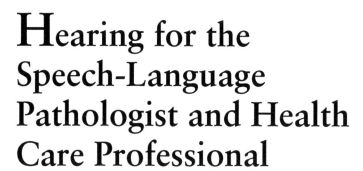

Hearing for the Speech-Language Pathologist and Health Care Professional

Lida G. Wall, PhD

Chair, Department of Speech and Hearing Science,
The Ohio State University, Columbus

Butterworth–Heinemann

Boston   Oxford   Melbourne   Singapore   Toronto   Munich   New Delhi   Tokyo

Every effort has been made to ensure that the drug dosage schedules within this text are accurate and conform to standards accepted at time of publication. However, as treatment recommendations vary in the light of continuing research and clinical experience, the reader is advised to verify drug dosage schedules herein with information found on product information sheets. This is especially true in cases of new or infrequently used drugs.

Recognizing the importance of preserving what has been written, Butterworth–Heinemann prints its books on acid-free paper whenever possible.

Library of Congress Cataloging-in-Publication Data
Hearing for the speech-language pathologist and health care
  professional / [edited by] Lida G. Wall.
      p.   cm.
  Includes bibliographical references and index.
  ISBN 0-7506-9526-9 (alk. paper)
  1. Hearing disorders. 2. Hearing aids.   I. Wall, Lida G.
  [DNLM: 1. Hearing Disorders. 2. Hearing Aids.   WV 270 H43453
  1955]
RF290.H432   1995
617.8--dc20
DNLM/DLC
for Library of Congress   95–15261
                                                          CIP

British Library Cataloguing-in-Publication Data
A catalogue record for this book is available from the British Library.

The publisher offers discounts on bulk orders of this book.
For information, please write:

Manager of Special Sales
Butterworth–Heinemann
313 Washington Street
Newton, MA 02158-1626

10 9 8 7 6 5 4 3 2 1

Printed in the United States of America

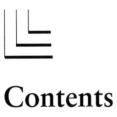

Contents

Preface   vii

Acknowledgments   ix

Contributors   xi

1 Anatomy and Physiology of the Hearing Mechanism   1
Sharmala V. Naidoo and Lawrence L. Feth

2 Disorders of Hearing in Children   39
Susan D. Dalebout

3 Disorders of Hearing in Adults   71
Lida G. Wall

4 Identification and Evaluation of Hearing Loss in Infants
and Preschool Children   103
Susan D. Dalebout

5 Hearing Screening for School-Aged Children, Adults,
and the Elderly   141
Lida G. Wall

6 Interpretation of Clinical Test Results   171
Kevin M. Fire

7 Hearing Aids   219
Stephanie A. Davidson

8 Assistive Listening Devices   265
Stephanie A. Davidson

9 Tactile Aids and Cochlear Implants   311
   Janet M. Weisenberger

10 Speech and Language Characteristics of Children and
    Adults with Hearing Impairments   337
    Lynne A. Davis

11 Intervention with Elderly   373
    Kevin M. Fire

12 Noise and Hearing Loss   401
    William Melnick

13 Central Auditory Processing Disorders in Children
    and Adults   415
    Jane A. Baran and Frank E. Musiek

    Index   441

Preface

This text is designed to benefit two specific groups: the working professional who needs a ready reference source and the speech-language pathologist in graduate school who needs to become acquainted with hearing and the profession of audiology. The text offers practical suggestions; informative explanations; and available resources for information about the physiology of the auditory system, hearing assessment, hearing disorders, hearing aids, hearing conservation, and aural rehabilitation for children and elderly that speech-language pathologists and health care professionals can readily use.

Speech-language pathologists receive training in a wide variety of speech and language disorders. Commonly, however, very few courses relative to hearing impairment and aural rehabilitation are sprinkled in the curriculum of study. While this may not be a problem for meeting licensure and certification requirements, it may become a problem for the speech-language pathologist in the workplace. It is likely that the speech-language pathologist, particularly in school or nursing home settings, will be considered to be the communication specialist. As the communication specialist, all questions or problems related to speech-language and *hearing* will be considered within the speech-language pathologist's area of expertise.

Although speech-language pathologists may not be directly involved in routine audiology activities, they will most certainly at some time be involved in providing services to individuals who have a hearing disorder. The ongoing relationship that the speech-language pathologist has with the client provides a ready communication path for giving information or answering questions about hearing disorders, follow-up recommendations, hearing conversation, hearing aids, assistive listening devices, and other sensory aids. If an audiologist is available for consultation, the problem for the speech-language pathologist is minimized. In many circumstances, however, an audiologist is not always readily available for interaction.

Educators and health care professionals, on the other hand, may learn some basic information about anatomy and hearing impairment in their curriculum of study, but it is unlikely they will receive instruction regarding management techniques for children or adults with a hearing loss. In addition, these profession-als rarely receive information about assistive listening devices, hearing aids, or tactile and sensory aids in spite of the fact they will frequently encounter individuals with hearing loss in the classroom or clinic.

We hope *Hearing for the Speech-Language Pathologist and Health Care Professional* will prove to be a valuable resource for the practicing speech-language pathologist, the educator, and the health care professional who need the information to review with clients. We also hope it will be useful as a textbook for speech-language pathologists taking an overview course in hearing.

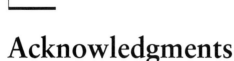

Acknowledgments

Little did I realize, when I couldn't say no to Charlena Seymour, how many hours would be required to write and edit a book on audiology for speech-language pathologists, educators, and health care professionals. My commitment to this project has been both rewarding and frustrating. I found it was very difficult to condense the field of audiology to necessary and useful topics that would benefit speech-language pathologists, educators, and health care professionals. I hope that the selected topics will provide useful and practical information needed for the practice of speech-language pathology and a ready reference for health care professionals and educators.

A few students, who responded to requests for assistance, deserve mention for their contribution to the project. Colleen Noe, a graduate teaching assistant who is now proficient in typing APA reference format, deserves a particular thanks. Without her dedicated help, the reference sections for each chapter might have been shambles, along with the project. Champa Sreenivas, a graduate research assistant, quickly learned the secrets of scanning illustrations and modifying them on MacDraw. The illustrations were done quickly and well. Beth Fuleky and Mary Light are to be thanked for finding all of the "missing" references.

Marcia Woodfill, a lecturer in the Department of Speech and Hearing Science at The Ohio State University and an audiologist at the AG Bell School for the Deaf in Columbus was very helpful in her contributions to Chapter 10, Speech and Language Characteristics of Children and Adults with Hearing Impairments. Her contributions on the psychology of deafness and cochlear implants were much appreciated. I'm sure I ruined more than one day in her life during the past year requesting just one more thing.

A special thanks goes to Ann Lambert, the department secretary and fiscal officer, and Vic Wall, my husband. Both individuals efficiently and without complaint completed all of those tasks I left undone.

Finally, I would like to thank my colleagues for taking the time to contribute to the book. They too were unable to say no and for that I am very grateful. Each of the contributors took time to write a chapter or two in spite of the fact that they were already heavily involved in other teaching and research projects. I cannot thank them enough for taking on one more responsibility.

Contributors

Jane A. Baran, Ph.D.
Professor
Department of Communication
  Disorders
University of Massachusetts
Amherst, MA

Susan D. Dalebout, Ph.D.
Assistant Professor
Communication Disorder Program
Curry School of Education
University of Virginia
Charlottesville, VA

Stephanie A. Davidson, Ph.D.
Assistant Professor
Department of Speech and Hearing
  Science
The Ohio State University
Columbus, OH

Lynne A. Davis, Ph.D.
Clinical Associate, Audiology
Massachusetts Eye and Ear
  Infirmary
Boston, MA

Lawrence L. Feth, Ph.D.
Professor
Department of Speech and Hearing
  Science
The Ohio State University
Columbus, OH

Kevin M. Fire, Ph.D., CCC-A
Associate Professor
Department of Communication
  Disorders
University of North Dakota
Grand Forks, ND

William Melnick, Ph.D.
Professor Emeritus
Department of Speech and Hearing
  Science
Department of Otolaryngology
The Ohio State University
Columbus, OH

Frank E. Musiek, Ph.D.
Professor
Departments of Otolaryngology
  and Neurology
Dartmouth Medical School
Hanover, NH

Director
Deparment of Audiology
Dartmouth-Hitchcock Medical
  Center
Lebanon, NH

Sharmala V. Naidoo, Ph.D.
Senior Research Associate
Hearing and Research
House Ear Institute
Los Angeles, CA

Lida G. Wall, Ph.D.
Professor and Chair
Department of Speech and Hearing
  Science
The Ohio State University
Columbus, OH

Janet M. Weisenberger, Ph.D.
Professor
Department of Speech and Hearing
  Science
The Ohio State University
Columbus, OH

Hearing for the Speech-Language Pathologist and Health Care Professional

1 ⫾

Anatomy and Physiology of the Hearing Mechanism

Sharmala V. Naidoo and Lawrence L. Feth

It is not unusual for situations to arise where speech-language pathologists, health care professionals, and educators need to understand the evaluation of auditory function and the benefits and limitations of hearing aids, assistive listening devices, and perhaps even cochlear implants. A basic understanding of the anatomy and physiology of the auditory system is a prerequisite for comprehension of diagnostic tests and of remedial measures and sensory aids. This chapter is an overview of the structure (anatomy) and function (physiology) of the human auditory system with an emphasis on recent developments in the field.

TERMINOLOGY

Anatomy

The human auditory system comprises the auditory periphery and the central auditory system (Figure 1.1). The peripheral auditory system consists of the outer, middle, and inner ear, and the cochlear nerve. The central auditory system includes the brainstem nuclei, thalamic nuclei, and the auditory cortex.

Acoustics and Auditory Perception

In introductory courses to audiology, one learns that when an object vibrates it sets molecules of air into motion. If the range of vibration is between 20 and 20,000 cycles per second, the movements of air particles may be picked up by the human ear and interpreted as sound. Sound is often described by its pitch and loudness. These terms are subjective descriptors of the physical dimensions of frequency and intensity, respectively. The frequency of sound is the number of vibrations per second. The more vibrations per second, the higher the frequency, which is measured in hertz (Hz). A young human listener is capable of hearing sound within the frequency range of 20 to 20,000 Hz.

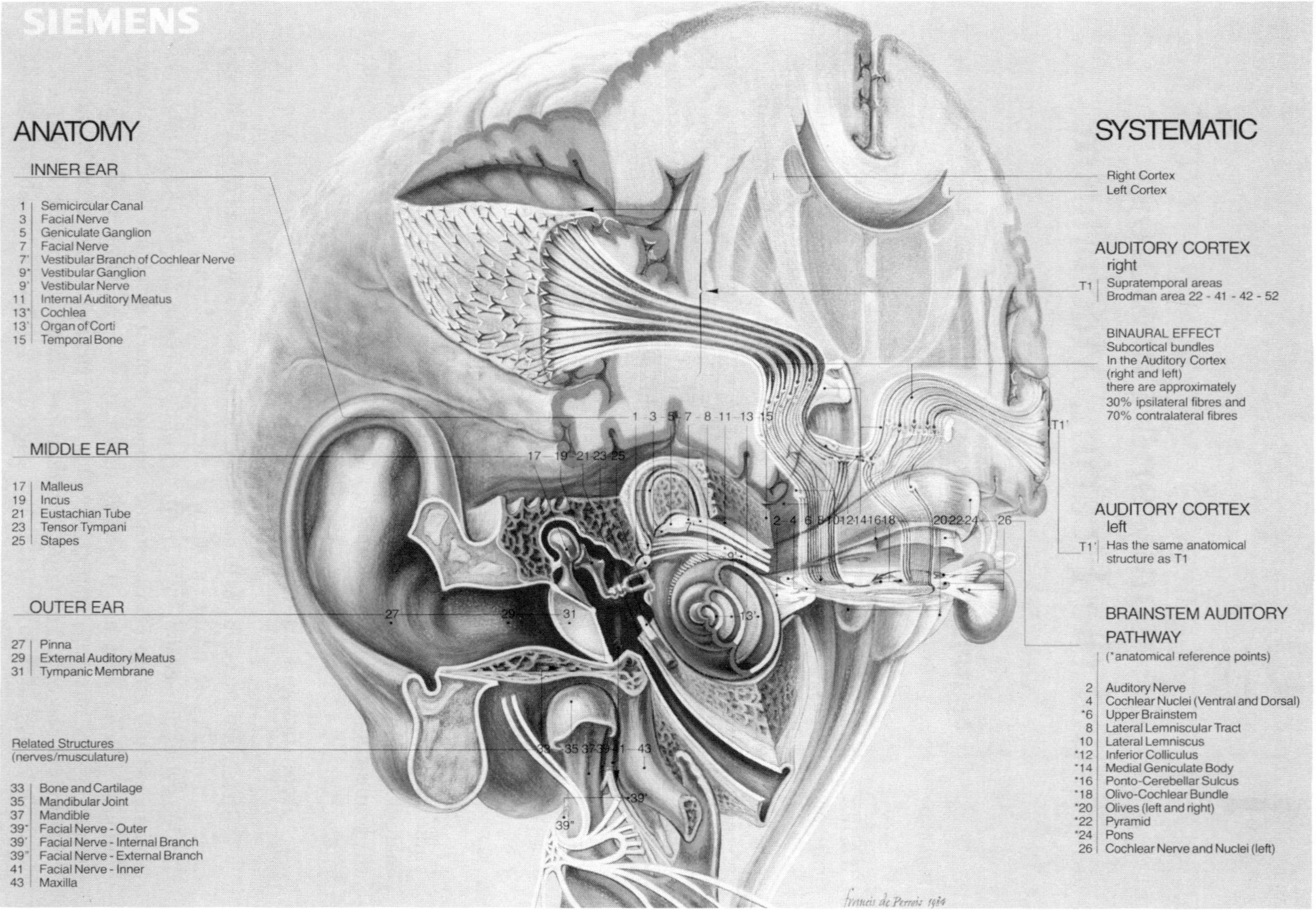
SIEMENS
ANATOMY
INNER EAR
1 Semicircular Canal
3 Facial Nerve
5 Geniculate Ganglion
7 Facial Nerve
7' Vestibular Branch of Cochlear Nerve
9* Vestibular Ganglion
9' Vestibular Nerve
11 Internal Auditory Meatus
13* Cochlea
13' Organ of Corti
15 Temporal Bone
MIDDLE EAR
17 Malleus
19 Incus
21 Eustachian Tube
23 Tensor Tympani
25 Stapes
OUTER EAR
27 Pinna
29 External Auditory Meatus
31 Tympanic Membrane
Related Structures
(nerves/musculature)
33 Bone and Cartilage
35 Mandibular Joint
37 Mandible
39* Facial Nerve - Outer
39' Facial Nerve - Internal Branch
39" Facial Nerve - External Branch
41 Facial Nerve - Inner
43 Maxilla
SYSTEMATIC
Right Cortex
Left Cortex
AUDITORY CORTEX
right
T1 Supratemporal areas
Brodman area 22 - 41 - 42 - 52
BINAURAL EFFECT
Subcortical bundles
In the Auditory Cortex
(right and left)
there are approximately
30% ipsilateral fibres and
70% contralateral fibres
T1'
AUDITORY CORTEX
left
T1' Has the same anatomical
structure as T1
BRAINSTEM AUDITORY
PATHWAY
(*anatomical reference points)
2 Auditory Nerve
4 Cochlear Nuclei (Ventral and Dorsal)
*6 Upper Brainstem
8 Lateral Lemniscular Tract
10 Lateral Lemniscus
*12 Inferior Colliculus
*14 Medial Geniculate Body
*16 Ponto-Cerebellar Sulcus
*18 Olivo-Cochlear Bundle
*20 Olives (left and right)
*22 Pyramid
*24 Pons
26 Cochlear Nerve and Nuclei (left)
francis de Perrois 1984

FIGURE 1.1 Anatomy of the human hearing mechanism from pinna to cortex.

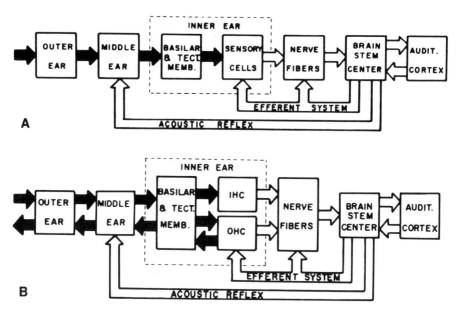

FIGURE 1.2A, B   (A) Classical view of sound energy and information flow in the auditory system.   (B) Contemporary view of the transmission of sound energy through the auditory system. This view includes a reverse flow of acoustic energy from the outer hair cells to the external ear canal.

(Adapted from Dallos, 1988. Reprinted by permission of the American Speech-Language-Hearing Association.)

The second dimension of sound is intensity. The ratio of the most intense to the weakest sound an average listener is capable of listening to is 10^{14}:1. This means one would have to deal with extremely large numbers if a direct measure of intensity were used. The use of the logarithmic scale of intensity, expressed in decibels sound pressure level (dB SPL) or decibels hearing level (dB HL) provides a solution to the problem. The average level at which a human listener barely perceives sound (threshold of hearing) is 0 dB HL, and the dynamic range between threshold of hearing and loudness discomfort level (LDL, the most intense sound a listener can tolerate) is 120 to 140 dB.

Physiology

Figure 1.2A shows the classical view of sound energy and information flow in the auditory system. With this model of hearing, sound energy is carried through the ear canal to the tympanic membrane. The vibrations are transmitted to the ossicles of the middle ear and the movement of the stapes footplate in the oval window induces a sound wave within the fluids of the cochlea. The wave sets the

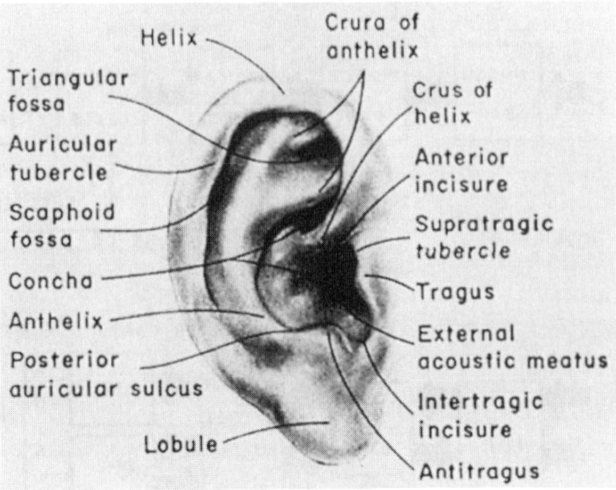

FIGURE 1.3

Parts of the pinna.

(Reprinted from Anson and Donaldson, 1967, with permission from WB Saunders, Philadelphia, Pa.)

basilar membrane and tectorial membrane into motion. The mechanical activity of the basilar membrane and tectorial membrane is delivered to the sensory cells and from there conducted as nerve impulses through the nerve fibers en route to the brainstem and ultimately to the auditory cortex. The auditory efferent system, within the confines of this model, is believed to originate in the brainstem and proceed through the nerve fibers to the sensory cells.

The contemporary view (Figure 1.2B) incorporates two new theories. First, the model indicates an involvement of the outer hair cells in the enhancement of the basilar membrane displacement. Second, the model depicts a reverse flow of acoustic energy from the cochlea to the outer ear.

The contemporary view of the auditory system is discussed in more detail through the course of the chapter. The goal is to reacquaint the reader with the basic anatomy and physiology of the auditory system and introduce the current view of cochlear mechanisms.

THE AUDITORY PERIPHERY

The Outer Ear

The external ear, also known as the auricle or pinna, lies at a 30-degree angle to the side of the head. The core of the external ear is fibrous cartilage (called the auricular cartilage). It is covered tightly by skin and has very little fat except at the lobule. The cartilage is continuous with the cartilaginous skeleton of the ear canal. Three muscles hold the pinna to the temporal bone: the anterior, superior, and posterior auricularis. The parts that compose the pinna are shown in Figure 1.3.

The pinna is innervated by the fifth (trigemenal), the seventh (facial), ninth (glossopharyngeal), and tenth (vagus) cranial nerves. The blood supply to the pinna is the external carotid artery. The auricle plays an important role in localization of high-frequency sounds in the vertical plane and for front-back localization. It is also an important appendage for placement of behind-the-ear (BTE) hearing aids.

The External Auditory Meatus

Sound that impinges on the pinna is channeled into the ear though the external auditory meatus. The ear canal is about 25 mm long in adults. The average width is 7 mm, but the width varies greatly throughout the length of the canal. The opening of the external auditory meatus is oval, and it takes on a curved shape up to the eardrum. The first lateral 10 mm (or one-third) is cartilage and is covered by skin 1 mm thick. This cartilaginous portion can be changed in shape and diameter. During an otoscopic examination the pinna can be pulled up and back to straighten it and obtain a clearer view of the tympanic membrane. The medial portion of the external auditory meatus is bony, and the skin is 0.2 mm thick. The same skin forms the outer layer of the tympanic membrane. The inferior external auditory meatus is innervated by the tenth cranial nerve, and the superior part by the fifth cranial nerve.

In the course of an otoscopic examination cerumen may be encountered within the external auditory meatus. The glands that produce cerumen are the sebaceous glands or ceruminous glands. These glands are located in the lateral one-third to one-half of the ear canal and are not found near the tympanic membrane. There are 1000 to 2000 of these glands within the external auditory meatus. Cerumen is acidic and sticky, may vary in color (light yellow to dark black), and can commonly be mistaken for blood. Cerumen plays an important role within the ear canal by keeping the external auditory meatus moist, inhibiting the formation of bacteria, and preventing insects and foreign objects from migrating too far into the ear canal. Cerumen often moves down the ear canal naturally and carries debris with it.

The ear canal has an acoustic effect, which is displayed as a filter transfer function. In other words, sound pressure at the eardrum is increased as much as 17 dB at 2700 Hz because of effects attributable to the head, body, concha, and pinna (Figure 1.4). At the end of the ear canal is the eardrum (or the tympanic membrane), which separates the outer from the middle ear.

The Middle Ear

The middle ear is an air-filled cavity that includes the tympanic membrane, three ossicles, middle ear muscles and ligaments, and the eustachian (auditory) tube (Figure 1.5). The six walls that make up the middle ear cavity are the superior tegmental wall, the inferior jugular wall, the lateral wall, the posterior mastoid wall, the anterior carotid wall, and the medial labrynthine wall.

The tympanic membrane is cone-shaped. A common observation during otoscopy is a cone-of-light, which is a reflection of otoscopic light from the umbo

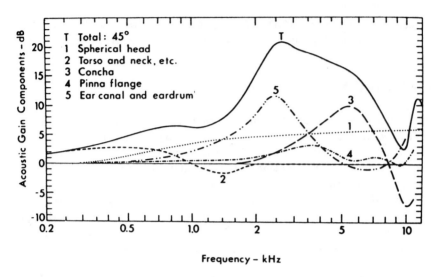

FIGURE 1.4 Filter transfer function of the external ear shows average pressure gain in the human ear canal.

(Reprinted from Shaw, 1974, with permission of authors and Springer-Verlag, Berlin.)

to the edge of the anterior inferior quadrant. There are three layers of the tympanic membrane: the lateral cutaneous layer, the fibrous middle layer or the lamina propria, and the mucous inner layer, which is continuous with the lining of the middle ear. The pars tensa makes up most of the tympanic membrane and provides the necessary tension. The superior section consists of the pars flaccida, which is triangular in shape and is known as Shrapnell's membrane. A normal tympanic membrane is translucent, and the ossicles are visible behind it. At times blood vessels that are part of the blood supply may be seen running across the tympanic membrane.

The middle ear cavity is comprised of three sections: the attic or epitympanic recess, the tympanic cavity, which houses the ossicles, and the hypotympanum or lower part of the tympanic cavity. The lining of the middle ear is a mucous membrane continuous with the lining of the aditus to the mastoid area and the eustachian tube. The middle ear communicates with the mastoid area via the aditus. The eustachian tube extends from the anterior wall of the middle ear (a few millimeters off the floor of the cavity) down to the nasal portion of the pharynx. The trigemenal nerve innervates the eustachian tube. The function of the eustachian tube is to equalize the air pressure in the middle ear with that of the external air pressure. Its functioning is often disrupted in the presence of upper respiratory difficulties and congestion.

There are three ossicles in the middle ear: the malleus (hammer), the incus (anvil), and the stapes (stirrup). The malleus is the largest and heaviest of the three ossicles and is connected to the incus by a ball-and-socket joint. The stapes is the smallest bone; its head is connected to the lenticular process of the incus through

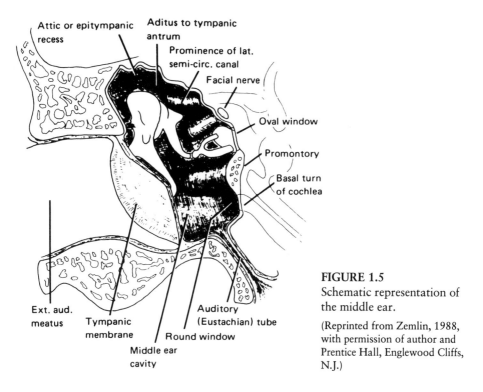

Attic or epitympanic recess

Aditus to tympanic antrum

Prominence of lat. semi-circ. canal

Facial nerve

Oval window

Promontory

Basal turn of cochlea

Ext. aud. meatus

Tympanic membrane

Auditory (Eustachian) tube

Round window

Middle ear cavity

FIGURE 1.5
Schematic representation of the middle ear.

(Reprinted from Zemlin, 1988, with permission of author and Prentice Hall, Englewood Cliffs, N.J.)

the incudostapedial joint, which is extremely vulnerable to damage. The two muscles in the middle ear are: the tensor tympani and the stapedius.

Function of the Middle Ear

One of the roles of the middle ear is impedance matching. Sound travels from the ear canal to the tympanic membrane, which is set into vibration. The vibrations are conducted through the air-filled canal of the outer ear via the ossicles to the oval window (through the stapes footplate) and into the fluid-filled cochlea of the inner ear. There is an impedance mismatch between the air-filled canal of the outer ear and the fluid-filled inner ear. In the absence of the middle ear, 99.9 percent of the sound would be reflected and only 0.1 percent would be transmitted through the oval window. This is a potential loss of 30 dB. The middle ear improves the transfer of energy from the air medium to the fluid medium. The middle ear acts as a sound-pressure transformer (not an amplifier) to overcome the potential loss in sound energy that would occur as a result of the impedance mismatch. The transformation occurs primarily through two mechanisms. First, the ratio of the area of the tympanic membrane to the area of the stapes footplate (17:1) amounts to an increase of approximately 25 dB in sound pressure within the middle ear. Second, the lever action of the malleus and the incus (1.3:1) is equivalent to a small but important increase of 2dB in sound pressure.

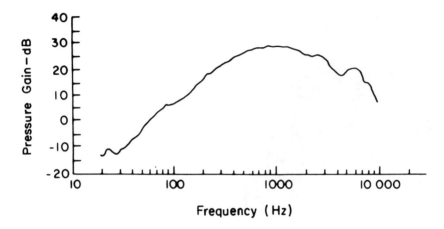

FIGURE 1.6 Transfer function of the middle ear.

(Reprinted from Nedzelnitsky, 1980, with permission of the author and the American Institute of Physics, Woodbury, N.Y.)

The increase in sound pressure is not uniform across all frequencies (Figure 1.6). It depends on the acoustic filtering of the middle ear. The compliance of the tympanic membrane and the enclosed air in the middle the ear cavity results in a decrease of sound pressure at the low frequencies, and the mass of the tympanic membrane and ossicles filters and reduces the response for the high frequencies. This means that the middle ear resonates at 800 to 1000 Hz (Figure 1.6).

Another role of the middle ear is related to the muscles. These muscles were previously considered to have a protective function. The stapedius muscle in particular was observed to contract in response to intense sounds of 90 dB SPL and greater. However, the time delay between the onset of an intense sound and the resultant contraction of the muscle is 120 to 150 msec. This is well beyond the reaction time necessary to protect the ear from damage due to intense impulse sounds. Furthermore, when the muscles contract only low-frequency sounds are attenuated. A more feasible explanation of middle ear muscle function is that the acoustic reflex is necessary for attenuation of low-frequency sounds emitted during chewing and vocalization (Simmons, 1964). The attenuation of intense low-frequency sounds could also result in decreased upward spread of masking (low-frequency sounds influencing high-frequency sounds) under difficult listening conditions.

The Inner Ear

After an air-conducted signal reaches the stapes footplate, the footplate vibrates in the oval window that leads to the inner ear. During bone conduction, the skull is set into vibration with a concomitant movement of the fluids within

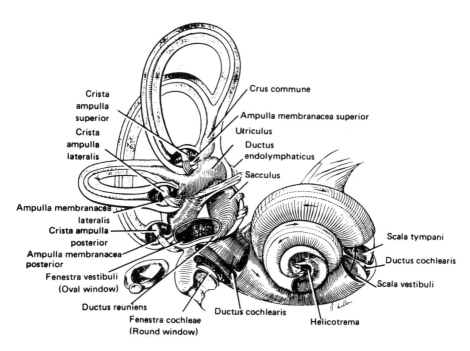

FIGURE 1.7 The vestibular and cochlear components of the inner ear.
(Reprinted with permission from Abbott Laboratories, North Chicago, Ill.)

the cochlea. The cochlea is the most important component of the peripheral auditory system. It is enclosed within a system of cavities within the temporal bone. Until recently, a traditional view of cochlear functioning persisted. However, advanced imaging techniques and the ability to record sound emitted by the cochlea have revealed new insights into inner ear anatomy and physiology. These findings have disputed some of the traditional views of cochlear transduction, namely that (1) the basilar membrane is broadly tuned and is functionally smooth; (2) hair cells are totally passive and are only involved in mechanical transduction; (3) transduction is a passive process and no energy is generated by the cochlea, and (4) energy absorption by the cochlea is essentially complete.

Structure of the Inner Ear

The inner connecting cavities in the temporal bone form the bony labyrinth. Inside the bony labyrinth are the organs of hearing and balance (Figure 1.7). In the bony labyrinth and conforming to its shape is the membranous labyrinth, which contains its own fluid and houses the sensory organs and all sensory cells. The cochlea (the organ of hearing) is a spiral-shaped structure with a base and an apex. An uncoiled representation of the cochlea often demonstrates the relation of frequencies from base (high frequencies) to apex (low frequencies). The membra-

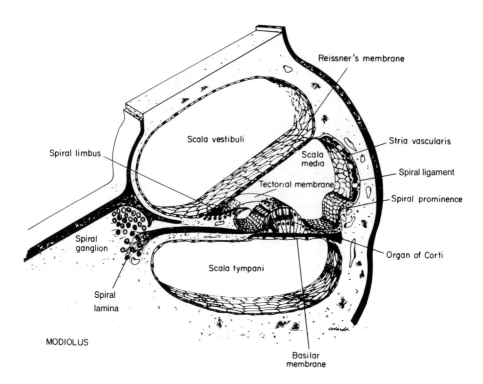

FIGURE 1.8 Cross-section of the cochlear duct shows the organ of Corti situated in the scala media on the basilar membrane.

(Reprinted from Bloom and Fawcett, 1986, with permission of WB Saunders, Phildelphia, Pa.)

nous labyrinth is formed by two membranes attached to the outer wall of the bony cochlea. The floor of the cochlear duct is formed by the osseous spiral lamina and the basilar membrane.

The characteristics of the basilar membrane play an important role in cochlear function. On one end it attaches to the wall of the bony cochlea via the osseous spiral lamina, and on the opposite end it attaches to the bony wall of the cochlea via the spiral ligament (Figure 1.8). Thus the basilar membrane and the osseous spiral lamina separate the scala tympani from the scala media. The roof of the cochlear duct is separated from the scala vestibuli by Reissner's membrane, which forms the top of the cochlear duct. Toward the apex of the cochlea, the scala media becomes smaller and narrower, the osseous spiral lamina becomes narrower, and the basilar membrane widens.

The cochlear duct is lined on its outer edge with the stria vascularis, which supplies blood and nutrients to the cochlea and may be responsible for the manufacture of endolymph. The blood supply to the cochlear duct comes from the labyrinthine artery, which emerges through the internal auditory meatus together with the nerve fibers which exit the temporal bone. A branch of this is the cochlear

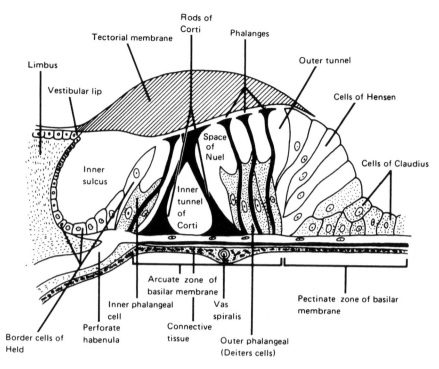

FIGURE 1.9 Supporting structures in the inner ear.

(Reprinted from Zemlin, 1988, with permission of Prentice Hall, Englewood Cliffs, N.J.)

artery, which supplies the stria vascularis with blood. The venous blood leaves the cochlea through the internal auditory vein, which also exits through the internal auditory meatus.

On top of the basilar membrane is the organ of Corti, which runs through the entire length of the cochlear duct. The organ of Corti consists of supporting structures, sensory cells, and nerve fibers. The supporting structures are the pillars of Corti, Deiter cells, cells of Hensen, cells of Claudius, and border cells of Held.

The pillars (or rods) of Corti are triangular and are positioned in the middle of the organ of Corti. The pillars act as a brace and support the other structures. Between the braces is the tunnel of Corti, which is an open space filled with fluid through its entire length (Figure 1.9). The Deiter cells provide most of the support for the outer hair cells and the inner hair cells. The cell bodies sit on top of the basilar membrane and are called the outer pharyngeal and inner pharyngeal cells. Growing out of the cells are the pharyngeal or phalangeal processes, which are slender pillars that run to the top of the organ of Corti and form the upper shelf called the reticular lamina. The cells of Hensen lie on the outside of the outer hair cells and act to support the hair cells. The cells of Claudius provide support for the cells of Hensen. The border cells of Held support the inner hair cells.

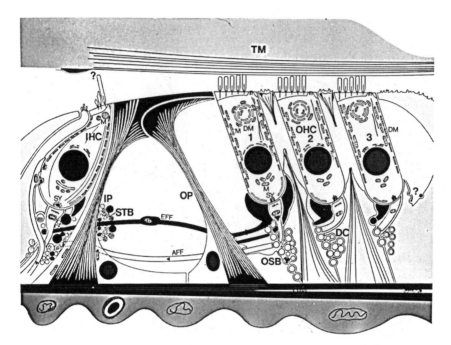

FIGURE 1.10 Schematic of hair cells in organ of Corti resting on the basilar membrane.

(Reprinted from Engström and Engström, 1988, courtesy of Widex Hearing Aid Co., Inc., Stockholm, Sweden.)

The Tectorial Membrane

The tectorial membrane consists of cell-like structures above the organ of Corti; it is made up of fine filaments. The membrane is attached to the spiral limbus on the modiolus side. The opposite end is thought to be attached by fibers to the Hensen cells. The function of the tectorial membrane is to interact with the cilia of the outer hair cells, which in turn begins the transduction process within the hair cells.

Hair Cells in the Organ of Corti

Outer Hair Cells   Two types of hair cells are found in the organ of Corti, namely the outer hair cells and the inner hair cells. Three rows of cylindrical outer hair cells are distributed throughout the scala media (Figure 1.10). The diameter of each outer hair cell is approximately 5 microns. The length of the outer hair cells changes from the base of the cochlea (20 microns) to the apex (50 microns). In other words, the outer hair cells become longer toward the apex of the cochlea. The cells are anchored at the top by the reticular lamina and at the bottom by the Deiter cells. The entire cell body is not supported but is surrounded by endolymph. The upper end of the outer hair cells, which fits into the reticular lamina, is covered

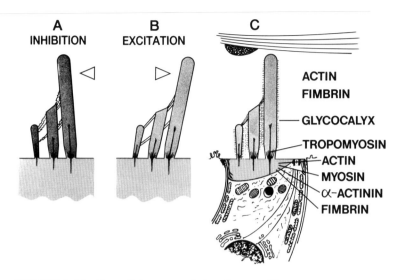

FIGURE 1.11 Cross-links among hair cell stereocilia.

(Reprinted from Engström and Engström, 1988, courtesy of Widex Hearing Aid Co., Inc., Stockholm, Sweden.)

with a thick rigid layer called the cuticular plate. Out of each hair cell through the plate project 100 to 200 stereocilia. The stereocilia and cuticular plate are composed of actin filaments and contain the proteins fimbrin, alpha-actinin, myosin, tropomyosin, and spectrin (Pickles, 1988). The three to four rows of stereocilia form a W pattern. These rows are graded in height. Only the tops of the stereocilia of the tallest row contact the bottom surface of the tectorial membrane. Specialized cross-links (Figure 1.11) between the tips of the shorter cilia and the sides of the taller ones play a role in the gating mechanism during mechanical transduction.

Inner Hair Cells   There are only about 3500 inner hair cells (relatively few compared with the outer hair cells). The inner hair cells are flask-shaped and totally surrounded by their supporting cells. About 60 cilia emerge from the top of each of the inner hair cells. They are coarser, stiffer, and stronger than those on the outer hair cells. There are three rows of cilia that are not neatly graded. There is no evidence that these cilia make contact with the tectorial membrane (Figure 1.10).

Cochlear Mechanics

Basilar Membrane Traveling Wave
Sound waves that enter the ear are transmitted from the tympanic membrane across the ossicles of the middle ear, where the sound pressure is transformed to match the impedance of the inner ear. The oval window membrane is set into vibration, and a pressure wave is initiated within the fluids of the cochlea (if the incoming sound is a 1000 Hz tone, the stapes moves in and out 1000 times per second). The traveling wave response of the basilar membrane moves from the base

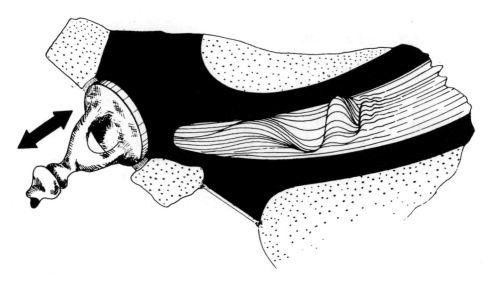

FIGURE 1.12A Schematic of the traveling wave in the cochlea.

(Reprinted from Dallos, 1988, with permission of American Speech-Language-Hearing Association.)

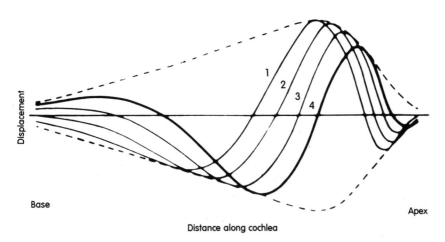

Base

Apex

Distance along cochlea

FIGURE 1.12B Traveling waves in the cochlea as first shown by von Békésy (1960).

(Reprinted from *Experiments in hearing* by von Békésy, 1960, with permission of McGraw-Hill, New York, N.Y.)

to the apex of the cochlea (Figure 1.12A) irrespective of the conductive pathway (air conduction or bone conduction). As the traveling wave moves up the basilar membrane, different portions of the basilar membrane move up and down at

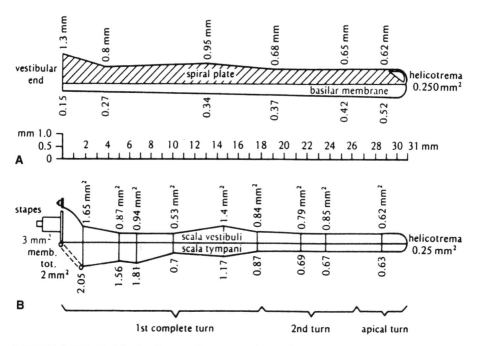

FIGURE 1.13A, B The basilar membrane is wider at the apical end and (A) the scalae are smaller at the apex than at the basal end (B).

(Reprinted from Yost, 1994, with permission from Academic Press, San Diego, Calif.)

various times. The magnitude of the displacement of the membrane changes as the traveling wave traverses the length of the basilar membrane. The envelope of the traveling wave (Figure 1.12B) provides a clear indication of the movement of the basilar membrane.

The width and stiffness of the basilar membrane are two important characteristics that determine the point of maximum displacement for any incoming sound. The basilar membrane is narrower and stiffer at the base and wider and more compliant at the apex of the cochlea, hence this structure responds to low frequencies more efficiently at the apex, whereas a high-frequency sound causes maximum displacement at a point near the base of the basilar membrane (Figure 1.13A, B).

It is worth noting that sounds of low frequency travel through the high-frequency region (basal end) of the cochlea before reaching their point of maximum displacement. In cases of intense low-frequency stimulation, the high-frequency region of the basilar membrane is also set in motion, a phenomenon that partly explains the upward spread of masking. After it reaches its peak, the traveling wave decays rapidly, which provides an asymmetric shape to the displacement envelope (Figure 1.12B). The mapping of frequency to specific locations on the basilar membrane in an orderly manner is termed *tonotopic organization* (Figure 1.13C).

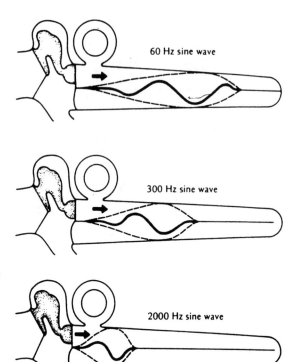

FIGURE 1.13 C
Behavior of the traveling wave
at different frequencies and its
dependence on basilar membrane stiffness gradient.

(Adapted from Zemlin, 1988,
by Yost, 1994. Reprinted with
permission from Prentice Hall,
Englewood Cliffs, N.J.)

Tonotopic (or cochleotopic) organization is maintained within the various
nuclei in the brainstem and in the auditory cortex. The distinctive mark of the
cochlea is the traveling wave with its sharply tuned tuning curve. The traveling
wave moves along the basilar membrane and takes time to reach the point of
maximum displacement. The time taken for the traveling wave to reach maximum
displacement is inversely proportional to the frequency of the incoming sound.
That is, low frequencies, which have their maximum displacement near the apex
of the cochlea (Figure 1.14), take longer than high frequencies, which have their
maximum displacement near the base.

Hair-Cell Excitation
When the basilar membrane is activated and a traveling wave is propagated,
the tectorial membrane moves across the top of the stereocilia of the outer hair
cells in a shearing motion causing displacement of the cilia (Figure 1.11 [A, B] and
Figure 1.15). When the stereocilia are displaced toward the tallest cilia, an
excitatory process is triggered within the outer hair cells. The mechanisms believed
to culminate in action potentials (electrical impulses) traveling centrally in the
eighth nerve are discussed in the following section.

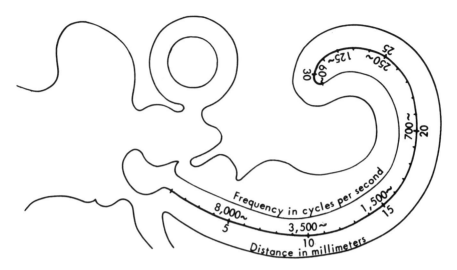

FIGURE 1.14 Relationship between frequency and distance in millimeters along the basilar membrane.

(Reprinted from Zemlin, 1988, with permission of Prentice Hall, Englewood Cliffs, N.J.)

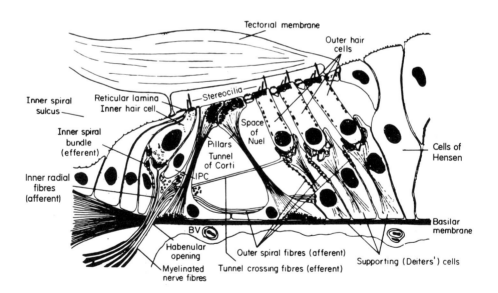

FIGURE 1.15 Cross-section of the organ of Corti.

(Adapted from Ryan and Dallos, 1984, with permission of Little, Brown, Boston, Mass.)

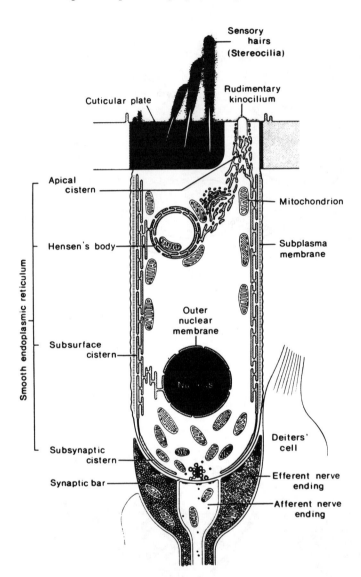

FIGURE 1.16 Schematic of an outer hair cell.

(Reprinted from Lim, 1986, with permssion of author and publisher.)

Role of the Outer Hair Cells

Outer hair cells (Figure 1.16) differ from inner hair cells in cell wall structure, their innervation pattern, and neurotransmitters. The structure of the outer hair cell membrane, in particular the sliding filaments, is conducive to mechanical hydraulic activity, which enables the outer hair cells to contract up to 30,000 times

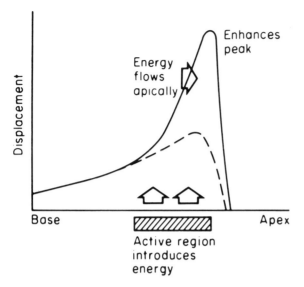

Displacement

Enhances peak

Energy flows apically

Base

Apex

Active region introduces energy

FIGURE 1.17
Enhancement of the initial traveling wave, possibly through active mechanical processes of the outer hair cell.

(Reprinted from Pickles, 1988, with permission of author and Academic Press Ltd, London.)

per second. That is far quicker than the rate of muscle fibers (300 times per second). This means that the outer hair cells are motor cells and are mechanically active, contradicting the traditional view of passive hair cells.

Two types of outer hair cell motility have been described in the literature—slow and fast motility. Slow motility is thought to be related to efferent nerve action and involves lengthwise contractions. Fast motility is believed to enhance the traveling wave and acts as a mechanical amplifier. For an incoming sound, the outer hair cell acts to enhance basilar membrane movement in a local region. In this manner the outer hair cells effect the fine tuning of the magnitude and phase of the traveling wave (Figure 1.17). Thus, displacement of a localized area on the basilar membrane is mechanically sharpened. When the outer hair cells are damaged or destroyed, the result is a broadly tuned basilar membrane and a concomitant hearing loss.

Once the traveling wave is initiated, the greater the movement of the tectorial membrane, the greater is the displacement of the stereocilia. The tips of the outer hair cells are embedded in the tectorial membrane (the inner hair cells have no contact with the tectorial membrane). Links between the stereocilia facilitate radial (or side-to-side) motion. When the stereocilia are pushed toward the tallest cilia, gating occurs; that is, ions enter the hair cell (Figure 1.18).

An electrochemical gradient is set up so that there is a difference in the voltage between the top and the bottom of the hair cell. A receptor potential then triggers the expansion and contraction of the hair cell. It is important to remember that no afferent (sensory) nerve impulses are sent to the brain from the outer hair cells.

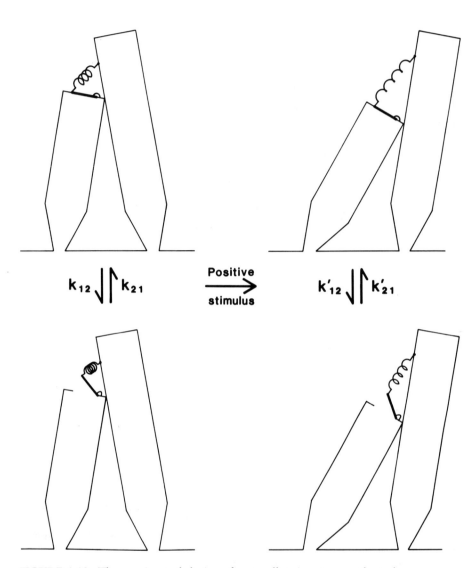

FIGURE 1.18   The opening and closing of pores allow ions to pass through mechanoelectrical transduction channels.

(Reprinted from Hudspeth, 1985, with permission of A. J. Hudspeth and *Science.* Copyright 1985 by the AAAS.)

Role of Inner Hair Cells

The inner hair cells (Figure 1.19) show no evidence of the motile properties of the outer hair cells. They do, however, resemble outer hair cells because of the presence of stereocilia. The inner hair cells are the only sense organs within the

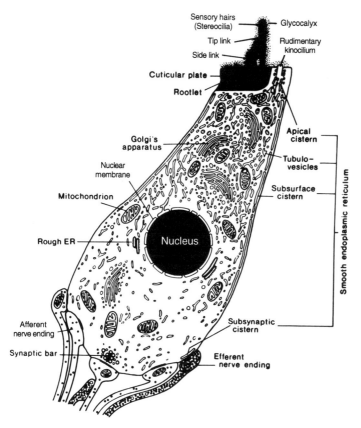

FIGURE 1.19 Schematic of an inner hair cell.
(Reprinted from Lim, 1986, with permission of author and publisher.)

cochlea. Ten to 20 afferent nerve fibers are attached to each inner hair cell. It is postulated that because the inner hair cells are not in contact with the tectorial membrane, direct movement of the basilar membrane and tectorial membrane and resultant motility of the cochlear fluid between the stereocilia is insufficient to induce motion of the cilia at levels within 30 dB of threshold. So how are the inner hair cell stereocilia deflected? The classical view of cochlear mechanics considered both inner hair cells and outer hair cells as passive; however, new developments in auditory physiology contradict that view.

The active cochlea theory discussed up to this point indicates that after the excitation phase of the outer hair cells (when the stereocilia of the outer hair cells move toward the tallest cilium), the outer hair cells move. It is this motility of the hair cells that amplifies and sharpens the initial movement of the basilar membrane. The result is an increase in the motion of the fluid surrounding the stereocilia of the inner hair cell and a displacement of inner hair cell cilia near the point of maximum displacement of the basilar membrane, that is, at a region corresponding to a specific frequency. This leads to hair-bundle coupling, gating, and establishment of an electrochemical gradient within the inner hair cell. Transmitter substances are eventually released into the synaptic cleft of the afferent nerve endings. The role of the outer hair cells is analogous to a parent's pushing a small child on a swing. The child's movement depends on the assistance of the parent.

In summary, evidence of outer hair cell motility has challenged the traditional view of the passive role of the outer hair cells. It is now known that the outer hair cells and inner hair cells can be differentiated in structure and function and that they play different important roles in the sensory processing of sound.

Another traditional view of cochlear transduction has been contradicted. It was previously postulated that energy absorption in the cochlea is essentially complete; in other words, the system is perfectly damped and no energy is reflected. This view has been in essence coupled with the view that the basilar membrane is functionally smooth and that its properties do not vary greatly from point to point. The basilar membrane may be highly irregular, and thresholds may change considerably within a few Hertz. This discovery has led to the use of the term *microstructure* of the audibility curve.

Otoacoustic Emissions

In 1978, Kemp reported that the human ear is capable of producing sound in response to acoustic stimulation—evoked otoacoustic emmissions (OAEs)—and of emitting sound in the absence of any auditory stimulation (spontaneous OAEs). The presence of OAEs has been attributed to the motility of the outer hair cells (Kemp, 1978) in conjunction with the activation of the cochlear efferent system. It is conceivable that the mechanisms responsible for nonlinearity and sharp-tuning within the basilar membrane have been related to the production of the emissions (Dallos, 1988). The additional energy is believed to be produced by the motility of the outer hair cells in the inner ear. It can be recorded using a very sensitive microphone in the ear canal (Figure 1.20A).

OAEs are generally classified as spontaneous OAEs or evoked OAEs. Spontaneous OAEs are narrow bands of acoustic energy that are produced in the absence of external stimulation. There are three subcategories of evoked OAEs. Transient evoked otoacoustic emmissions (TEOAE) are generated in response to brief acoustic signals such as clicks or tone bursts. Stimulus-frequency otoacoustic emissions (SFOAE) are a result of a low-level continuous tone swept across a frequency range. Distortion product otoacoustic emissions (DPOAE) are elicited in the presence of two continuous pure tones. The most common DPOAE measured (and of the most diagnostic significance) in human ears is the cubic difference tone. If the stimulating tones are delivered at frequencies F1 and F2, the cubic difference tone is found at frequency $2f_1-f_2$ (Figure 1.20B).

The recording of OAEs (see Figure 1.20C on page 24) is a simple noninvasive method of rapidly obtaining objective information about the status of the periph-

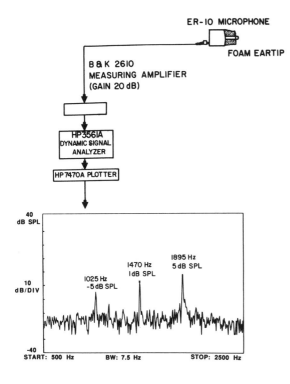

FIGURE 1.20A
Recording equipment for spontaneous otoacoustic emissions.

(Reprinted from Martin et al, 1990, with permission of authors and publisher.)

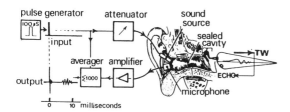

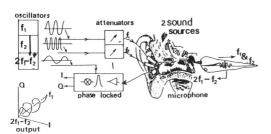

FIGURE 1.20B
Top—A basic transient OAE detector system. *Bottom*—A system for recording of distortion product otoacoustic emissions.

(Reprinted from Kemp et al, 1990, with permission of publisher.)

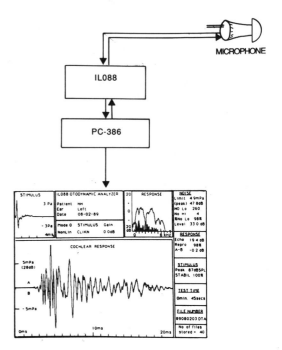

FIGURE 1.20C
Transient emissions showing
frequency measured using
spectrum and emission waveform in the time domain.
Patient record and stimulus
are shown at the top center.

(Reprinted from Kemp et al,
1990, with permission of
publisher.)

eral auditory system. Emissions in human ears are generally reduced or absent in the presence of temporary or permanent sensorineural hearing loss, for example, hearing loss due to acoustic overstimulation or to ototoxic drugs (Figure 1.21).

One of the advantages of OAE testing is the role in isolating the sensory component of a sensorineural hearing loss (Robinette, 1992). Collet et al (1993) showed that click-evoked OAEs were absent when hearing loss at the best hearing frequency exceeded 40 dB HL. OAEs, especially transient evoked OAEs and distortion product OAEs, have been used to screen newborns, obtain audiometric information in difficult-to-test clients, and to diagnose and monitor changes in progressive or recuperating dysfunctions of the ear (presbycusis, Ménière's disease, and middle ear pathology).

The Cochlear Nerve

A tone produces a maximum of basilar membrane displacement at a site along its length that depends on the frequency of the tone. The intensity of the tone determines the size of the displacement. When the displacement is of sufficient magnitude, the inner hair cells are activated to release a transmitter substance at

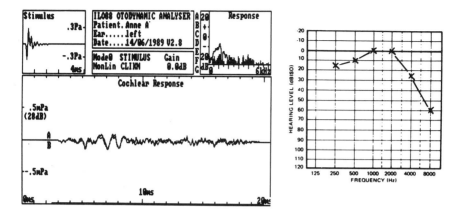

FIGURE 1.21 Emissions from a patient with a high-frequencty hearing loss. (Reprinted from Kemp et al, 1990, with permission of publisher.)

their bases. This substance may then excite the postsynaptic membrane of the eighth-nerve dendrites supplied to each inner hair cell. The sensitivity of the ear to very weak sounds is enhanced by the mechanical amplification affected by the motion of nearby outer hair cells. It is estimated that outer hair cell activity makes the normal ear 30 to 40 dB more sensitive than it would be in the absence of this action. Because outer hair cell action is restricted to a narrow region around the frequency of maximum response, frequency selectivity is also enhanced.

The auditory nerve fibers pass from the modiolus to the internal auditory meatus, where they join the vestibular branch to form the eighth cranial nerve. The facial nerve (seventh cranial nerve) also passes through the internal auditory meatus. Each neuron in the auditory branch of the eighth cranial nerve consists of a cell body, a dendrite that receives information from an inner hair cell in the cochlea, and the axon that carries information from the excited cell body to the next neural unit (Figure 1.22).

In the auditory periphery, the dendritic endings that attach to the inner hair cells travel through the habenula perforata (small openings in the bony spiral lamina) toward the modiolus. This portion of the auditory nerve fiber is unmyelinated. The dendrites are supplied by cell bodies that form the spiral ganglion (in Rosenthal's canal in the modiolus). The axons from each cell body exit through the internal auditory meatus as part of the eighth cranial nerve and proceeds to the cochlear nucleus into the brainstem.

There are two types of auditory neurons in the spiral ganglion, type I and type II. Type I neurons supply myelinated, bipolar dendrites that make up 95 percent of the fibers in the Organ of Corti. They are believed to synapse only with inner hair cells. Each inner hair cell is innervated by about 20 afferent dendrites.

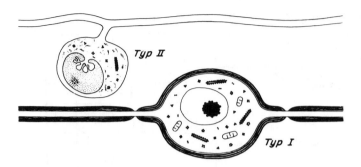

FIGURE 1.22   A typical bipolar sensory neuron.

(Reprinted from Spoendlin, 1978, with permission of author and
Academic Press, Ltd, London.)

Each neuron supplies a dendrite to only one inner hair cell. The remaining 5 percent of afferent fibers are from smaller type II cells. They supply unmyelinated (outer spiral bundle), monopolar dendrites that cross the tunnel of Corti and synapse onto six to ten outer hair cells (Figure 1.23). The afferent fibers conduct sensory information from the inner hair cells toward the central auditory nervous system. The efferent fibers primarily carry information from the level of the olivo-cochlea bundle to synapse onto the outer hair cells.

Each dendrite of afferent peripheral auditory neurons has two portions: an unmyelinated part and a myelinated portion. A graded electrical potential (generator potential) proportional to the stimulus strength is established in the unmyelinated portion of the dendrite (where the dendrite synapses onto the inner hair cell). Each neuron has a threshold of firing, so the generator potential must exceed a critical level to elicit a response in the axon of the nerve fiber. The response in the axon, however, is not graded but occurs in the form of neural spikes that function according to the all-or-none principle. Once the spike potential is initiated, the spike travels the entire length of the neuron to the next point of synapse in the central auditory nervous system.

CENTRAL AUDITORY NERVOUS SYSTEM

The central nervous system (CNS) consists of the brain and the spinal cord (Figure 1.24). The brain includes the cerebrum, cerebellum, and brainstem. The eighth-nerve afferent auditory fibers enter the brainstem at the junction of the medulla and the pons, where they synapse onto cell bodies of second-order neurons in the cochlear nucleus (Figure 1.25). There are parallel pathways from each ear that conduct sensory information contralaterally and ipsilaterally up the central auditory system.

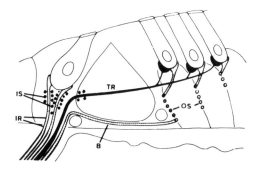

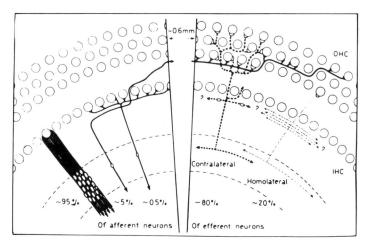

FIGURE 1.23 *Top*—Afferent and efferent innervation of the organ of Corti. *Bottom*—Arrangement of nerve fibers to the inner and outer hair cells.

(Reprinted from Spoendlin, 1975, with permission of publishers.)

Cochlear Nucleus

All afferent nerve fibers from the cochlea synapse within the cochlear nucleus. The cochlear nucleus is divided into three sections: anterior-ventral cochlear nucleus, posterior-ventral cochlear nucleus, and dorsal cochlear nucleus. Each of these sections exhibits tonotopic organization (Figure 1.26). On entering the cochlear nucleus, eighth-nerve fiber branches to the anterior-ventral cochlear nucleus, which relays afferent information, and to the posterior-ventral cochlear nucleus and the dorsal cochlear nucleus, where more complex processing occurs.

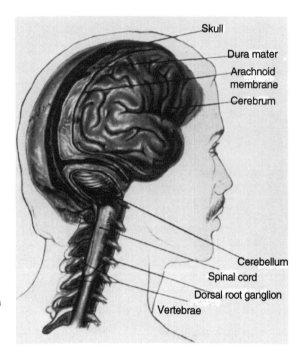

FIGURE 1.24
Relation of the brain and spinal cord to the head and neck.

(Reprinted from Carlson, 1991, with permission of author and publisher. Copyright © 1991 by Allyn and Bacon, Boston, Mass.)

The axons of these second-order neurons proceed to the ipsilateral and contralateral superior olivary complex, or nuclei of the lateral lemniscus, or to the inferior colliculus.

Superior Olivary Complex

The superior olivary complex is a collection of nuclei in the brainstem above the cochlear nuclei. Third-order neurons and the auditory efferent nerve fibers arise from the superior olivary complex. The lateral and medial nuclei are the major divisions of the superior olivary complex (Figure 1.27).

A third nucleus is the trapezoid body. The lateral nucleus and medial nucleus receive nerve fibers from both ears, making the superior olivary complex the first binaural processing center in the central auditory nervous system. This is important for sound localization, which is accomplished through comparisons of interaural time and intensity cues. The lateral nucleus of the superior olivary complex is the largest nucleus and is tonotopically organized, especially in the high frequencies; it is consequently involved in comparisons of interaural intensity differences. The medial nucleus of the superior olivary complex, on the other hand, is sensitive to low- to mid-frequency signals and interaural time differences. The medial nucleus

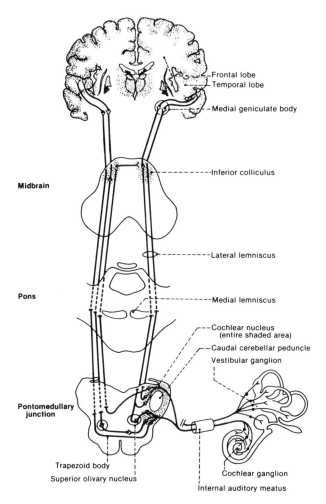

FIGURE 1.25
Cochlear pathways of the eighth cranial nerve.

(Reprinted from De Myer, 1988, with permission of Williams & Wilkins, Baltimore, Md.)

of the superior olivary complex receives direct fibers from the ipsilateral and contralateral anterior-ventral cochlear nuclei and proceeds to the ipsilateral inferior colliculus via the lateral lemniscus tract. The fibers from the lateral nucleus of the superior olivary complex proceed to the inferior colliculus ipsilaterally and contralaterally.

Olivo-Cochlear Bundle

The efferent auditory nervous system transmits information from higher centers of the central auditory nervous system to lower areas. The olivo-cochlear bundle is one such pathway (Figure 1.28).

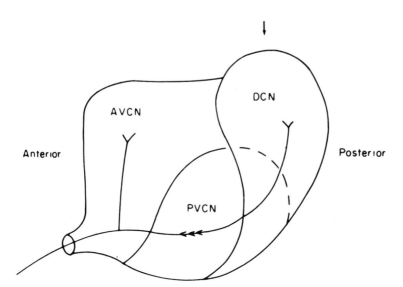

FIGURE 1.26 Schematic of saggital section of the cochlear nucleus of a cat. VCN, anterior-ventral cochlear nucleus; DCN, dorsal cochlear nucleus; PVCN, posterior-ventral cochlear nucleus.

(Reprinted from Pickles, 1988, with permission of author and Academic Press Ltd, London.)

   The efferent fibers that originate bilaterally in the superior olivary complex are either crossed (fibers from the contralaral nucleus) or uncrossed (fibers from the ipsilateral nucleus). Ten to 25 percent of the fibers form the uncrossed olivo-cochlear bundle and arise almost exclusively from the ipsilateral lateral nucleus. The remaining units of the olivo-cochlear bundle make up the crossed olivo-cochlear bundle. These fibers arise from the large cell bodies of the medial nucleus. The endings of the uncrossed olivo-cochlear bundle terminate onto the dendrites of the afferent fibers supplied to the inner hair cells on the same side of the head. The fibers of the crossed olivo-cochlear bundle attach directly onto the outer hair cells in the contralateral cochlea. Each outer hair cell has six to ten efferent fibers supplied to it, the number of efferent fibers decreasing from base to apex. The threshold of the efferent fibers is higher than that of the afferent fibers; that is, it takes more sound pressure to activate the efferent fibers. The effect of the efferent fibers is inhibitory. Activation of the efferent fibers decreases the whole-nerve action potential and inhibits the activity of the afferent nerve fibers.

   The hypotheses are that the olivo-cochlear bundles (1) improve the signal-to-noise ratio (S/N) to assist the listener in extracting the signal from a background of noise, (2) may help to protect the cochlea from acoustic trauma, (3) may control the mechanical state of the cochlea, and (4) may play a role in attention (Pickles, 1988).

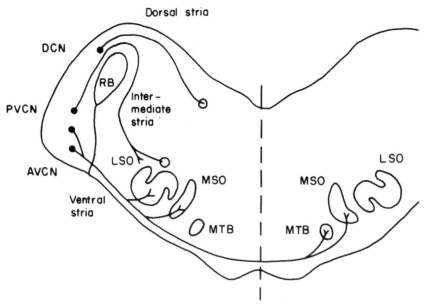

FIGURE 1.27 Three main outflows of the cochlear nucleus on a transverse section of a brainstem of a cat. RB, restiform body; AVCN, anteroventral cochlear nucleus; DCN, dorsal cochlear nucleus; MSO, medial nucleus of the superior olive; LSO, lateral nucleus of the superior olive; MTB, medial nucleus of the trapezoid body; PVCN, posteroventral cochlear nucleus.

(Reprinted from Pickles, 1988, with permission of author and Academic Press Ltd, London.)

Inferior Colliculus

Afferent nerve fibers from the cochlear nucleus and the superior olivary complex have their next synapse in the inferior colliculus. The inferior colliculus together with the superior colliculus are in the midbrain (Figure 1.29 on page 33).

The superior colliculus plays a role in vision and in mapping of audiovisual space. The inferior colliculus is tonotopically organized and receives input bilaterally from the superior olivary complex and contralaterally from the dorsal cochlear nucleus. Complex analyses of signals occur in the inferior colliculus, some fibers may fire to certain features of the signal. Interaural time and intensity cues for bilateral localization are also processed here. Zrull and Coleman (1991) investigated a model for the development and recovery of function in the central auditory system. They grafted fetal rat tissue from the inferior colliculus into lesioned areas of the inferior colliculi of adult rats. The results indicated that most of the grafts from the fetal tissue formed neural connections similar to those in the adult rat inferior colliculus before the lesions were made. Further research is needed to establish restored function of afferent neural inputs to the cortex and

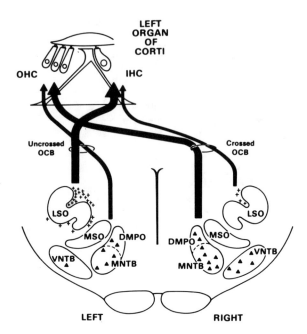

FIGURE 1.28
The olivo-cochlear bundle.
OCB, olivo-cochlear bundle;
LSO, lateral nucleus of superior
olive; MSO, medial nucleus of
superior olive; DMPO, dorsal
periolivary nucleus; MNTB,
medial nucleus of trapezoid
body; VNTB, ventral nucleus
of trapezoid body.

(Reprinted from Gelfand, 1990,
with permission of Marcel Dekker,
New York, N.Y.)

its implications for recovery of auditory function in areas of lesions in the human central auditory nervous system.

Medial Geniculate Body of the Thalamus

Fibers from the inferior colliculus synapse within the medial geniculate body in the thalamus. The medial geniculate body receives input from the ipsilateral and possibly from the contralateral inferior colliculus. Fibers leave the medial geniculate body to synapse ipsilaterally with the auditory cortex (anterior transverse temporal lobe, or Heschl's gyrus). The medial geniculate body is sensitive to differences in time and intensity cues and is involved in speech processing.

Auditory Cortex

The nerve fibers from the medial geniculate body proceed to the auditory cortex, which is the highest level of the auditory pathway. Ipsilateral ascending fibers proceed to the ipsilateral temporal lobe. The main areas for auditory processing in the temporal lobe are usually coded by a letter and a roman numeral, such as AI, also known as the Heschl gyrus or the transverse gyrus (Figure 1.30). Most of the cells in AI respond to sound. There are six layers of cells, layer four being especially concentrated with cells that are responsive to sound. Cells

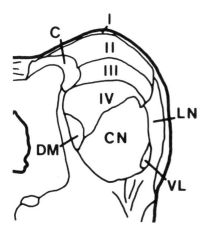

FIGURE 1.29
Transverse section of the inferior colliculus as defined by Morest and Oliver (1984).

(Adapted from Pickles, 1988, with permission of author and Academic Press Ltd, London.)

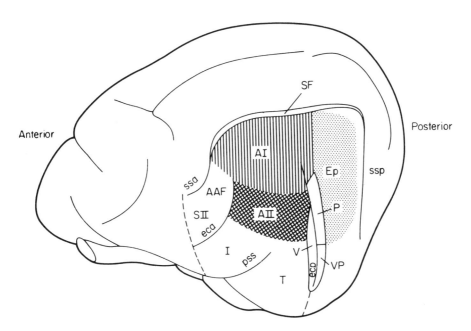

FIGURE 1.30 The cortical auditory areas in the cat. AI, primary auditory cortex; AII, secondary auditory cortex; AAF, anterior auditory field; Ep, posterior ectosylvian field; P, posterior field; VP, ventral posterior field; SII, secondary somatosensory area; I, insular area; T, temporal area; SF, suparasylvian fringe area; ssa and ssp, anterior and posterior suprasylvian sulci; eca and ecp, anterior and posterior ectosylvian sulci; pss, pseudosylvian sulcus.

(Adapted from Pickles, 1988, with permission of author and Academic Press Ltd, London.)

organized in columns along isofrequency strips across the AI are believed to play a role in frequency analysis. On the other hand, cells involved in time-intensity analyses are arranged in layers. Tuning curves from some of the AI region are sharply tuned, others are broadly tuned at high intensities, and yet others are multipeaked. The AI is also involved in binaural and temporal processing of information.

The role of the auditory cortex is integrative; more complex processing of sound requires increased involvement of the auditory cortex. According to Heffner and Heffner (1990), auditory cortical lesions in primates affect detection and localization of sound and identification of speech sounds. The AII (auditory cortex, secondary area) does not receive any ascending fibers from the medial geniculate body of the thalamus. Many of the inputs to the AII arise from the AI. The cells in the AII are not well organized tonotopically for frequency, and many cells exhibit broad tuning curves. Some cells that respond to sound may also be stimulated by information from other senses, such as vision and somatosensation.

Interhemispheric Connections

The left and right hemispheres of the brain are connected by a tract of fibers called the corpus callosum. The two auditory cortices are linked via the auditory pathway of the corpus callosum. The role of the interhemispheric connection is to provide redundancy for complex processing. Although the both cortices communicate with each other, there is some specialization of function. For example, most people process speech in the left hemisphere and process nonverbal sound such as music in the right hemisphere.

In summary, the route of an incoming sound stimulus has been delineated from the external ear canal through the cochlea and to the high centers in the brain. New developments in understanding the structure and function of the auditory system, such as the active role of outer hair cells and the generation of OAEs, have been described. As new discoveries about the auditory system are reported, additional questions arise such as: Is it possible to restore hearing? In this age of technological advances, is sensory hearing loss reversible?

HAIR-CELL REGENERATION

A hearing loss occurs when there is damage to the receptor cells as a result of exposure to ototoxins, acoustic trauma, or temporal bone fracture. The exact relation between amount of hair-cell loss and magnitude of hearing loss has not been established (Weisleder & Rubel, 1993). In mammals the full complement of inner and outer hair cells is present at birth. According to Weisleder and Rubel (1993), until recently it was believed that any hair-cell loss during the course of life was permanent and irreversible. Birds, fish, and amphibians, however, continually grow and regenerate hair cells throughout their life time. Investigations by Weisleder and Rubel (1992) in birds demonstrated that the vestibular system of birds is able to regenerate hair cells postnatally after exposure to aminoglycosides. Several questions (Weisleder & Rubel, 1993) emerge from these revolutionary findings:

What cells are responsible for renewed growth of hair cells?
What triggers the response? Do the new hair cells resemble previously undamaged hair cells?
Do mammals demonstrate similar regeneration?
What are the implications for humans?

It has been postulated that supporting cells are involved in regeneration of hair cells (Corwin, 1992; Corwin & Warchol, 1991; Forge et al, 1993; Warchol et al, 1993; Weisleder & Rubel, 1992). When the link between the stereocilia and supporting structures is severed, the supporting cells are triggered to repair the damaged links. In cold-blooded vertebrates, supporting cells can divide into either additional supporting cells or into hair cells to replace damaged cells. It is not clear what cells are responsible for regeneration in birds. It is believed that regeneration occurs either by involvement of cells outside the sensory epithelium or by proliferation of supporting cells.

Research in the area of hair-cell regeneration demonstrates that after partial or total elimination of hair cells, hair cells can regenerate on the periphery of the cochlea until they are of a normal number, density, and type. Normal connection to the brain is made through regeneration of efferent and afferent fibers (Weisleder & Rubel, 1993). Experiments that utilized evoked potentials indicated appropriate recovery and function of the acoustic nerve. Furthermore, behavioral measurements in starlings, after exposure to gentamycin, demonstrated recovery of threshold responses. There are, however, some shortcomings, especially the abnormal orientation of new stereociliary bundles. It is believed that this abnormality could lead to hearing loss.

In conclusion, hair-cell regeneration has been found in birds after exposure to ototoxic drugs and noise damage. Hair-cell regeneration leads to sensory and perceptual recovery in some animals. However, there is insufficient information regarding complex sound perception. Mammals have an auditory epithelium different from that of lower vertebrates (Manley, 1990); however, the vestibular epithelium is morphologically similar in all vertebrate classes. Research in regeneration demonstrates recovery of hair cells in the utricle, cristae, and sacculi of guinea pigs and in the vestibules of adult humans in vitro after exposure to aminoglycosides (Warchol et al, 1993). There is a need for extensive experimentation into the proliferation of hair cells in the organ of Corti. Further research is required to determine the nature of the signals responsible for proliferation of new hair cells, and whether these signals can be stimulated in the inner ear of humans (Weisleder & Rubel, 1993).

CONCLUSION

The following is a summary of what is known and what is still unknown about the auditory system.

1. It is now known that the basilar membrane displacement is much more sharply tuned than was once believed. Because of the active mechanical filtering effected by the outer hair cells, there is no need for neural sharpening.

2. Outer hair cells are mechanically active and may sharpen the response to sound of the basilar membrane. The outer hair cells are possibly affected by the cochlear efferent system.

3. The basilar membrane is functionally highly irregular, and thresholds change significantly within a few hertz, resulting in a microstructure of the audibility curve.

4. The cochlea may function as a spontaneous source of acoustic energy in people with normal hearing. This process is believed to be related to the motility of the outer hair cells. The exact mechanisms for generation of OAEs is yet to be discovered. OAEs have contributed to our understanding of how the medial olivo-cochlear efferent system influences the receptor potentials of the inner hair cells (Brown et al, 1983). There is a need to determine whether the different types of OAEs are indicative of similar or unique stages of processing (Probst et al, 1991).

5. It is possible to restore normal neuronal connections in the lesioned inferior colliculus of an adult rat by means of fetal rat tissue obtained from the caudal tectum. It is unknown whether this results in restoration of normal auditory processing. The implications for lesions in the human central auditory nervous system, likewise, are not known.

6. There is evidence of hair cell regeneration in the vestibular organs of birds. The regeneration is primarily due to the proliferation of supporting cells. This may have implications for restoration of hearing and balance in humans. There is a need to identify what initiates hair cell regeneration in mammals and whether it can be stimulated in the damaged cochleae of humans.

REFERENCES

Abbott Laboratories (1946). *An atlas of some pathologial conditions of the eye, ear, and throat*. North Chicago: Abbott.

Anson, B. J., & Donaldson, J. A. (1981). *The surgical anatomy of the temporal bone* (3rd ed.). Philadelphia: Saunders.

Bloom, W. & Fawcett, D. W. A. (1986). *Textbook of histology* (11th ed.) Philadelphia: Saunders.

Brown, M. C., Nuttall, A. L., & Masta, R. I. (1983). Intracellular recordings from cochlear inner hair cells: Effects of stimulation of the crossed olivo-cochlear efferents. *Science*, 222, 9-72.

Carlson, N. C. (1991). *Physiology of behavior* (4th ed.). Boston: Allyn and Bacon.

Carpenter, M. B. (1991). *Core text of neuroanatomy* (4th ed.). Baltimore: Williams & Wilkins.

Collet, L., Levy, V., Veullet, E., Truy, E., & Morgan, A. (1993). Click-evoked otoacoustic emissions and hearing thresholds in sensorineural hearing loss. *Ear and Hearing, 14,* 141-143.

Corwin, J. T. (1992). Regeneration in the auditory system. *Experimental Neurology, 115,* 7-1.

Corwin, J. T., & Warchol, M. E. (1991). Auditory hair cells: Structure, function, development and regeneration. *Annual Review of Neuroscience, 14,* 301-333.

Dallos, P. (1988). Cochlear neurobiology. *Asha, 35,* 50-56.

De Myer, W. (1988). *Neuroanatomy* (from the National medical series for independent study). Baltimore: Williams & Wilkins.

Engström, H., & Engström, B. (1988). *The ear: With some notes on the structure of the human ear.* Stockholm, Sweden: Widex.

Forge, A., Lin, L., Corwin, J. T., & Nevill, G. (1993). Ultrastructural evidence for hair cell regeneration in the mammalian inner ear. *Science, 259,* 1616-1619.

Gelfand, S. A. (1990). *Hearing: An introduction to psychological and physiological acoustics* (2nd ed.). New York: Marcel Dekker.

Heffner, H. E., & Heffner, R. S. (1990). Role of primate auditory cortex in hearing. In *Comparative perception. Vol. II. Complex signals.* New York: Wiley.

Hudspeth, A. J. (1985). The cellular basis of hearing. *Science, 230,* 745-752.

Kemp, D. T. (1978). Stimulated acoustic emissions from within the human auditory system. *Journal of the Acoustical Society of America, 64,* 1386-1391.

Kemp, D. T., Ryan, S., & Bray P. (1990). A guide to the effective use of otoacoustic emissions. *Ear and Hearing, 11,* 93-105.

Lim, D. J. (1986). Effects of noise and ototoxic drugs at the cellular level in the cochlea: A review. *American Journal of Otolaryngology, 7,* 73-99.

Manley, G. A. (1990). *Peripheral hearing mechanisms in reptiles and birds.* Berlin: Springer-Verlag.

Martin, G. K., Probst, R., & Lonsbury-Martin, B. L. (1990). Otoacoustic emissions in human ears. Normative findings. *Ear and Hearing, 11,* 106-120.

Morest, D. K., & Oliver, D. L. (1984). The neuronal architecture of the inferior colliculus in the cat defining the functional anatomy of the auditory midbrain. *Journal of Comparative Neurology, 222,* 209-236.

Nedzelnitsky, V. (1980). Sound pressures in the basal turn of the cat cochlea. *Journal of the Acoustical Society of America, 68,* 1676-1689.

Pickles, J. 0. (1988). *An introduction to the physiology of hearing* (2nd ed.). London: Academic Press.

Probst, R., Lonsbury-Martin, B., & Martin, G. K. (1991). A review of otoacoustic emissions. *Journal of the Acoustical Society of America, 89,* 2027-2061.

Robinette, M. S. (1992). Clinical observations with transient evoked otoacoustic emissions with adults. *Seminars in Hearing, 13,* 23-36.

Ryan, A. F., & Dallos, P. (1984). Physiology of the cochlea. In J. L. Northern (Ed.), *Hearing disorders* (2nd ed.) (pp. 253-266). Boston: Little, Brown.

Shaw, E. A. G. (1974). The external ear. In W. D. Kiedel & W. D. Neff (Eds.), *Handbook of sensory physiology*, Vol. 5, part 1 (pp. 455-490). Berlin: Springer-Verlag.

Simmons, F. B. (1964). Perceptual theories of middle ear muscle function. *Annals of Otology, Rhinology, & Laryngology, 73,* 724-739.

Spoendlin, H. (1975). Neuroanatomical basis of cochlea coding mechanisms. *Audiology, 14,* 383-407.

Spoendlin, H. (1978). Afferent innervation of the cochlea. In R. Naunton & C. Fernandez (Eds.), *Evoked electrical activity in the auditory nervous system*. London: Academic Press.

von Békésy, G. (1960). *Experiments in hearing* (translated and edited by E. G. Wever). New York: McGraw-Hill.

Warchol, M. E., Lambert, P. R., Goldstein, B. J., Forge, A., & Corwin, J. T. (1993). Regenerative proliferation in inner ear sensory epithelia from adult guinea pigs and humans. *Science 259,* 1619-1622.

Weisleder, P., & Rubel, E. W. (1992). Hair cell regeneration in the avian vestibular epithelium. *Experimental Neurology, 115,* 2-6.

Weisleder, P., & Rubel, E. W. (1993). Born again hair cells: Regeneration studies. Presented at the 5th Annual Convention of the American Academy of Audiology, April 15-18, Phoenix.

Yost, W. A. (1994). *Fundamentals of hearing: An introduction* (3rd ed.). San Diego: Academic Press.

Zemlin, W. R. (1988). *Speech and hearing science: Anatomy and physiology* (3rd ed). Englewood Cliffs: Prentice Hall.

Zrull, M. C., & Coleman, J. R. (1991). Structural features of neurons in whole grafts of the rat inferior colliculus. *Hearing Research, 55,* 117-132.

SUGGESTED READING

Dallos, P., & Martin, R. L. (1994). The ear: The new theory of hearing. *Hearing Journal, 47,* 41-42.

Hudspeth, A. J., & Markin, V. S. (1994). The ear's gears: Mechanoelectrical transduction by hair cells. *Physics Today, 47,* 22-28.

Lipscomb, D., & Martin, R. L. (1994). The ear: A capsule reintroduction to the ear. *Hearing Journal, 47,* 28-30.

Martin, F. N. (1991) *Introduction to audiology* (4th ed.). Englewood Cliffs: Prentice Hall.

Moore B. C. J. (1989). *An indroduction to the psychology of hearing* (3rd ed.). London/San Diego: Academic Press.

Northern, J. L. (Ed.) (1992). Otoacoustic emissions. *Seminars in Hearing, 13.*

2

Disorders of Hearing in Children

Susan D. Dalebout

After the identification of a hearing loss, it is the physician's responsibility to determine its cause and to decide if medical or surgical intervention is indicated. Therefore, it is imperative that any infant or young child identified as having a hearing impairment be referred for medical evaluation and diagnosis, concurrent with the initiation of aural habilitation measures. It is important that the cause of the hearing loss be determined because such knowledge may allow the clinician to predict progression of the hearing loss, predict that additional disorders are likely to be present or to manifest later in life, and to develop an appropriate intervention plan. Determination of causal factors also allows for effective genetic counseling when appropriate and may serve to diminish parental anxiety and feelings of guilt. Unfortunately, however, in approximately one-third of all cases of congenital hearing loss, no cause can be identified (Levine, 1989; Salamy & Eldredge, 1991). Many of these cases are likely to be of genetic or viral origin.

This chapter provides basic information for speech-language pathologists, other health care professionals, and educators regarding the causes of peripheral hearing loss in children. The chapter is not exhaustive; it addresses the causes of hearing loss most commonly encountered in pediatric patients. Techniques for evaluating the hearing of infants and young children are covered extensively in Chapter 4.

CONDUCTIVE HEARING LOSS

A conductive hearing loss occurs when something interferes with the conduction of energy through the external auditory canal, the middle ear, or both, into the inner ear (cochlea). Pathologic conditions may involve the outer ear (pinna or auricle), the external auditory canal, the tympanic membrane, the middle ear cavity, the ossicles or any of the other structures within the middle car cavity, the mastoid air cell system, or the eustachian tube. The cochlea and the auditory nerve (cranial nerve VIII), which compose the sensorineural mechanism, are normal in a purely conductive hearing loss. Therefore, a person with such a hearing loss exhibits normal pure–tone thresholds by bone conduction and abnormal thresholds by air conduction. This difference is referred to as an *air-bone gap*. Conductive hearing losses generally do not exceed 60 to 70 decibels hearing level (dB HL) because sound intensities beyond this level set the bones of the skull into vibration, resulting in hearing by bone conduction. Unlike sensorineural hearing losses, conductive hearing losses frequently are amenable to medical or surgical treatment. Conductive hearing losses are particularly prevalent among neonates, infants, and young children. Some of the more common causes of pediatric conductive hearing loss are described herein.

Congenital Malformations of the Outer and Middle Ear

The external and middle ear develop from the same embryonic tissue; therefore, it is not surprising that congenital defects of the external and middle ear often occur together and frequently occur in combination with congenital defects of other embryologically related systems. Thus, it is important that any child observed to have absent, malformed, or misplaced pinnae be referred for both audiologic and medical evaluation. Ballenger (1985a) and others (eg, Hawke & Jahn, 1987) have reported that because the inner ear develops from entirely different tissue, it rarely is influenced by maldevelopment of the outer or middle ear. However, Meyerhoff (1986) reported that approximately 30 percent of patients with malformations of the pinna and external auditory canal have an associated sensorineural hearing loss. According to Meyerhoff, ears with more severe malformations also tend to have the highest incidence of sensorineural loss.

Genetic defects sometimes cause congenital anomalies of the outer or middle ear, but intrauterine influences during the first trimester of pregnancy are responsible in a considerable number of cases. Unilateral involvement is reported more often than bilateral involvement; boys are affected more often than girls in a ratio ranging from 2:1 to 5:1 (Ballenger, 1985a); and the right side is affected more often than the left side (Meyerhoff, 1986). Some congenital defects impair hearing, whereas others have little effect on hearing but may cause emotional distress because of disfigurement. However, the most urgent problem is always improving hearing when it is impaired. It has been demonstrated that sound deprivation early in life may result in deficient language, speech, and auditory skills even after hearing is regained. Evidence (Bess et al, 1986; Bess & Tharpe, 1984) has shown that even unilateral hearing losses can be educationally handicapping, and most otologists now agree that given adequate cochlear function, surgical correction of unilateral anomalies is of sufficient value to warrant the chance of failure and the surgical risks involved (Ballenger, 1985a).

The following congenital malformations of the pinna and external auditory canal are among those most frequently observed in children.

Protruding Ears

By far the most common deformity is the protruding ear, a congenital malformation that can be recessively or dominantly inherited (Tardy, 1985). Because in humans the pinna plays only a minimal role in hearing (that of localization and direction of sounds from the environment into the external auditory canal), it is only because of the potential psychologic effect on the patient that protruding ears assume clinical significance. Fortunately, this deformity can be corrected simply and satisfactorily with surgical intervention at an early age.

Microtia and Anotia

The pinna may be malformed, small (microtia), or both, or it may be absent (anotia). Although microtia and anotia occur bilaterally in 15 to 20 percent of cases (Bess & Humes, 1990), both conditions more commonly occur unilaterally. When the conditions do occur bilaterally, the degree of deformity may differ on the two sides (Hawke & Jahn, 1987). As with other congenital anomalies of the ear, these conditions occur more often in boys than in girls. Meyerhoff (1986) reported that microtia and anotia occur twice as often on the right side. Congenital malformations of the pinnae may be isolated but more often are associated with atresia, middle ear anomalies, or various syndromes. Thus, audiologic evaluation is important, even though malformations of the pinnae do not in themselves result in impaired hearing. For information regarding syndromes associated with malformations of the pinnae, the reader is referred to Gerber (1990) and Northern and Downs (1991).

Although plastic surgery, in which a new pinna is grafted onto the head, often is recommended, the success of these procedures is limited when the deformity is severe. An alternative to surgery is the use of a plastic pinna, which can be affixed to the head with an adhesive. Ballenger (1985a) reported that plastics are available that imitate skin texture closely and that nonirritating glues provide firm attachment of the prosthesis to the skin. Growth of the head requires that the prosthesis be replaced periodically. It is important that when both options are viable, the patient and the parents be allowed to make the choice between surgery and a prosthesis. In some instances, after a trial period with a prosthesis, surgical treatment is chosen because of the difficulties inherent in the daily application of a prosthesis and attendant skin care.

Aural Atresia and Stenosis

The outer portion of the external auditory canal is supported by a framework of cartilage and is lined with relatively thick skin that contains hair follicles and many sebaceous and cerumen-producing glands. The deeper portion of the canal is supported by a framework of bone and is lined with thin skin that essentially lacks glands and hair follicles. Congenital atresia is the condition in which the cartilaginous portion, the bony portion, or the entire external auditory canal has never formed properly. The canal may be partially developed or completely replaced by an atresia plate formed of bone or fibrocartilaginous tissue (Hawke & Jahn, 1987; Harris & Endres, 1990).

Atresia is relatively common, with an incidence of approximately 1 in 10,000 live births (Meyerhoff, 1986). Between 60 and 70 percent of cases occur in boys, and there is a slight preponderance to the right ear (Harris & Endres, 1990). The disorder is bilateral in approximately 25 percent of cases (Harris & Endres, 1990). In about 92 percent of cases there is some degree of coexisting auricular malformation that ranges from a minimal alteration to complete anotia (Harris & Endres, 1990). More important from a diagnostic standpoint, however, are the 8 percent of patients with normal auricles.

In atresia, the degree of hearing loss is directly related to the area and structures involved. The loss may be mild if only the cartilaginous portion of the canal is affected but is more severe if the bony portion is closed or middle ear structures are involved. When atresia is associated with anomalies of the tympanic membrane and middle ear, the maximum (approximately 70 dB HL) conductive hearing loss may occur. In the case of unilateral malformation, early provision of sound to the affected ear is not as urgent as when there is bilateral involvement; however, the apparently normal ear must be evaluated within the first few months of life, because occult malformations accompanied by appreciable hearing loss occur in as many as 10 percent of apparently unaffected contralateral ears (Harris & Endres, 1990). For children with bilateral atresia, early fitting with bone conduction hearing aids is essential.

Harris and Endres (1990) reported that in bilateral atresia, one ear generally is corrected between the ages of 4 and 6 years, provided that sensorineural function is adequate. They suggested that the second ear be corrected once the first has stabilized, but not earlier than 1 year after the first surgery. Harris and Endres cautioned that a child with bilateral atresia who has had one ear corrected is not the same as a patient with unilateral atresia. This is because the corrected ear is considerably less stable than a normal ear, and generally complete closure of the air-bone gap cannot be achieved. The potential for normal hearing is best when only the cartilaginous portion of the canal is involved and the middle ear and tympanic membrane are normal. In some cases it is preferable to treat the child with hearing aids rather than surgery. This decision is the responsibility of the physician, the child, and the parents. However, if surgical intervention is postponed or fails to bring hearing into the normal range, it is the responsibility of the audiologist to recommend appropriate amplification.

A condition that sometimes is confused with atresia is stenosis, a marked narrowing of the external auditory canal. Stenotic external auditory canals do not produce hearing loss in the same manner as atresia does; however, a very narrow canal may easily become occluded by cerumen or debris, resulting in a temporary conductive hearing loss.

Imaging techniques, such as high-resolution computed tomography (CT), have dramatically improved the preoperative assessment of patients with aural atresia. The thickness and nature of the atretic plate can be determined, as can the status of middle ear structures (Hawke & Jahn, 1987). However, although these techniques can delineate fine structures in the tympanic cavity and inner ear, they cannot be used to determine whether or not an ossicular chain is functional, nor can they be used to rule out sensorineural involvement (Hawke & Jahn, 1987). Audiologic testing, including air- and bone-conducted auditory brainstem response (ABR) audiometry are helpful in this regard.

Foreign Bodies in the External Auditory Canal

Children frequently place foreign objects in their external auditory canals. If the object is pushed beyond the junction of the cartilaginous and bony portions of the canal, swelling at the isthmus formed by this junction may trap the object. The problem may be compounded if an unskilled person has unsuccessfully attempted to remove the object, producing local trauma and more swelling. When the object is lodged beyond the isthmus, removal may be difficult and may even require surgery under general anesthesia. Temporary hearing loss may be caused by swelling in the canal.

Cerumen in the External Auditory Canal

Some people produce cerumen (earwax) in excess. Moreover, in some people spontaneous extrusion does not occur or is inefficient. Factors that predispose to cerumen impaction may include small or collapsing ear canals, unusual properties of the cerumen itself, increased production of cerumen, an inefficient self-cleaning mechanism, or a combination of these factors (Bergstrom, 1990).

Cerumen is known to have protective qualities. It is toxic to insects and has been shown to possess bactericidal properties (Boies, 1989). It provides lubrication and acts as a vehicle for the movement of epithelial debris and contaminants away from the tympanic membrane and toward the outer portion of the external canal.

Perhaps the greatest danger associated with excess cerumen involves unskilled attempts to remove it. Cotton-tipped applicators are a major source of lacerated ear canals, perforated tympanic membranes, and occasional sensorineural hearing loss that occurs when displaced ossicles are accidentally forced into the inner ear (Northern & Downs, 1991). Attempts to clean the ear canal, particularly with implements such as cotton swabs, may result in cerumen being impacted or pushed from the cartilaginous canal into the bony canal, where removal is more difficult. If a cerumen plug is so tightly impacted that it cannot be removed without excessive pain, the problem usually can be resolved by instructing the patient to use ceruminolytic drops for several days before attempts at removal are renewed (Meyerhoff, 1986).

The amount of hearing loss caused by impacted cerumen is related to the amount of canal occlusion. When the canal becomes occluded, hearing loss may result. However, even when a large amount of cerumen is present, hearing remains essentially normal as long as a tiny opening exists between the tympanic membrane and the outside environment. Losses that result from occluding cerumen can range from very mild to moderately severe (Martin, 1991). Treatment of excessive or impacted cerumen is removal by a professional. It may involve the use of instruments, suction, or irrigation.

Otitis Externa

Otitis externa is an infection of the skin that lines the external auditory canal. A condition known as swimmer's ear, the most common type of otitis externa, sometimes develops in people who have had water trapped in their ears after swimming, particularly in hot, humid weather. The entrapment of water is common because cerumen is hygroscopic, or highly absorbent of water. Cerumen expands as it absorbs water, occluding the canal and trapping water behind the occlusion.

The bony portion of the external canal is unique in that it is the only place in the body where skin lies directly over bone with no subcutaneous tissue (Boies, 1989). Thus, this area is extremely sensitive and swelling is very painful because there is no room for expansion. In addition to the extreme pain caused by swelling, symptoms of otitis externa may include itching, discharge, elevated body temperature, and hearing loss. The hearing loss results from extensive swelling and consequent occlusion of the canal.

The source of otitis externa is most commonly bacterial infection; however, the cause may less frequently be fungal. According to Bergstrom (1990), the most important aspect of management is thorough cleaning of the ear canal to remove all debris. A cotton or synthetic wick may be required to dilate the meatus and carry medication into the canal (Hawke & Jahn, 1987; Bergstrom, 1990; Ballenger, 1985b). The patient should be warned of the possibility of future episodes, especially after swimming.

External otitis frequently is found in users of hearing aids. The presence of an occluding earmold results in increased moisture in the ear canal, which seems to predispose external otitis (Northern & Downs, 1991). The use of open-style or vented earmolds helps to prevent this condition by allowing air to ventilate the canal.

Collapsing Ear Canals

Occasionally during hearing assessment the pressure of an earphone against the side of the head moves the pinna forward and causes the soft cartilaginous portion of the ear canal to close, producing what appears to be a conductive hearing loss of 15 to 30 dB HL. This condition is thought to occur in about 3 percent of patients who undergo hearing evaluations (Bess & Humes, 1990). Although the condition is more prevalent in the elderly it does affect children, particularly neonates. Canal collapse presumably occurs due to a structural deficiency in the surrounding fibroelastic cartilage (Hawke & Jahn, 1987). To prevent canal collapse during audiometric testing, the external canal is kept open by inserting a small piece of plastic tubing, a hearing aid earmold, or an immittance probe tip into the opening of the canal.

Perforations of the Tympanic Membrane

Perforations may result from the development of excessive pressure in the middle ear during an acute episode of otitis media, trauma with an object such as a cotton swab or hairpin, or a violent pressure change in the external auditory canal, as in the case of an explosion at close range or a slap on the ear. Participation in water sports (eg, diving or water-skiing) is another source of traumatic perforations that occur as a result of sudden pressure changes in the ear canal. In these cases, the inward displacement of the column of air normally contained in the external auditory canal ruptures the tympanic membrane.

In the case of traumatic perforations, there is severe pain at the time of the injury; however, this pain abates quickly. The pain is accompanied by bleeding, which stops spontaneously. The amount of hearing loss varies as a function of the size and location of the perforation.

Because they affect healthy tissue, traumatic perforations tend to heal spontaneously more often than perforations that result from disease (Martin, 1991). Moreover, perforations in the inferior quadrants of the tympanic membrane tend to heal more rapidly than those in the superior quadrants because, in part, normal epithelial migration is more active in the inferior quadrants (Martin, 1991). Clean, traumatic perforations are treated by protecting the ear from water and administering systemic antibiotics if there is persistent pain or inflammation (Paparella et al, 1989). When spontaneous healing does not occur, repair requires unrolling and stimulating the edges of the perforation, then covering it with a material suitable for patching. This technique typically is repeated a number of times before healing is complete. When patching is not effective, surgery (ie, myringoplasty) may be required. Of greatest concern are perforations due to injuries that also cause damage to the ossicular chain, the temporal bone or both. Such damage is suspected when hearing loss greater than 25 dB HL and vertigo are present (Paparella et al, 1989). The presence of these symptoms constitutes a true otologic emergency, and immediate exploration of the middle ear and ossicular chain is necessary (Paparella et al, 1989).

Longitudinal Temporal Bone Fractures

Temporal bone fractures are divided into two general types: longitudinal fractures and transverse fractures. Approximately 80 percent of temporal bone fractures are longitudinal, whereas approximately 20 percent are transverse

(Hawke & Jahn, 1987; Levine, 1989). Transverse fractures tend to be more serious, and typically are associated with a loss of consciousness. Longitudinal fractures frequently result in tympanic membrane perforation, bleeding from the ear, and conductive hearing loss, conditions that are relatively infrequent in the case of transverse fractures, in which the hearing loss tends to be sensorineural and profound. Longitudinal fractures result in injury to the facial nerve 10 to 20 percent of the time, but spontaneous recovery of function is common (Meyerhoff, 1986). The treatment of longitudinal temporal bone fractures is observation for at least 6 weeks (Hawke & Jahn, 1987). If the patient continues to experience hearing loss after this 6-week period, the clinician should turn his or her attention to the middle ear and rule out ossicular damage (Hawke & Jahn, 1987).

Otitis Media

Garrard and Clark (1985) described otitis media as an inflammation of the middle ear that may result in a transient or permanent hearing loss. The middle ear can be described as an irregularly shaped air-filled space within the petrous portion of the temporal bone between the tympanic membrane and the inner ear.

Prevalence and Predisposing Factors

It has been reported that excluding the common cold, otitis media is the most common problem seen in a pediatric office (Paparella et al, 1989; Klein, 1991). Garrard and Clark (1985) indicated that otitis media is responsible for 33 to 50 percent of all patient visits to physicians during the first year of life. Teele, Klein, and Rosner (1989) reported that by the age of 3 years, approximately 70 percent of all children have experienced one or more episodes of otitis media, and approximately 30 percent have experienced three or more episodes. Similarly, Northern and Downs (1991) reported that approximately 50 percent of all children have had one episode of otitis media by the age of 1 year, and by the age of 2 years the number increases to 75 percent. Bluestone and Klein (1990c) suggested that by 3 years of age children may be categorized into three groups of approximately equal size relative to acute infections of the middle ear. One group is free of ear infections, a second group may have occasional episodes of otitis media, and a third group is otitis prone, or subject to repeated episodes of acute middle ear infection. Otitis media is undoubtedly the most common cause of hearing loss among children.

A number of factors have been associated with an increased risk for otitis media. The single most important factor is the age of the child. Otitis media is most common during the first 2 years of life, particularly the second 6-month period of life (Klein, 1991), and decreases in prevalence thereafter. Although there is a secondary increase in incidence in the age range of 5 to 6 years (when children begin school), otitis media is relatively uncommon in children older than 7 years (Bluestone & Klein, 1990c). The inverse relationship between age and prevalence probably is related to three factors: young children are more susceptible to upper respiratory infections, eustachian tube function is less competent in young children, and young children have less mature immune systems.

A related predisposing factor is the age at which children experience their initial episode of otitis media. Children who experience an episode during their first 12 to 18 months are more likely to go on to have severe and recurrent disease than those who experience their first episode later (Teele et al, 1980). Like the association between age and prevalence, the association between age at initial episode and recurrence of the disease may be related to the immaturity of a young child's immune system. However, it is also possible that children who are anatomically and physiologically predisposed to middle ear disease are likely to have episodes earlier in life than those who are not. Alternatively, it may be that otitis media in infancy damages the middle ear mucosa, leading to recurrent infections (Bluestone & Klein, 1990c).

Otitis media appears to be more prevalent in boys than in girls (Paparella et al, 1989; Klein, 1991). The disease occurs more frequently in late winter and early spring, a pattern that parallels peaks in upper respiratory infections, and effusions (accumulations of fluid) tend to persist longer during the winter months (Bluestone & Klein, 1990c). Middle ear disease is more common in whites than in blacks and is particularly common among Native Americans. Differences in the length, width, and angle of the eustachian tube have been reported among racial groups, implicating an anatomic basis for racial predisposition to, or protection from, otitis media (Bluestone & Klein, 1990c). The disease has been reported to be more prevalent among children of lower socioeconomic status, children of parents with less education, children of parents with relatively lower income, children from large families, children who attend day care centers where they are exposed to more upper respiratory infections at a younger age, children who come from families in which there are other members with histories of otitis media, children with allergies, children with cleft palate, and children with Down syndrome. It is becoming apparent that smoking in the home is an important predisposing factor.

There is some evidence that breast-fed babies have a decreased risk for recurrent otitis media, at least during the first year of life. A number of possible explanations for this hypothesis have been suggested (Bluestone & Klein, 1990c). For example, immunologic factors may be provided in breast milk that reduce an infant's susceptibility to viral and bacterial infections; allergy to one or more components in cow's milk or formula may result in an alteration of the mucosa of the eustachian tube and middle ear in bottle-fed infants; the facial musculature of breast-fed infants may develop differently from that of bottle-fed infants, resulting in improved eustachian tube function and drainage of middle ear fluids in breast-fed infants; or aspiration of fluids into the middle ear may be more likely during bottle feeding because bottle feeding requires a higher negative intraoral pressure than does breast feeding. Finally, breast-fed infants tend to be maintained in a more upright position than bottle-fed infants, who often are placed in a reclining position that may encourage reflux of milk through the wide, horizontal infant eustachian tube into the middle ear (Bluestone & Klein, 1990c). Of course, any combination of these factors may be involved.

A final element that may be considered in the context of predisposing factors is eustachian tube competence. The eustachian tube connects the middle ear cavity with the nasopharynx (back of the nose) and is intimately related to diseases of both (Paparella et al, 1989). According to Bluestone and Klein (1990c), abnormal function of the eustachian tube appears to be the most important factor in the pathogenesis of middle ear disease. A child with a poorly functioning eustachian tube is highly likely to experience recurrent episodes of otitis media or persistent negative pressure in the middle ear.

The eustachian tube normally is closed; however, it is opened periodically by active muscular contraction of the tensor veli palatini muscle during swallowing and, less frequently, yawning and opening of the jaws (Paparella et al, 1989). The functions of the eustachian tube are ventilation of the middle ear cavity so that the air pressure on both sides of the tympanic membrane can be equalized, drainage and clearance of secretions produced within the middle ear into the nasopharynx, and protection of the middle ear from contamination by nasopharyngeal secretions. The most important of these functions is ventilation of the middle ear. In its normal state, the middle ear cavity is air-filled. However, air constantly is absorbed by the middle ear tissues and must be replenished regularly. This is accomplished when the eustachian tube opens and allows a small bubble of air into the cavity. When the eustachian tube is not functional, air that has been absorbed cannot be replenished and the pressure within the middle ear space becomes negative relative to atmospheric pressure.

Bluestone and Klein (1990c) reported that eustachian tube obstruction can be functional, mechanical, or both. According to Bluestone and Klein (1990c), functional obstruction results from persistent collapse of the eustachian tube due to increased compliance, an abnormal opening mechanism, or a combination of these factors. Functional obstruction is particularly common in infants and young children because of maturational differences. For example, the eustachian tube in infants is short, wide, and situated in an almost horizontal plane relative to the base of the skull (Paparella et al, 1989). As the child grows, the tube elongates, narrows, and develops a more downward course. Moreover, the eustachian tube in infants is more compliant because of the decreased stiffness of supporting cartilage. In addition, there appear to be marked differences in the craniofacial base, which render the tensor veli palatini muscle less efficient before puberty. All of these factors work together to make eustachian tube dysfunction more likely in infants and young children.

An example of an abnormal opening mechanism, the second cause of functional obstruction noted by Bluestone and Klein (1990c), is seen in cases of cleft palate, a condition in which eustachian tube dysfunction results from poor anchorage of the tensor veli palatini muscle (Paparella et al, 1989). Poor attach-ment prevents the muscle from exerting sufficient contraction strength on the eustachian tube orifice to open it during swallowing (Paparella et al, 1989). The inability of the tube to open results in inadequate ventilation of the middle ear, and inflammation ensues. Thus, the prevalence of middle ear disease in children with cleft palate is extremely high.

Bluestone and Klein (1990c) specified that mechanical obstruction may be intrinsic or extrinsic. Intrinsic obstruction most commonly is a result of inflammation within the eustachian tube due to infection or allergy. Extrinsic obstruction could be a result of increased pressure exerted on the tube by a tumor or an adenoid mass.

The prevalence of otitis media has accelerated dramatically during the last 50 years. Downs (1987) attributed the increase to two primary factors: the advent of antibiotics and the increasing number of mothers who work outside the home, necessitating the placement of infants and very young children in day care centers, a practice that has been demonstrated to be a risk factor in the development of recurrent otitis media. Although antibiotics have reduced the serious complications of bacterial otitis media, such as mastoiditis, meningitis, and other dangerous secondary infections, middle ear disease today presents in a chronic and insidious form that often causes hearing loss. The use of antibiotics arrests the acute infectious stage and prevents the development of a full-fledged suppurative process with a spontaneous perforation but also predisposes to the development of subclinical forms of infection, such as otitis media with effusion (Hawke & Jahn, 1987). Treatment of the effusion, which often remains in the middle ear for days, weeks, or months after the acute infection has been resolved with antibiotics, is unsatisfactory. Teele, Klein, and Rosner (1980) reported that after the onset of an episode of acute otitis media, 70 percent of children examined still had effusion 2 weeks later, 40 percent had effusion 1 month later, 20 percent had effusion 2 months later, and 10 percent had effusion 3 months later. Similar reports of persistent middle ear effusion following an episode of acute otitis media have been noted in other studies. The morbidity of persistent effusion usually means the presence of hearing loss. Therefore, young children who experience recurrent episodes of otitis media may have reduced or fluctuant hearing sensitivity during a large portion of their early, developmentally critical years.

Classification of Subtypes

A current hypothesis is that the different clinical subtypes of otitis media form a continuum and are dynamically interrelated. At any specific point on the continuum a particular clinical entity can be identified, whereas at another point a different entity may be present in the same patient (Northern & Downs, 1991). The various subtypes of otitis media generally are classified on the basis of their time course or the nature of the fluid they produce. For example, Northern and Downs (1991) suggested a classification scheme in which the general categories are otitis media without effusion, otitis media with effusion, and otitis media with perforation. Each of these categories may be subclassified by duration into acute (0 to 21 days), subacute (22 days to 8 weeks), and chronic (lasting more than 8 weeks). In otitis media with effusion and otitis media with perforation, the fluid or discharge may be characterized as serous (a thin, watery liquid), purulent (a pus-like liquid), or mucoid (a thick, viscid, mucus-like liquid).

It is often difficult to determine by physical examination the specific type and stage of otitis media at a given time. A more definitive diagnosis can be made when the physician also has knowledge about the condition of the middle ear before the onset of the present illness. In this way, a clear idea of where the current episode falls on the diagnostic continuum emerges and treatment can be better tailored to the patient.

Although the terms used to classify the various subtypes of otitis media are used inconsistently in the literature, the entities described here enjoy some degree of acceptance. However, many classification schemes do exist and many different terminologies are employed.

Otitis Media Without Effusion

In certain cases, inflammation of the middle ear mucosa and tympanic membrane is present without evidence of a middle ear effusion. This condition usually is present in the early stages of acute otitis media but also may be found in the resolution stage or may even be chronic (Bluestone & Klein, 1990c).

Acute Otitis Media

Acute otitis media is an active infection of the middle ear space of relatively brief duration. The associated effusion can be described as infectious, suppurative, or purulent, all terms associated with the presence of pus. An episode typically lasts less than 3 weeks, after which the condition resolves or progresses into another clinical subtype. Most acute otitis media infections are caused by bacteria (Paparella et al, 1989). Symptoms may include pain (otalgia), fever, irritability, loss of appetite, vomiting, and diarrhea.

Most cases of acute otitis media arise from upper respiratory infections that move from the nasopharynx to the middle ear via the eustachian tube. Bluestone and Klein (1990c) described a pattern that begins with congestion of the respiratory tract mucosa (including the nasopharynx, eustachian tube, and middle ear) due to infection or allergy. The congestion of the mucosa in the eustachian tube results in obstruction of the narrowest portion of the tube (the isthmus), rendering it dysfunctional. With the tube unable to open, secretions of the middle ear mucosa have no egress and accumulate in the middle ear. Finally, microbial pathogens (bacteria in most cases) that may be present in the middle ear proliferate in the secretions and result in a suppurative and symptomatic otitis media.

Without treatment, the tympanic membrane is likely to rupture with subsequent drainage of purulent material. After perforation, the pain resolves dramatically, although drainage persists. The perforation generally heals spontaneously over the next 4 to 5 weeks. With antibiotic treatment, however, the natural progression to spontaneous perforation is less likely to occur. Instead, the suppuration is arrested, with either complete resolution of the infection or subsequent development of otitis media with effusion.

Otitis Media with Effusion

Also known as serous otitis media, secretory otitis media, or nonsuppurative otitis media, otitis media with effusion is characterized by a thin fluid in the middle ear space. This condition often follows an episode of acute otitis media, particularly if only antibiotics have been used to treat it. In this case, the antibiotic may have destroyed the invading bacteria, but the fluid, rendered noninfectious, may remain in the middle ear for weeks or months. Although the infection is asymptomatic during this time, hearing is likely to be impaired. Thus, the most important distinction between otitis media with effusion and acute otitis media is that the signs and symptoms of acute infection (eg, otalgia and fever) are lacking; however, hearing loss is likely to be present in both conditions (Bluestone & Klein, 1990c).

Otitis media with effusion also may develop independently of acute otitis media, in which case eustachian tube dysfunction is at fault. The eustachian tube may be dysfunctional because of anatomic or physiologic immaturity, inflammation and swelling due to upper respiratory infection or allergies, or enlarged adenoids at the orifice. In any case, it does not open to provide adequate aeration of the middle ear space. The air in the middle ear is absorbed by the tissues that line the cavity, and the pressure within the cavity becomes negative relative to atmospheric pressure. The tympanic membrane becomes retracted (drawn in by the negative pressure) and vibrates less efficiently, perhaps causing a slight hearing loss. If the negative pressure persists, the tissues of the middle ear are stimulated to secrete a serous fluid. This fluid cannot drain because of the incompetence of the eustachian tube, and hearing loss results. Moreover, the fluid acts as a ready medium for subsequent infection (acute otitis media). This condition is the most prevalent cause of hearing loss among school-aged children (Paparella et al, 1989).

Both acute otitis media and otitis media with effusion may be described as recurrent; that is, the ear alternates between a diseased condition and a healthy state. The ear also may alternate between recurrent episodes of acute otitis media and otitis media with effusion, with or without disease-free periods.

Chronic Otitis Media

The term *chronic* sometimes is used as a time-related adjective; however, *chronic otitis media* more typically refers to a distinct clinical entity that usually falls into the suppurative category. Chronic otitis media may persist for months or years despite vigorous and appropriate medical treatment, during which hearing probably does not return to normal. The condition generally is defined by the presence of a persistent tympanic membrane perforation, drainage, and hearing loss.

In chronic otitis media, suppuration has produced irreversible damage to the middle ear mucosa and underlying bone (Schloss, 1990); however, the disease can be considered active or inactive at a given point in time (Paparella et al, 1989). The term *active* refers to the presence of infection with steady purulent drainage. The bacteria present are usually quite different from those that cause acute otitis media (Hawke & Jahn, 1987). *Inactive chronic otitis media* refers to complications from a previously active infection that has resolved; drainage is scant (Paparella et al, 1989).

Complications and Sequelae of Otitis Media

The term *sequelae* refers to unfavorable conditions that occur as consequences of a disease. With the exception of hearing loss, medical sequelae of otitis media are unusual today. Medical complications can be divided into those that occur within the middle ear and temporal bone (intratemporal complications) and those that occur within the intracranial cavity. It should be noted that although these conditions are considered here as sequelae of otitis media, they may develop from other causes as well. Intratemporal complications include hearing loss, perforation of the tympanic membrane, adhesive otitis media, chronic suppurative otitis media, mastoiditis, cholesteatoma and retraction pocket, tympanosclerosis, ossicular discontinuity or fixation, petrositis, labyrinthitis, and facial paralysis. In children, the more common intracranial complications associated with otitis media are meningitis and development of a brain abscess. A brief description of each of these conditions follows.

Intratemporal Complications

Hearing Loss Hearing impairment is the most prevalent complication of otitis media. The hearing loss typically associated with otitis media with effusion, the most common type of otitis media in children, is a mild to moderate conductive loss in the range of 15 to 40 dB HL (Bluestone & Klein, 1990b). This degree of hearing loss makes it likely that morphological markers and voiceless consonants will be missed, especially in adverse listening situations. Perhaps more important, the loss tends to fluctuate, which means that a young child may be receiving an inconsistent auditory signal during the critical period for speech and language development.

The hearing loss is influenced more by the quantity than the quality of fluid in the middle ear (Bluestone & Klein, 1990b). Ears filled with thin fluid are impaired to approximately the same degree as ears filled with gel-like fluid (Bluestone & Klein, 1990b). Friel-Patti et al (1987) reported that the mean air-conduction threshold for the frequencies of 250 to 4000 Hz in ears with thick effusion was 30.8 dB HL, whereas in ears with thin effusion, the mean air-conduction threshold was 26.8 dB HL. Normal hearing generally is restored with resolution of the effusion. However, on occasion, permanent conductive hearing loss develops as a result of irreversible changes associated with recurrent or chronic otitis media (eg, adhesive otitis media, ossicular discontinuity or fixation, persistent perforation). In this case, the maximum conductive hearing loss may result. Severe negative pressure that results in atelectasis of the tympanic membrane also may cause conductive hearing loss in the absence of effusion (Bluestone & Klein, 1990b).

Sensorineural hearing loss may occur as a result of otitis media, presumably due to the spread of infection through the round window membrane or the occurrence of a perilymphatic fistula (opening or hole in the bone of the labyrinth), resulting in labyrinthitis. Sensorineural hearing loss is more frequently a complication of chronic suppurative otitis media than of acute otitis media.

Perforation of the Tympanic Membrane The effect of a small perforation on hearing, regardless of the location of the perforation and in the absence of other abnormalities of the middle ear, is not clinically significant (Bluestone & Klein, 1990b). However, a large perforation can be associated with a conductive hearing loss of 20 to 30 dB HL (Bluestone & Klein, 1990b).

Adhesive Otitis Media Adhesive otitis media develops as a result of healing after recurrent inflammation of the middle ear and mastoid process (Bluestone & Klein, 1990b). There may be a proliferation of fibrous tissue within the middle ear, accompanied by severe retraction of the tympanic membrane and negative pressure within the middle ear space (Northern & Downs, 1991). Nonsuppurative effusion may become gel-like and form adhesions on the ossicles, impeding their movement and permanently impairing hearing. Persistent negative pressure may cause a retraction pocket (pouch or sac) to form in the superior portion of the tympanic membrane, in which case the development of a cholesteatoma is probable.

Chronic Suppurative Otitis Media Chronic suppurative otitis media is a stage of ear disease in which there is chronic inflammation of the middle ear and mastoid process and in which a perforation of the tympanic membrane, discharge, and hearing loss are present. Mastoiditis is invariably a part of the pathologic process.

Mastoiditis Before antibiotics were widely used, acute mastoid osteitis (inflammation of bone) was a common suppurative complication of acute otitis media that sometimes resulted in death (Bluestone & Klein, 1990b). The mastoid air-cell system, located posterior to the middle ear cavity, consists of a series of small air cells that are interconnected with each other and with the middle ear. Thus, because of the proximity of the mastoid to the middle ear cleft, most cases of suppurative otitis media are associated with inflammation of the mastoid air cells. Acute mastoiditis is a natural extension of the pathologic process in acute otitis media. Acute mastoiditis usually resolves as the acute infection of the middle ear resolves.

Similarly, chronic suppurative otitis media is invariably associated with chronic mastoiditis. The chronic infection at this stage may be brought under control by medical treatment; however, when there is extensive granulation tissue (a vascularized form of connective tissue associated with inflammatory reaction) and osteitis in the mastoid, mastoidectomy (surgical hollowing out of the mastoid, removing the bony partitions that form the mastoid cells) usually is necessary, especially if cholesteatoma is present (Bluestone & Klein, 1990b).

Cholesteatoma and Retraction Pocket An acquired cholesteatoma is a cyst-like growth of squamous epithelium (skin) that occurs in the middle ear. Cholesteatomas most commonly develop when functional obstruction of the eustachian tube results in negative middle ear pressure, which causes severe retraction and atelectasis of the tympanic membrane. Atelectasis is a condition in which sustained negative pressure causes the eardrum to lose its elasticity and to become flaccid. When the atelectasis becomes severe and localized (usually in the posterosuperior quadrant), a retraction pocket, or pouch-like invagination in the tympanic membrane, may form. Infection causes this pocket to migrate further into the middle ear, where it grows by a process of shedding and re-encapsulating debris. As it enlarges and migrates inward, the cholesteatoma destroys bone (including the ossicles) and other tissues in its path. Less commonly, acquired cholesteatomas develop when skin from the external auditory canal grows into the middle ear through a perforation of the tympanic membrane. In either case, damage to the middle ear and surrounding structures can be severe, the risk of intracranial complications is great, and surgical intervention is indicated. Unfortunately, recurrence of cholesteatoma is common among children (Northern & Downs, 1991).

Tympanosclerosis Tympanosclerosis is the formation of hyalinized (glass-like), calcified scar tissue on the tympanic membrane. The scarring process is pathologic. Conductive hearing loss may occur if tympanosclerotic plaques envelop the ossicles; this condition is uncommon in infants and children. Tympanosclerosis involving only the tympanic membrane does not appreciably affect hearing. Surgical correction is not indicated, because removal of large tympanosclerotic plaques may result in permanent perforation, and even in the absence of perforation, the pathologic scarring process will be repeated.

Ossicular Discontinuity and Fixation Ossicular interruption may occur as a result of osteitis secondary to chronic inflammation of the middle ear or destruction associated with a cholesteatoma. Ossicular fixation may be a result of adhesive otitis media or tympanosclerosis.

Petrositis Petrositis is a rare suppurative complication in which infection extends from the middle ear and mastoid process into the petrous portion of the temporal bone. Like mastoiditis, petrositis may be acute or chronic. In the acute form, there is an extension of acute otitis media and mastoiditis into the pneuma-tized petrous air cells. The condition usually resolves with resolution of the acute otitis media and mastoiditis. Chronic petrous osteomyelitis (inflammation of the deepest portion of the bone) can be a complication of chronic suppurative otitis media or cholesteatoma, or both, and is more common than the acute type (Bluestone & Klein, 1990b). The infection may persist for months or years with mild and intermittent signs and symptoms, or it may spread to the intracranial cavity and cause one or more of the suppurative intracranial complications of ear disease, such as meningitis.

Labyrinthitis This complication of otitis media occurs when infection spreads from the middle ear or the meninges into the cochlea and vestibular apparatus. The most common route of entry from the middle ear is the round window, although other routes include the oval window or a labyrinthine fistula. The signs and symptoms include sudden, progressive, or fluctuating sensorineural hearing loss, vertigo, or both, in association with otitis media or its complications (Bluestone & Klein, 1990b). Suppurative labyrinthitis can lead to complete loss of cochlear and vestibular function.

Facial Paralysis Facial paralysis may occur during an episode of acute otitis media when the facial nerve is exposed to purulent material through a congenital dehiscence (split or opening) of the bony facial canal, which travels through the middle ear. Facial paralysis is a relatively common complication of acute otitis media in infants and children and usually improves rapidly with myringotomy and the administration of antibiotics (Bluestone & Klein, 1990b; Meyerhoff, 1986). Chronic otitis media causes facial paralysis by a different mechanism (Paparella et al, 1989). Granulation tissue or a cholesteatoma may cause pressure on the nerve and toxic products may be released. (Paparella et al, 1989). Antibiotics neither eliminate nor ameliorate this process, and surgical intervention is indicated (Paparella et al, 1989; Bluestone & Klein, 1990b). The prognosis for the return of function is poor (Meyerhoff, 1986).

Intracranial Complications
There has been an overall decline in the incidence of suppurative intracranial complications of otitis media since the advent of antibiotics (Bluestone & Klein, 1990a). Today, these complications more often occur in conjunction with chronic suppurative otitis media and mastoiditis than with acute otitis media.

Meningitis Meningitis is an inflammation of the meninges, the membranes that cover the brain and spinal cord. Before the use of antibiotics, meningitis sometimes occurred as a result of infection from the middle ear and mastoid spreading to the meninges. Today, infection spread by this route is rare. Instead, the most common route now involves the spread of infection from the upper respiratory tract to the meninges via the bloodstream (Bluestone & Klein, 1990a). Still, meningitis remains the most common intracranial complication of acute otitis media in children (Meyerhoff, 1986).

Brain Abscess Of all age groups, infants and children have the highest incidence of brain abscesses (Bluestone & Klein, 1990a). However, the incidence of brain abscess, in general, has decreased considerably in the antibiotic era (Bluestone & Klein, 1990a). An abscess of the brain may follow directly from acute or chronic middle ear and mastoid infection or may follow the development of an adjacent infection, such as lateral sinus thrombosis, petrositis, or meningitis (Bluestone & Klein, 1990a). When caused by the extension of a middle ear and mastoid infection, the dura mater (tough, fibrous membrane covering the brain) that overlies the infected mastoid process can be invaded along vascular pathways or by adherence to infected bone (Bluestone & Klein, 1990a). Alternatively, chronic otitis media or mastoiditis may lead to erosion of the tegmen tympani (thin shelf of bone separating the middle ear cavity from the brain), with resultant inflamma-tion of the dura and invasion of pathogenic organisms. Ultimately, brain tissue is invaded and the various stages of abscess formation take place.

Treatment of Otitis Media

Treatment of children with otitis media is either medical or surgical. With appropriate antibiotic therapy, the condition of most children with acute otitis media improves considerably in 48 to 72 hours; however, complete clearing of the effusion may take 6 weeks or longer (Bluestone & Klein, 1990c). If complete resolution is observed and the episode represents the only known attack, the patient may be discharged. However, if bouts are frequent and close together, prevention of further attacks is desirable and the patient requires further evaluation. Manage-ment options at this stage commonly include (a) antibiotic treatment of each episode, (b) antibiotic prophylaxis, and (c) myringotomy with tympanostomy tube insertion (Bluestone & Klein, 1990c). Antibiotic prophylaxis implies the use of drugs in anticipation of infection, whereas antibiotic treatment implies the use of drugs after infection has taken place or when signs of infection are present. For example, antibiotic prophylaxis might involve the administration of antibiotics in low dosage for periods of up to 6 months during the autumn, winter, and spring seasons.

Myringotomy is a procedure in which an incision is made in the tympanic membrane, either to provide ventilation to the middle ear, to permit drainage of middle ear fluid, or to obtain cultures (Paparella et al, 1989). In children, the procedure most often is performed under general anesthesia. In fact, myringotomy with insertion of tympanostomy tubes currently is the most common surgical procedure performed in children that requires general anesthesia (Bluestone & Klein, 1990c).

Tympanostomy tube insertion involves placement of a small tube in the myringotomy incision. The pressure equalization ("pe") tube acts as a vent to allow air into the middle ear; that is, the tube temporarily performs the ventilating function of the dysfunctional eustachian tube. Ventilation of the middle ear relieves the negative pressure and prevents the redevelopment of effusion, unless an acute infection develops.

According to Paparella et al (1989), the decision to proceed to surgery is not based solely on the duration of ear disease. Severity of the hearing impairment and the frequency and severity of preceding episodes also are considered. For example, a child with a thin fluid, minimal hearing loss, or unilateral ear disease may be treated with a more conservative approach (ie, antibiotic therapy) for a longer time. On the other hand, thinning of the tympanic membrane, a deep retraction pocket, significant hearing impairment, or delayed speech and language development may be indications to proceed to myringotomy sooner.

The insertion of tympanostomy tubes often provides immediate restoration of hearing. The tubes are left in place until spontaneously extruded, usually a period of 6 to 12 months. Myringotomy incisions without tube placement often heal within 48 hours. Unfortunately, because of continuing eustachian tube dysfunction and consequent recurrence of effusion, some children require reinsertion of tubes after extrusion or the insertion of special tubes designed to stay in the ear for longer than 1 year. The disadvantage of these longer-lasting tubes has been the persistence of a perforation after extrusion. In addition to the inherent surgical risks, the greatest disadvantage of tympanostomy tubes, in general, is the need to keep the middle ear dry. Water from bathing or swimming should not be allowed to enter the middle ear through the tube, because contamination often results in acute otitis media and discharge.

Indications for myringotomy with insertion of tympanostomy tubes include the presence of otitis media with effusion that has been unresponsive to antibiotic therapy for at least 3 months; recurrent episodes of acute otitis media in spite of continuous prophylactic antibiotics; persistent pain after 48 hours of antibiotic treatment; persistent negative middle ear pressure and resultant atelectasis of the tympanic membrane, especially with retraction into the posterior superior quadrant; potential development of complications such as labyrinthitis, facial paralysis, or meningitis; or development of otitis media in an immunosuppressed patient (Paparella et al, 1989). Finally, tympanostomy tubes are indicated for children who have recurrent acute episodes superimposed on persistent otitis media with effusion. Antibiotic prophylaxis should be considered only for children who have no evidence of a middle ear effusion between acute attacks (Bluestone & Klein, 1990c).

Infrequent complications of tympanostomy tube insertion include scarring of the tympanic membrane, tympanosclerosis, and localized or diffuse membrane atrophy, with or without retraction pockets. A frequent complication is an infection with otorrhea (drainage) through the tube. Much less commonly, a perforation may remain at the insertion site after extrusion of the tube, a cholesteatoma may develop, or the tube may extrude into the middle ear. For the tube to function properly it must remain patent. Blockage of the tube with blood, mucus, or other debris may lead to a return of the effusion and the need for tube removal and replacement.

A management option sometimes recommended as an alternative or adjunct to surgical intervention is the fitting of hearing aids on children who have persistent hearing loss due to middle ear disease. This may include cases in which surgery has not restored hearing to normal, or in which reconstructive surgery must be postponed until a child grows older. Children with recurrent middle ear disease in conjunction with cleft palate or Down syndrome are particularly good candidates for amplification because they tend to have persistent middle ear disease and hearing loss, despite aggressive medical treatment. However, all children who have early recurring episodes of otitis media that result in fluctuating hearing loss are at risk for a variety of developmental difficulties, including those involving speech and language, auditory skills, attention, and academic achievement. Although research findings are not conclusive, evidence strongly suggests that an early history of recurrent otitis media may result in such difficulties for some children. Of special concern are children who have frequent bouts of otitis media between birth and

2 years of age, a particularly common time of occurrence, because this period is especially critical for the acquisition of language. Thus, provision of amplification may be most important during the earliest years of development.

SENSORINEURAL HEARING LOSS

People with sensorineural hearing loss demonstrate impaired hearing sensitivity by both air conduction and bone conduction. The degree of hearing loss shown by air- and bone-conduction thresholds is approximately the same. That is, air- and bone-conduction thresholds are interwoven; there is no air-bone gap. In a pure sensorineural loss, the outer and middle ear systems function normally. Instead, the pathologic condition or damage affects the sensory receptors in the cochlea, the neural pathways that lead from the cochlea to higher centers in the auditory system, or both sensory and neural structures. Unlike conductive hearing loss, which often is medically or surgically treatable, sensorineural hearing loss typically is permanent. For children with sensorineural hearing loss, treatment usually involves the use of amplification systems and placement in intervention programs.

Some of the more common causes of sensorineural hearing loss in children are described herein. The term *prenatal* refers to an influence that affects the fetus before birth. The term *congenital* refers to a condition that is present at birth. The term *perinatal* refers to the period extending from shortly before birth to soon after birth. A condition acquired later in life is said to be acquired postnatally.

Prenatal Causes of Sensorineural Hearing Loss

Genetic Hearing Loss

Approximately 50 percent of all severe to profound childhood deafness of the sensorineural type is genetic, making it the single most common cause of congenital or early-onset sensorineural hearing loss (Stewart, 1987; Bess & Humes, 1990; Levine, 1989). It is estimated that there are 150 to 175 different types of genetic syndromes that include hearing loss as a primary feature (Bess & Humes, 1990). In addition, about 16 types of genetic deafness are known to occur without any associated anomalies (Bess & Humes, 1990). For information regarding syndromes of genetic or chromosomal origin, the reader is referred to Gerber (1990) and Northern and Downs (1991).

Like many other traits, genetic hearing loss is known to follow dominant, recessive, sex-linked, and polygenic inheritance patterns. Autosomal dominant inheritance is believed to account for less than 10 percent of all genetically inherited hearing losses. Autosomal recessive inheritance accounts for most instances of genetic hearing loss; approximately 90 percent of all genetic hearing losses are of the autosomal recessive type (Northern & Downs, 1991). Only 2 to 3 percent of genetic deafness is associated with sex-linked inheritance (Bess & Humes, 1990).

Finally, hearing loss can be attributable to many different gene pairs, and it is likely that there are cases in which multiple genes contribute to deafness. This is known as polygenic inheritance. The incidence of deafness transmitted by this pattern is not known.

Prenatal and Perinatal Viral Infections

Some infections contracted by a mother during pregnancy can have adverse effects on the auditory function of the fetus. Most notable are the TORCH infections. In the acronym, *T* represents toxoplasmosis; *O*, other (syphilis); *R*, rubella; *C*, cytomegalovirus (CMV) infection; and *H*, herpes simplex virus infection. These infections are difficult to diagnose because they present with minimal nonspecific symptoms, yet they can cause devastating developmental complications in a fetus. Moreover, a subclinical infection can result in the same serious consequences as one that is clinically apparent (Northern & Downs, 1991). Fetal viral infections may kill or destroy cells, or they may decrease the rate at which each cell can divide and reproduce by mitosis (Martin, 1991). In addition, as maternal body temperature increases in response to a viral (or other) infection, the oxygen required by the fetus increases dramatically (Martin, 1991). Consequent oxygen deprivation in the fetus may result in damage to cells.

There is no consistent pattern in the sensorineural hearing losses attributed to TORCH complex infections. The hearing loss may range from mild to profound and may be unilateral or bilateral but is likely to be progressive. Virus excretions may remain active for several years after birth, contributing to the degenerative process (Northern & Downs, 1991).

Toxoplasmosis

Toxoplasmosis is a parasitic infection that is transmitted from the mother to the fetus via the placenta. It is thought that the maternal infection results from eating undercooked meat or from making contact with cat feces. The mother often has no symptoms. According to Gerber (1990), approximately one-third of women who contract toxoplasmosis during the first trimester of pregnancy have babies who die in utero, and approximately one-half have babies who are severely handicapped. The risk to the fetus posed by the maternal virus diminishes as the pregnancy proceeds. If exposed in the third trimester, most babies will suffer no consequences (Gerber, 1990). Still, about 30 to 40 percent of infected women have infected infants, making toxoplasmosis one of the most common causes of birth defects in the United States (Gerber, 1990). According to Bess and Humes (1990), approximately 17 percent of infected newborns exhibit a sensorineural hearing loss, which is typically mild to moderate in degree and progressive.

Syphilis

Unlike the other TORCH complex infections, which are of viral origin, syphilis is produced by a bacterium that can pass through the placental barrier.

Bacteria generally do not cross the placental barrier because of their relatively large size; however, the bacterium that causes syphilis is extremely small. Although in Western countries congenital syphilis is now relatively rare, it continues to be one of the most important contributors to perinatal mortality and morbidity in many parts of the world (Northern & Downs, 1991).

Prenatally contracted syphilis is transmitted to the child by intrauterine infection from the mother, who has contracted it as a sexually transmitted disease. The congenital disease may manifest anytime between birth and the sixth decade of life. If the onset is early, the associated hearing loss tends to be profound, bilateral, sensorineural, and of sudden onset. Poor auditory function and limited success with amplification can be expected as a result of neural atrophy (Northern & Downs, 1991). If the onset is in adulthood, the hearing loss tends to be asymmetric and fluctuating and may appear gradually or suddenly. Congenital syphilis may result in a multitude of central nervous system abnormalities, including mental retardation (Northern & Downs, 1991). Treatment involves the administration of large doses of penicillin at birth or in utero when an infected mother is identified. The bacterium that causes syphilis does not pass to the fetus before the fourth month of gestation; therefore, the importance of early treatment is obvious (Gerber, 1990).

Rubella
Rubella infects the mother by the respiratory route and is carried by the bloodstream to the placenta and to the fetus. Maternal infection poses the greatest danger to the fetus if contracted during the first trimester of pregnancy. Maternal symptoms may be very mild; in fact, the mother may be unaware that she has contracted the disease. The child may exhibit a number of deficits, including mental retardation and cardiac, visual, and hearing abnormalities. The associated hearing loss most typically is severe to profound, bilateral, and sensorineural with a flat, sloping, or bowl-shaped configuration. The rubella virus may remain in the tissues of the cochlea after birth, resulting in a progressive hearing loss. This means that the infant also may pass the infection to others, including pregnant women (Northern & Downs, 1991).

Maternal rubella has been largely eradicated by widespread vaccination programs, and only occasionally do new cases appear. Recent estimates are that rubella now accounts for less than 5 percent of all deafness (Carter & Wilkening, 1991). Northern and Downs (1991) expressed concern, however, that with a decrease in public awareness regarding rubella, there may also be a decrease in the number of immunizations. A related concern is that in some women, the vaccine seems to provide immunity for only 8 to 12 years. Thus, women who were vaccinated during their prepuberty years may again become susceptible during their child-bearing years (Northern & Downs, 1991).

Cytomegalovirus Infection
CMV, a member of the herpes group of viruses, is the most common viral disease among newborns and the most common viral cause of mental retardation

(Gerber, 1990). It is also the most common viral cause of hearing loss (Northern & Downs, 1991). CMV infections generally are innocuous; most people have had a CMV infection by the time they reach adulthood. In 1975, Marx reported that 80 percent of the population of the United States carries antibodies for CMV by the age of 35 to 40 years. This does not mean that all of these individuals have contracted a CMV infection, only that they have been exposed to the virus and have developed antibodies (Gerber, 1990).

Most people pass through a CMV infection with no known symptoms. However, although antibodies are then established, the virus itself remains in the cells of the body in an inactive state, perhaps for the remainder of an individual's life (Northern & Downs, 1991). Unfortunately, the inactive virus can be reactivated under certain circumstances, including pregnancy, during which time the reactivated virus is excreted in bodily fluids such as urine, saliva, feces, blood, semen, and cervical secretions (Northern & Downs, 1991).

The generalized, herpes-like viral infection of infants most typically is contracted prenatally or postnatally from the mother, although it also can be contracted perinatally in conjunction with passage through the birth canal. Approximately 20 percent of infants infected in utero sustain damage; however, infants who contract CMV at birth or later (eg, from infected breast milk) usually suffer no sequelae (Gerber, 1990).

The incidence of congenital CMV infection has been reported to be 0.5 to 1.5 percent of all live births (Gerber, 1990). According to Gerber, very few infants born with a CMV infection have observable symptoms. In other words, approximately 1 in 100 infants is born with an active CMV infection but appears normal at birth (Northern & Downs, 1991). Ten to fifteen percent of these infants will develop central nervous system disabilities, including hearing loss, developmental delay, psychomotor retardation, and intellectual problems (Northern & Downs, 1991). Most asymptomatic congenital CMV infections are undetected, and the resultant hearing losses are incorrectly attributed to unknown or genetic causes.

Approximately 1 infant in 1000 live births shows evidence of CMV disease at birth (Northern & Downs, 1991). When the disease is clinically detectable at birth, approximately 80 percent of the infants who survive have sequelae related to the central nervous system. Approximately 10 to 25 percent of infants with symptomatic CMV infections have sensorineural hearing loss severe enough to be handicapping. (Northern & Downs, 1991). Infants identified with CMV-related hearing losses show nonspecific sensorineural audiometric configurations. The associated hearing loss ranges from mild to profound and can be progressive.

Gerber (1990) suggested that a relatively new problem may be the association of CMV with acquired immunodeficiency syndrome (AIDS) in infants. As a consequence of the immunosuppression that results from AIDS, AIDS-infected infants are at increased risk for CMV and other viral infections. In fact, CMV may infect nearly all patients with AIDS.

Herpes Simplex Virus

Herpes simplex virus infection is rapidly becoming one of the most common sexually transmitted diseases; no cure or effective treatment is currently available (Northern & Downs, 1991). The virus can be passed to the fetus in utero or, more commonly, during the birth process. Few infants who survive prenatal infection do so without complications, one of which may be sensorineural hearing loss. As is the case with CMV infection, hearing loss is more likely to occur when the virus is contracted prenatally than when it is acquired perinatally or postnatally.

Acquired Immunodeficiency Syndrome

It has been reported that 30 to 50 percent of infants born to mothers with AIDS or HIV (human immunodeficiency virus) infection become infected (Gerber, 1990). According to Gerber, mothers of AIDS-infected infants may not show overt evidence of infection at the time of delivery but may simply be at risk for the development of symptomatic illness at a later time. Although perinatal transmission (eg, via the birth canal or breast milk) has been reported, the risk is low compared with that of intrauterine transmission.

Children with AIDS are more vulnerable to opportunistic and severe infections than adult patients with AIDS because of the immaturity of their immune systems; these infections include upper respiratory infections and middle ear disease. In addition, Real, Thomas, and Gerwin (1987) reported the occurrence of sudden-onset sensorineural hearing loss.

Postnatal Viral Infections

Some common childhood viral infections, including mumps, chickenpox, measles, influenza, and herpes zoster (Levine, 1989), can produce sensorineural hearing loss if the infection enters the inner ear through the blood supply or nerve fibers. Mumps, for example, is a common cause of unilateral sensorineural hearing loss. The associated hearing loss can vary from a mild, high frequency loss to a profound hearing loss. The onset is usually sudden. Measles may result in a sensorineural hearing loss that is likely to be severe to profound, bilateral, and high-frequency in configuration. The onset is often sudden and may not begin until some time after the other symptoms have disappeared (Martin, 1991).

The natural response to infection is the elevation of body temperature. When fevers become excessive, cells, including those of the cochlea, may be damaged (Martin, 1991). Sometimes children run high fevers with no apparent cause but with a resultant hearing loss. In such cases it is difficult, if not impossible, to determine whether the hearing loss is a result of the fever or a result of the initial cause of the fever.

Infections of the middle ear can, on occasion, gain access to the inner ear. Metabolic products can pass from the middle ear into the cochlea by a variety of routes, most notably through the round window. This process can occur in acute otitis media, but is seen more often in conjunction with chronic otitis media.

Perinatal Causes of Sensorineural Hearing Loss

Asphyxia

A common cause of damage to the cochlea and the central nervous system is asphyxia, or oxygen deprivation. Asphyxia is the most frequent cause of brain damage in the perinatal period; it occurs in more than 1 percent of all live births (Gerber, 1990). Asphyxia alters the metabolism of cells, resulting in damage or destruction. It often occurs in conjunction with low birthweight and prematurity, making it difficult to separate these factors as causes of hearing loss.

Low Birthweight

According to Bach et al (1985), there are two types of low birthweight infants: the premature infant who is the expected size for its fetal age and the small-for-gestational-age infant who is born on time but did not grow properly in utero. The latter category can be further divided into cases of primary and secondary growth deficiency. Primary growth deficiency involves chromosomal defects, genetic disorders, and inborn errors of metabolism. The growth failure is intrinsic to the fetus. In secondary growth deficiency, the genetic coding is normal, but the fetus is affected by its environment. The growth deficiency is secondary to a problem outside the fetus that limits its capacity for growth. For example, abnormal delivery of nutrients, hormones, or oxygen to the cells can result in secondary growth deficiency (Bach et al, 1985). Both prematurity and growth deficiency increase an infant's risk for hearing loss and other congenital defects.

Prematurity

Infants delivered before 37 weeks gestation are considered to be premature (Northern & Downs, 1991). However, although the incidence of hearing loss is clearly higher among preterm infants than among full-term infants (Northern & Downs, 1991), a number of factors associated with prematurity also have been associated with sensorineural hearing loss. Thus, it may be difficult to ascertain the origin of a hearing loss in a premature infant. For example, asphyxia, hyperbilirubinemia, bacterial and viral infections, the use of ototoxic medication, and meningitis are all conditions associated with both prematurity and sensorineural hearing loss (Ruben, 1990; Northern & Downs, 1991).

Ruben (1990) reported that the incidence of prematurity in a clinical outpatient population is approximately 10 percent, but is as high as 23 percent in a population of deaf children. Moreover, Ruben reported that the chance of a premature infant being deaf is 20 times greater than that of a child with normal birthweight. The hearing loss typically associated with prematurity is bilateral, severe, high-frequency, and sensorineural. These children have a high percentage of additional handicaps.

Hyperbilirubinemia

Hyperbilirubinemia (jaundice) occurs when there is an excess of bilirubin (a red bile pigment formed from hemoglobin) in the blood (Northern & Downs, 1991). As described by Northern and Downs, with the breakdown of red blood cells, unconjugated bilirubin routinely is released into the plasma serum. Unconjugated bilirubin is then bound to plasma albumin and transported to the liver where an enzyme conjugates it. That is, the potentially toxic unconjugated bilirubin is joined with a substance in the body to form a detoxified product. The now conjugated bilirubin normally is excreted through the small intestine. When it cannot be conjugated because of inadequate liver function, massive breakdown of red blood cells, or both, bilirubin builds up in the blood until it crosses the plasma membrane and is deposited in the brain. This condition is known as kernicterus. Kernicterus causes motor and sensory deficits, mental retardation, and death (Northern & Downs, 1991). Most infants with kernicterus die during the first week of life; 80 percent of those who survive have complete or partial deafness (Northern & Downs, 1991). Audiometric findings may show mild to profound sensorineural hearing loss, often characterized by a "cookie-bite" configuration.

Rh (or ABO) incompatibility between mother and child may be associated with hyperbilirubinemia (Northern & Downs, 1991). Rh incompatibility is a danger when a fetus whose blood contains a protein molecule, called the Rh factor, is conceived by a mother in whom the factor is absent. After delivery of a first child, the mother's body produces an antibody for protection against the harmful effects of the Rh factor. The number of antibodies produced increases with each succeeding pregnancy, until a sufficient number is present to damage the developing red blood cells of a fetus. Damage to fetal red blood cells can reduce the oxygen available to body parts, including the cochlea.

Hearing losses that result from Rh incompatibility occur less frequently than they once did because physicians have learned to predict and prevent disorders with maternal immunization and infant blood transfusion after birth. The incidence and sequelae of Rh incompatibility have dropped by 80 percent since 1970 because of the use of these preventive measures (Gerber, 1990). A more conservative approach used with infants at lower risk than those for whom transfusion is indicated is phototherapy. Phototherapy is a procedure in which the infant is placed under a bank of lights that have the property of causing excess bilirubin to exude through the skin.

Complications of Rh incompatibility account for about 3 percent of all cases of profound sensorineural hearing loss among school-aged deaf children (Northern & Downs, 1991). This number is expected to decrease to 1 percent in the future (Northern & Downs, 1991).

Postnatal Causes of Sensorineural Hearing Loss

Meningitis

Pappas (1985) defined meningitis as an inflammation of the meninges and their circulating fluid (cerebrospinal fluid) that may extend to the brain itself. Although most cases are acquired peri- or postnatally, meningitis also can be contracted in utero as a result of a maternal infection. Meningitis develops in approximately 1 of every 2500 live births and is a leading cause of acquired hearing loss in infants and children (Northern & Downs, 1991). Since the advent of antibiotics, the mortality rate has decreased, resulting in a statistical increase in the number of survivors with sensorineural hearing loss. Ruben (1990) suggested that hearing loss secondary to meningitis may account for 4 to 7 percent of all cases of childhood hearing loss. Stein et al (1990), however, reported that bacterial meningitis was the etiologic factor in 21 percent of the hearing impaired children they studied.

Although meningitis occurs more commonly as a viral disease, most of the cases that cause neurologic sequelae are of bacterial origin (Pappas, 1985). Microscopic examination of the cerebrospinal fluid, achieved by lumbar puncture, is necessary for diagnosis. When the specific bacterial agent involved is known, the infection can be treated with specific antibiotics. Symptoms include fever, headache, neck stiffness, irritability, altered consciousness, and vomiting. In the preantibiotic era, meningitis often developed as a result of invasion of the meninges by an infection of the middle ear. Today, the most common pathway is the bloodstream and the most common site of the original infection is the upper respiratory tract.

Hearing loss varies in amount, symmetry, and configuration; however, complete hearing loss, sometimes due to the ossification of cochlear structures, tends to occur more often than is the case with hearing losses due to other causes. Hearing may fluctuate for as long as 3 months after recovery from the infection and occasionally has been reported to return to normal (Pappas, 1985). Northern and Downs (1991) suggested, however, that documented hearing improvement occurs only in isolated cases. Improved hearing levels following meningitis may be related to inaccurate behavioral results obtained during the acute stage of the disease or to resolution of a transient conductive component of the hearing loss. However, because as many as 50 percent of the cases of hearing loss associated with meningitis are unstable, close audiologic monitoring of hearing and amplification is critical.

Survivors of meningitis, even those without hearing loss or other neurologic deficits, may function at lower levels than their peers because of a number of additional handicaps that affect learning. Moreover, the acquired loss of hearing secondary to meningitis may, in some ways, be worse (ie, more traumatic) than a congenital hearing loss. That is, the acquired hearing loss is the loss of a known quantity that results in sudden isolation. Such a loss is likely to be frightening, and adjustment is likely to be difficult.

Northern and Downs (1991) reported that the number of children who suffer hearing loss due to meningitis is expected to decrease sharply as a result of the development of a protective vaccine. According to Northern and Downs, the vaccine is recommended for all children at 2 years of age, and at 18 months of age for those children who are at increased risk for meningitis, such as children in day care or children with other underlying diseases. Unfortunately, the vaccine is not effective in infants. Vaccines capable of inducing antibodies in infants are under study (Stein et al, 1990).

Ototoxicity

Some drugs, including some used to treat meningitis, are known to produce a severe, high-frequency sensorineural hearing loss. Today, the largest and most commonly encountered group of ototoxic drugs are the aminoglycoside antibiotics, a group of antibiotics sometimes referred to as the *mycins*. This group includes dihydrostreptomycin, streptomycin, neomycin, kanamycin, and gentamycin. There are considerable differences in individual susceptibility to ototoxic drugs. Factors that may sensitize the cochlea and increase the ototoxic effects of the aminogly-cosides include age, health, heredity, impaired renal function, the use of more than one ototoxic drug simultaneously, the use of increased daily doses for extended periods of time, hyperthermia, dehydration, and concurrent noise exposure (Hawke & Jahn, 1987; Northern & Downs, 1991).

The initial cochleotoxic effect of the aminoglycosides occurs in the basal turn of the cochlea and consequently affects the high-frequency range of hearing (Hawke & Jahn, 1987). Careful and regular monitoring of auditory function and serum antibiotic levels should enable the physician to predict when ototoxic effects will occur. The use of ultra high-frequency audiometry allows the early detection of cochlear toxicity in the frequency range between 8000 and 20,000 Hz and should allow cessation of treatment with consequent preservation of hearing in the frequencies necessary for communication (Hawke & Jahn, 1987).

The most common situations in which sensorineural deafness results from the use of these drugs are when an overdose is unintentionally given, when there is unrecognized renal impairment, or when the drug is used to preserve life, even with knowledge of possible cochlear damage (Ruben, 1990). Some medications (eg, neomycin) may continue to cause irreversible hearing loss even after the first signs of destruction are noted and the drug is discontinued (Ruben, 1990). Others, such as ethacrynic acid, typically cause a hearing loss that resolves when the medication is stopped (Ruben, 1990). A unique feature of dihydrostreptomycin is that its ototoxic effects may not manifest for weeks or months after its administration (Hawke & Jahn, 1987).

Ingestion of ototoxic drugs by pregnant women can result in a variety of congenital abnormalities, including hearing loss, as a result of passage of the drugs across the placenta (Northern & Downs, 1991). It seems that renal failure, concomitant use of diuretics, a prolonged course of drug therapy, or a combination of these elements are the most important factors in the development of fetal ototoxicity (Northern & Downs, 1991).

The evaluation of ototoxicity in infants is particularly difficult because these infants are likely to be receiving medical therapy for severe problems, including systemic infection; that may accompany low birthweight, jaundice, or other health disorders that are themselves associated with hearing loss (Northern & Downs, 1991).

Transverse Temporal Bone Fractures

Approximately one-fifth of all temporal bone fractures are of the transverse type. More force is required to produce these fractures than is required to produce longitudinal fractures, and loss of consciousness is probable. Transverse fractures may disrupt structures of the cochlea, the internal auditory canal, and the auditory nerve, often resulting in profound sensorineural hearing loss (Meyerhoff, 1986). The facial nerve is injured in as many as 50 percent of patients (Meyerhoff, 1986).

A hearing loss also may result from hemorrhage or concussion within the cochlea (Ballenger, 1985c). In this case, structures of the inner ear may be torn, stretched, or deteriorated due to the loss of oxygen after hemorrhage (Martin, 1991). Trauma to the skull may result in other complications, such as otitis media or meningitis, which may themselves be causes of hearing loss (Martin, 1991).

Noise-Induced Hearing Loss

As with adults, exposure to high-intensity noise can result in permanent hearing loss in children. Although children typically are not exposed to intense noise for prolonged periods of time, as are adults who are exposed to occupational noise, they sometimes are exposed to potentially damaging recreational noises (eg, those associated with hunting, riding on snowmobiles, and listening to music through stereo headphones). They also may suffer from acoustic trauma, damage that results from exposure to impulsive sounds, such as explosions. In the latter case, exposure can result in a tympanic membrane perforation, a high-frequency sensorineural hearing loss, or both, often with a characteristic acoustic trauma notch between 3000 and 6000 Hz. Children, and parents of children, with hearing losses that may be attributable to noise damage should be counseled vigorously about the hazards of continued exposure (see Chapter 12).

A possible cause of noise-induced hearing loss unique to neonates is the high sound level generated by incubators (Ruben, 1990). Although these sound levels do not exceed acceptable damage risk criteria for hearing loss (Williams-Steiger Occupational Safety and Health Act, 1970), they may constitute a factor that contributes to deafness in premature infants who may also be ill and receiving ototoxic medication (Ruben, 1990). Moreover, noise exposure is 24 hours per day over a period of several weeks to several months. In addition, it may be that infants and children are more susceptible to damage from noise than are adults.

Bess, Peek, and Chapman (1979) reported on incubator noise levels combined with different types of life-support equipment and the impulse noise produced by striking the side of the incubator or by opening and closing the doors of the storage unit. The life-support equipment increased the overall noise levels by as much as 15 to 20 decibels sound pressure level (dBA SPL); the impulse signals produced by striking the sides of incubators (a practice of physicians and nurses used to stimulate breathing in apneic infants) ranged from 130 to 140 dBA SPL. Opening and closing the storage unit doors produced peak amplitudes of 114 dBA SPL. These levels are potentially damaging.

MIXED HEARING LOSS

People with mixed hearing losses exhibit impaired hearing sensitivity by both air conduction and bone conduction; however, air-conduction thresholds are poorer than bone-conduction thresholds by at least 15 dB HL. That is, although both air-conduction and bone-conduction thresholds are outside the normal range, an air-bone gap exists. Sensorineural function is impaired to the degree demonstrated by bone-conduction thresholds, with a conductive component superimposed.

A mixed hearing loss occurs when both conductive and sensorineural pathologic conditions exist in the same ear. The conductive component may be medically or surgically correctable; however, hearing improves only to the level of the bone-conduction thresholds as sensorineural hearing losses generally cannot be remediated. An example of a mixed hearing loss might be found in a child with a stable sensorineural hearing loss of genetic origin who develops otitis media. The conductive hearing loss that is superimposed on the sensorineural hearing loss can be resolved with medical/surgical treatment of the otitis media; however, hearing improves only to the level of the bone-conduction thresholds that represent the stable sensorineural hearing loss.

REFERENCES

Bach, S., Ginsberg, L., Overbeck, A., Sparks, S., & Willis, C. (1985). Speech and language in genetic disorders. Presented at the American Speech-Language-Hearing Association Annual Convention, November 18-21, 1985, Washington, DC.

Ballenger, J. J. (1985a). Congenital malformations of the ear. In J. J. Ballenger (Ed.), *Diseases of the nose, throat, ear, head, and neck* (pp. 1217-1231). Philadelphia: Lea & Febiger.

Ballenger, J. J. (1985b). Diseases of the external ear. In J. J. Ballenger (Ed.), *Diseases of the nose, throat, ear, head, and neck* (pp. 1084-1097). Philadelphia: Lea & Febiger.

Ballenger, J. J. (1985c). Noninflammatory diseases of the labyrinth. In J. J. Ballenger (Ed.), *Diseases of the nose, throat, ear, head, and neck* (pp. 1247-1274). Philadelphia: Lea & Febiger.

Bergstrom, L. (1990). Diseases of the external ear. In C. D. Bluestone & S. E. Stool (Eds.), *Pediatric otolaryngology* (pp. 311-319). Philadelphia: Saunders.

Bess, F. H., & Humes, L. E. (1990). *Audiology: The fundamentals.* Baltimore: Williams & Wilkins.

Bess, F. H., Klee, T., & Culbertson, J. L. (1986). Identification, assessment and management of children with unilateral sensorineural hearing loss. *Ear and Hearing, 7,* 43-51.

Bess, F.H., Peek, B., & Chapman, J. (1979). Further observations on noise levels in infant incubators. *Pediatrics, 63,* 100.

Bess, F. H., & Tharpe, A. M. (1984). Unilateral hearing impairment in children. *Pediatrics, 74,* 206-216.

Bluestone, C. D., & Klein, J. O. (1990a). Intracranial suppurative complications of otitis media and mastoiditis. In C. D. Bluestone & S. E. Stool (Eds.). *Pediatric otolaryngology* (pp. 537-546). Philadelphia: Saunders.

Bluestone, C. D., & Klein, J. O. (1990b). Intratemporal complications and sequelae of otitis media. In C. D. Bluestone & S. E. Stool (Eds.). *Pediatric otolaryngology* (pp. 487-536). Philadelphia: Saunders.

Bluestone, C. D., & Klein, J. O. (1990c). Otitis media, atelectasis, and eustachian tube dysfunction. In C. D. Bluestone & S. E. Stool (Eds.). *Pediatric otolaryngology* (pp. 320-486). Philadelphia: Saunders.

Boies, L. R. (1989). Diseases of the external ear. In G. L. Adams, L. R. Boies, & P. A. Hilger (Eds.). *Boies fundamentals of otolaryngology: A textbook of ear, nose and throat diseases* (pp. 77-89). Philadelphia: Saunders.

Carter, B. S., & Wilkening, R. B. (1991). Prevention of hearing disorders: Neonatal causes of hearing loss. *Seminars in Hearing, 12,* 154-167.

Downs, M. P. (1987). The nature of otitis media. Presented at Michigan State University, February 6, 1987, East Lansing, Michigan.

Friel-Patti, S., Finitzo, T., & Hieber, J. P. (1987). Communication disorders screening in a pediatric practice. *Seminars in Hearing, 8,* 143-148.

Garrard, K. R., & Clark, B. S. (1985). Otitis media: The role of speech-language pathologists. *Asha, 27,* 35-39.

Gerber, S. E. (1990). *Prevention: The etiology of communicative disorders in children.* Englewood Cliffs: Prentice Hall.

Harris, J. P., & Endres, D. (1990). Surgery for congenital aural atresia. In G. B. Healy (Ed.), *Common problems in pediatric otolaryngology* (pp. 39-49). Chicago: Year Book.

Hawke, M., & Jahn, A. F. (1987). *Diseases of the ear.* Philadelphia: Lea & Febiger.

Klein, J. O. (1991). Prevention of acute otitis media. *Seminars in Hearing, 12,* 140-145.

Levine, S. C. (1989). Diseases of the inner ear. In G. L. Adams, L. R. Boies, & P. A. Hilger (Eds.), *Boies fundamentals of otolaryngology: A textbook of ear, nose and throat diseases* (pp. 123-141). Philadelphia: Saunders.

Martin, F. N. (1991). *Introduction to audiology.* Englewood Cliffs: Prentice Hall.

Marx, J. (1975). Cytomegalovirus: A major cause of birth defects. *Science, 190,* 1184-1186.

Meyerhoff, W. L. (1986). *Disorders of hearing.* Austin: Pro-Ed.

Northern, J. L., & Downs, M. P. (1991). *Hearing in children*. Baltimore: Williams & Wilkins.

Paparella, M. M., Adams, G. L., & Levine, S. C. (1989). Diseases of the middle ear and mastoid. In G. L. Adams, L. R. Boies, & P. A. Hilger (Eds.), *Boies fundamentals of otolaryngology: A textbook of ear, nose and throat diseases* (pp. 90-122). Philadelphia: Saunders.

Pappas, D. G. (1985). *Diagnosis and treatment of hearing impairment in children*. San Diego: College Hill.

Real, R., Thomas, M., & Gerwin, J.M. (1987). Sudden hearing loss and acquired immunodeficiency syndrome. *Otolaryngology—Head and Neck Surgery, 97*, 409-412.

Ruben, R. J. (1990). Diseases of the inner ear and sensorineural deafness. In C. D. Bluestone & S. E. Stool (Eds.), *Pediatric otolaryngology* (pp. 547-570). Philadelphia: Saunders.

Salamy, A., & Eldredge, L. (1991). Neonatal risk and hearing loss. *Seminars in Hearing, 12*, 146-153.

Schloss, M. D. (1990). Otorrhea. In C. D. Bluestone & S. E. Stool (Eds.), *Pediatric otolaryngology* (pp. 198-202). Philadelphia: Saunders.

Stein, L. K., Jabaley, T., Spitz, R., Stoakley, D., & McGee, T. (1990). The hearing-impaired infant: Patterns of identification and habilitation revisited. *Ear and Hearing, 11*, 201-205.

Stewart, J. M. (1987). Genetics of deafness: New prenatal diagnostic techniques. *Seminars in Hearing, 8*, 77-81.

Stewart, J.M. (1987). Genetics of deafness: New prenatal diagnostic techniques. *Seminars in Hearing, 8*, 77-81.

Tardy, E. M. (1985). Reconstruction of the outstanding ear. In J. J. Ballenger (Ed.), *Diseases of the nose, throat, ear, head, and neck* (pp. 1232-1246). Philadelphia: Lea & Febiger.

Teele, D. W., Klein, J. O., & Rosner, B.A. (1980). Epidemiology of otitis media in children. *Annals of Otology, Rhinology and Laryngology, 89*, 5-6.

Teele, D.W., Klein, J.O., & Rosner, B. (1989). Epidemiology of otitis media during the first seven years of life in children in greater Boston. *Journal of Infectious Disease, 160*, 83-94.

Williams-Steiger Occupational Safety and Health Act. (1970). PL 91-569.

3

Disorders of Hearing in Adults

Lida G. Wall

This chapter is designed to acquaint speech-language pathologists, educators, and health care professionals with hearing disorders that affect adults and with health problems that place adults at risk for hearing loss. Each disorder is described and the suggested management options are discussed; the location of the disorder within the auditory system is defined; and the type of hearing loss, conductive or sensorineural, associated with the disorder is discussed. Many hearing disorders are common to both children and adults; however, some hearing disorders occur more frequently in one of the groups relative to the other. The disorders covered in Chapter 2, such as atresia, stenosis, external otitis, and otitis media, are only briefly mentioned in this chapter. Disorders that occur more frequently in adults, such as temporal bone fractures, vestibular schwannomas, and multiple sclerosis, are covered in depth.

OUTER EAR DISORDERS

Outer ear disorders that occur in adults include deformities of the auricle and external ear canal, external otitis, cerumen occlusion, foreign body occlusion, cysts, and collapsed canal (Hawke & Jahn, 1987). Most of these disorders are not associated with a hearing impairment, except under the unusual circumstance of complete occlusion of the ear canal. If a hearing loss is present with an outer ear disorder, it is a conductive hearing loss. An audiogram for a conductive hearing loss (Chapter 6) shows normal bone-conduction thresholds that are better than air-conduction thresholds by 10 dB or more. The external ear disorders described in Chapter 2 are all conditions that may affect adults as well as children.

Atresia

A malformation of the cartilaginous portion of the auricle and of the ear canal during development may result in a condition known as atresia (Hawke & Jahn, 1987). The degree of malformation ranges from the presence of a small piece of external tissue with no recognizable features to partial or total absence of the external auricle (microtia). Frequently the malformation includes portions of the middle ear but only rarely is the inner ear involved (see Chapter 2). Atresia has an incidence of 1:10,000 to 1:20,000 (Frolsch & Sommer, 1991). The associated hearing impairment varies with the degree of malformation. The loss is conductive, unless the inner ear is involved, exhibiting up to a 50 dB air-bone gap.

Stenosis

Narrowing of the external canal opening is known as stenosis. No hearing impairment is associated with this condition, but because of the narrow opening, the canal may close when pressure is applied by the earphone to the auricle. Special care must be taken under these circumstances to prevent the false appearance of a hearing impairment during testing.

Cerumen Occlusion

Both ceruminous and sebaceous glands are located in the skin of the external canal, and secretions from these glands combine to lubricate the external auditory canal (Cohn, 1981). Excessive cerumen accumulation is a common problem, but the degree of the accumulation varies from one person to another. If the amount of cerumen is such that the ear cannot function in a self-cleaning manner, then accumulation of cerumen and possible occlusion of the canal may occur. Adults who wear hearing aids are particularly susceptible to cerumen occlusion of the ear canal because the earmold prevents the self-cleaning action of the ear canal. No hearing loss is evident with cerumen accumulation unless total occlusion occurs. In cases of total occlusion of the canal, a mild temporary conductive hearing loss may occur. Removal of cerumen may be necessary to alleviate the occlusion and associated hearing loss.

Ceruminoma

The most common tumor of the external canal is a ceruminoma, a term that has been used to describe a group of glandular tumors (Hawke & Jahn, 1987) located in the external canal. According to Hawke and Jahn, there are four types of ceruminomas. The first type (ceruminal adenoma) is a benign tumor of variable size in the external canal and is usually asymptomatic. The second type (ceruminal pleomorphic adenoma) is rare and is superficially comparable to ceruminal adenoma. This mixed-type tumor appears as a skin-covered mass in the external canal and is asymptomatic unless the opening of the canal is occluded. The third type of tumor is ceruminal adenocarcinoma, which is malignant. This tumor appears as a nodule in the ear canal and is likely to be associated with pain. Unless complete obstruction of the canal occurs, no hearing loss is apparent. The last type of ceruminoma is adenoid cystic carcinoma which is a rare, malignant tumor. The tumor is usually associated with pain, may appear similar to a polyp in the ear canal, and is frequently associated with chronic ear infections. The degree of canal obstruction varies.

In summary, then, depending on the type and size of the ceruminoma, the tumor may be asymptomatic or may have associated symptoms of pain and hearing loss. If the tumor is large, the most common symptom is a sensation of blockage; total obstruction of the opening of the canal, however, results in a hearing loss (Hawke & Jahn, 1987). Whenever a tumor or obstruction is observed in the ear canal, medical referral is imperative. Any change in a previously identified chronic ear infection or any onset of pain or bleeding associated with a chronic ear infection should prompt referral to a physician.

Perforation of the Tympanic Membrane

The incidence of traumatic ruptures of the tympanic membrane is estimated to be 1.4 per 100,000 people per year (Kristensen et al, 1989). Perforation of the tympanic membrane can result from otitis media, a traumatic injury, or other complicating injuries such as disruption of the ossicular chain. In most cases of traumatic perforation, the tympanic membrane heals naturally (Kristensen et al, 1989). If the perforation does not heal, however, tympanoplasty (surgical repair of the middle ear) or myringoplasty (surgical repair of the tympanic membrane) is necessary. Kirstensen et al (1989) determined from their series of case studies that no correlation could be made between cause, location, or size of the perforation and spontaneous healing. They did report, however, that loss of tissue and secondary infection contributed to the lack of spontaneous healing of the perforation. They also noted that patients younger than 30 years experienced spontaneous healing more frequently than patients older than 30 years. It is suggested that spontaneous healing time can be predicted to be 1 month for 10 percent of surface area lost to the perforation (Pahor, 1981).

Tympanic perforations not associated with a middle ear infection are caused by abrupt high-pressure changes in the ear canal or by objects inserted through the ear canal. The abrupt pressure change may be caused by an explosion, a slap against the ear, or a traumatic head injury. Perforations from objects are usually caused by items such as cotton-tipped applicators, bobby pins, or pencils may cause damage and disruption of the ossicular chain. Perforations due to abrupt pressure change or object injury frequently heal spontaneously within a month or two.

Work-related perforations from hot metals or liquids are less likely to heal spontaneously, and complications are possible (Hawke & Jahn, 1987).

Tympanosclerosis

Tympanosclerosis, which is a result of repeated ear inflammation and damage to the tissue, looks like white deposits (calcium) on the tympanic membrane and is usually not associated with a hearing loss (Hawke & Jahn, 1987). Tympanosclerosis may involve the ossicular chain and, as it increases, may begin to reduce the mobility of the ossicles. If the middle ear structures are involved and hearing is affected, surgical reconstruction or amplification may be the treatment of choice.

Otitis Externa

An inflammatory condition of the skin in the external ear canal or auricle is known as otitis externa (Cohn, 1981). The multiple causes of otitis externa range from infection to trauma with localized or diffuse involvement. The infection is most frequently due to bacterial or fungal infection. Otitis externa in the external canal may involve swelling of the skin caused by accumulation of tissue fluid; redness; shedding of epithelium; and discharge of pus (Hawke & Jahn, 1987).

It is not expected that a hearing loss will result from this inflammatory process. However, the pain associated with the infection may prevent audiometric testing. Pain and inflammation may prevent insertion of a hearing aid earmold during the acute state of the inflammation. Some patients may temporarily shift the hearing aid to the other ear. If the inflammation is chronic, changes in the external ear may, in rare cases, cause a conductive hearing impairment.

MIDDLE EAR DISORDERS

Middle ear disorders typically show a conductive hearing impairment on an audiogram; in other words, the air- and bone-conduction thresholds differ from each other The air-conduction responses indicate a greater impairment than the bone-conduction responses (air-bone gap), which would be expected to fall within the normal range (0 to 15 decibels hearing level [dB HL]). The air-bone gap can vary, and the threshold differences can be as great as 50 dB. Middle ear disorders alone can cause a conductive hearing impairment, but other auditory conditions (presbycusis, ototoxicity, noise-induced hearing loss) may co-exist in the inner ear. The combination of impairments (mixed hearing loss) can be seen on an audiogram. In mixed hearing losses, both air- and bone-conduction thresholds are impaired, and an air-bone gap of varying degree is present.

Otitis Media

Otitis media refers to infectious or inflammatory conditions that involve the middle ear space (Hawke & Jahn, 1987). Otitis media and its complications occur more frequently in children (see Chapter 2) but may occur in adults of any age.

Glomus Tumor

One of the more common neoplasms to occur in the middle ear space is a glomus tumor. Glomus tumors occur more commonly in women than men with a reported ratio of 3:1 or 4:1 (Alford & Guilford, 1962). It is rare that a glomus tumor would occur before adolescence. The tumor is most likely to occur in the middle years. No race differences are reported.

The origin and physiologic nature of this vascular tumor were not well understood when it was first described in the literature, and this resulted in lack of consistent terminology. The 1945 report in the literature by Rosenwasser suggests that glomus tumors arise from the glomus jugulare and are essentially blood-vessel tumors with interspersed epithelioid cells (Bratt et al, 1979). Glomus tumors now have been classified into tympanicum tumors, located primarily in the mastoid and middle ear region, and jugulare tumors, which originate from the jugular bulb (Glasscock et al, 1974; 1978).

A glomus tympanicum tumor arises from the glomus bodies, which are located on the floor or medial wall of the middle ear space (Bratt et al, 1979). The tumor expands through the middle ear space and may alter the function of the middle ear structures, resulting in a mild conductive hearing impairment and a pulsatile tinnitus, which are the early symptoms.

A glomus jugulare tumor, which develops from glomus bodies within the adventitia (outer covering) of the jugular bulb, may expand into the middle ear space and produce symptoms similar to those of a glomus tympanicum tumor. It may expand along the base of the skull and enter into the posterior cranial fossa, where it produces pressure on cranial nerves such as the glossopharyngeal, vagus, and spinal accessory nerves as they pass through the jugular foramen (Bratt et al, 1979). The symptoms produced are unique to the cranial nerve involved.

In spite of the complex array of symptoms produced, Bratt et al (1979) suggests that the following four characteristic symptoms may typify glomus tumors: (1) the tumor is very vascular and bleeds easily; (2) pulsatile tinnitus, synchronous with the heart rate, is produced as the tumor increases in size; (3) the tumor grows slowly (decades); and (4) an individual may have long-standing symptoms, which can recur after treatment. On occasion, the tumor expands rapidly and thus must be treated aggressively.

The seven most common complaints (Bratt et al, 1979) reported by patients include tinnitus, hearing loss, dizziness, ear pain, feeling of ear pressure, bleeding from the ear, and hoarseness. These symptoms vary with the type and size of the tumor. Audiometric results provide valuable information because the degree of impairment associated with the tumor may vary from mild to profound, and the type of hearing loss may be conductive, during the early stages, or mixed. Probably the most valuable audiometric information is determined with immittance measurements. The regular pulses associated with the vascularity of the tumor can be depicted on tympanometric tracings. As the blood pressure in the tumor increases and decreases in response to the heart contractions, these changes are seen as immittance changes that coincide with the heart rate.

Of the two types of glomus tumors, the jugulare tumor has a greater potential for causing a profound loss of hearing. The tumor may erode the petrous portion of the temporal bone, resulting in a sensorineural hearing impairment. As the tumor size and invasion increases, the degree of hearing loss increases. It is even possible for the acoustic nerve to be compressed in the internal auditory canal when the tumor invasion is extensive (Bratt et al, 1979).

Glomus tumors are managed with surgical removal when possible or with radiation therapy. A result of most of the surgical techniques is a moderate to profound hearing loss, even with reconstructive surgery. So an essential part of the care of patients with glomus tumors is monitoring hearing status for several months after treatment (Bratt et al, 1979). Hearing impairment that persists should be managed with the appropriate assistive listening device or hearing aid to assist the person with communication.

Otic Barotrauma

The eustachian tube serves to equalize the air pressure on both sides of the tympanic membrane. Failure of the eustachian tube to equalize the air pressure, which results in damage, is referred to as otic barotrauma (Hawke & Jahn, 1987). The eustachian tube under normal circumstances functions as a "flutter" valve that is inactive as air passes in one direction, from the middle ear space into the nasopharynx, but an active muscle contraction is needed for air to pass in the reverse direction, from the nasopharynx to the middle ear space (Hawke & Jahn, 1987). This contraction occurs when a person swallows or yawns; the tube is opened by the tensor veli palatini and levator palatini muscles.

Under conditions in which the atmospheric pressure may be changing (such as ascent or descent in an aircraft), the pressure in the middle ear space needs to adjust accordingly. For example, if the pressure within the middle ear space is less than the surrounding air pressure, the tympanic membrane is pushed medially. A yawn or swallow opens the tube and allows for pressure equalization and reduced membrane displacement. Conversely, if the pressure within the middle ear space is greater than the surrounding atmospheric pressure, the eustachian tube valve spontaneously opens, allowing air to flow into the nasopharynx and thus equalizes the pressure across the tympanic membrane (Hawke & Jahn, 1979).

These changes in air pressure occur during the descent of an aircraft or the ascent of a deep-sea diver. People with normally functioning eustachian tubes have no difficulty adjusting to the pressure changes, but people with blocked or poorly functioning eustachian tubes, usually due to an upper respiratory infection, may not be able to adjust to slow or abrupt pressure changes. Under such circumstances, and when a critical pressure differential is reached between the pressure in the middle ear space and atmospheric pressure, the tympanic membrane is displaced. If the tube is dysfunctional, that is, it cannot open to adjust to atmospheric pressure, negative middle ear pressure may continue, and a thin, serous fluid, present in the mucosa, fills the middle ear space (Hawke & Jahn, 1987). When the tympanic membrane is displaced, pain may result from pressure on the membrane. In some cases soft tissue near the opening of the eustachian tube may be drawn into the opening and block the normal closing function; edema of the mucosa may result.

For other cases of barotrauma, the pressure changes may be only minimal and associated with only mild discomfort. However, pressure changes can be great enough to cause rupture of the oval or round window and concurrent leakage of perilymph; sensorineural hearing impairment and dizziness may occur under these circumstances (Hawke and Jahn, 1987). Immediate medical attention is required.

Otosclerosis

The onset of otosclerosis is most common in white, young adults in the second or third decade of life (Hawke & Jahn, 1987). Twice as many women as men have the disease (Derlacki, 1984). The disease may involve only one ear initially, but as the disease progresses most (80 percent) patients exhibit bilateral involvement.

Otosclerosis involves destruction of normal bone and the development of new abnormal bone anywhere in the otic capsule. The destruction of bone is the initial stage of otosclerosis. As the normal bone is lost, the space left is filled with fibrous vascular tissue. At this stage of otosclerosis, the lesion (spaces filled with fibrous tissue) is soft and spongy (Hawke & Jahn, 1987). The second stage is characterized by active (immature bone formation) and quiescent (hardening of the bony growth) periods. During the active period, abnormal immature bone forms that is extremely vascular and spongy. The vascular state contributes to the red glow that can be visualized behind the tympanic membrane and is referred to as a Schwartze sign (Hawke & Jahn, 1987). During the inactive periods of the third stage, the bone becomes dense, gray, and hard (Derlacki, 1984).

Otosclerosis primarily involves the footplate of the stapes and is considered to be nonclinical until symptoms such as hearing loss arise (Hawke & Jahn, 1987). stapedectomy (replacement of the stapes by a prosthesis) is frequently the treatment of choice for the ear with the poorer thresholds. If both ears are affected, the second ear is not usually considered for surgery until at least 1 year after the operation on the first ear (Derlacki, 1984) to assure that good hearing is maintained in the repaired ear. Of course there is always a possibility of a recurrent conductive hearing loss due to prosthesis problems or to regrowth of abnormal bone. For some patients who do not elect to undergo surgical intervention, possibly because of other physical conditions, amplification can be an alternative. Amplification for otosclerosis is highly successful for aiding communication.

It is important for patients with otosclerosis that the history be carefully taken. Evidence of a progressive, conductive hearing impairment and a positive family history are good indicators of otosclerosis. The conductive hearing loss is usually bilateral but may occasionally be unilateral.

An audiogram associated with otosclerosis shows the air-conduction thresholds to be elevated across the frequency range with the greatest impairment in the lower frequency range (250 and 500 Hz) but normal bone-conduction thresholds for 500 Hz, 1000 Hz, and 4000 Hz. An impaired threshold for the bone-conduction response at 2000 Hz, also known as the Carhart notch, may be present. The impaired 2000-Hz bone-conduction threshold is a result of a mechanical effect associated with the fixation of the anterior portion of the stapes (Derlacki, 1984). Because the ossicular chain contributes to the bone-conduction response, it should be anticipated that there will be an improvement in the bone-conduction threshold as well as the air-conduction threshold after surgical treatment. Hearing thresholds may be returned to within 10 dB of the preoperative bone-conduction thresholds (Derlacki, 1984). Because otosclerosis may recur, the speech-language pathologist, educator, and health care professional should be alert to the possibility of change in hearing of a person previously identified to have the condition. Hearing should be screened periodically, or the patient should be referred for a complete hearing evaluation as needed.

COCHLEAR AND RETROCOCHLEAR DISORDERS

The most frequently encountered type of hearing impairment among adults is sensorineural hearing loss, which reflects damage to both the cochlea and the eighth cranial nerve. An adult with a sensorineural hearing loss can benefit from hearing aids, assistive listening devices, and adjustment of the work or home environment. However, some adults with sensorineural hearing impairment need medical treatment or surgical intervention for the impairment. After the medical intervention, decisions regarding hearing status and rehabilitation needs must be made.

Audiologic Pattern

The audiogram usually seen with a cochlear disorder has overlapping air- and bone-conduction symbols. In other words, responses from both threshold measurements should yield approximately the same hearing sensitivity on an audiogram. The shape or configuration of the audiogram may differ with each disorder. Some of the configurations suggest better hearing sensitivity in the low frequencies (falling configuration) and others suggest better hearing in the high frequencies (rising configuration). The degree of impairment for each disorder varies from mild to moderate to severe and may involve one or both ears. Although an audiogram may indicate that a sensorineural hearing impairment is present, it does not indicate where the impairment is located. Cochlear impairment is most likely to result from damage to the sensory cells. In many cases, degeneration of the neural fibers after sensory cell damage may also contribute to the sensorineural hearing loss. On the other hand, retrocochlear or eighth nerve impairments may result from tumors that arise on the vestibular portion of the eighth nerve and result in a sensorineural hearing loss. Further separation of the type of hearing impairment and location of the disorder can be assisted by special audiologic tests (see Chapter 6). The following hearing disorders may result in a sensorineural loss.

Vestibular Schwannoma (Acoustic Neuroma)

Acoustic neuroma is the term that has been applied to benign tumors that arise from Schwann cells (Monsell & Rock, 1990; Weaver & Staller, 1984), which form the neurilemmal sheath on the vestibular portion of the eighth cranial nerve. However, *acoustic neuroma* is no longer considered to be the appropriate term to use with eighth nerve tumors. In 1991 the National Institutes of Health (NIH) Consensus Development Conference on Acoustic Neuroma agreed that *vestibular schwannoma* is the preferred term because it more appropriately describes the cell type from which the tumor arises and denotes the general location as the vestibular portion of the eighth cranial nerve. Schwannoma is the most common of the eighth nerve tumors.

The occurrence of vestibular schwannomas in the general population is not known. The findings at postmortem temporal bone examinations (Welling et al, 1990) indicate that the incidence may be as high as 1.7 percent. According to the NIH (1991), this seems to be an overestimate of occurrence in the general population. Approximately 2000 to 3000 new cases are reported each year (NIH, 1991), which suggests an incidence of 0.8 to 1.0 per 100,000 population per year (Monsell & Rock, 1990; NIH, 1991) and indicates that vestibular schwannomas are a relatively rare hearing disorder.

Classification of Schwannomas

Vestibular schwannomas occur in a single, round, encapsulated mass and have a growth rate that is difficult to predict (NIH, 1991). Some tumors grow very slowly over several years, whereas others have a rapid growth rate. If the tumor is left untreated, the symptoms become progressively more severe and can result in death. The tumor initially is located in the internal auditory canal; as it continues to grow it erodes the bony canal and may eventually protrude into the cerebellar pontine angle, where it accounts for approximately three-fourths of all cerebellopontine angle tumors (Hawke & Jahn, 1987). As tumor growth progresses, it produces pressure on nearby structures within the brainstem, resulting in additional symptoms, which range from headaches, nausea, vomiting, ataxia, coma, and respiratory depression to death. Pressure on the cranial nerves produces various symptoms. Compression on cranial nerve V may produce facial numbness or pain; compression on cranial nerve VII may result in facial spasms, weakness, or paralysis. Compression on cranial nerve VI may cause double vision, and compression on cranial nerve IX, X, or XII results in swallowing or speaking difficulties (NIH, 1991).

The vestibular schwannoma is usually classified on the basis of size, location, and growth rate (NIH, 1991). In addition, classification of vestibular schwannomas can be based on whether the tumor is familial or sporadic (NIH, 1991). *Sporadic* means that no other family member has the disease and there is no family history of the disease. Most vestibular schwannomas are sporadic.

Neurofibromatosis Syndrome

Vestibular schwannomas, whether familial or sporadic, occur with neurofibromatosis syndrome. According to Parry (1990), neurofibromatosis comprises two autosomal dominant disorders, neurofibromatosis 1 and neurofibromatosis 2. These two disorders have in common the occurrence of neurofibromas but are technically different disorders; neurofibromatosis 1 is a peripheral form of the disorder, and neurofibromatosis 2 is a central form of the disorder. Both types of neurofibromatosis are genetically transmitted. The gene for neurofibromatosis 1 is on chromosome 17, and the gene for neurofibromatosis 2 is on chromosome 22 (Parry, 1990). Neurofibromatosis 2 is associated with bilateral schwannomas as part of the inherited syndrome; however, the more common condition, neurofibromatosis 1 (Recklinghausen disease) is rarely associated with vestibular schwannomas.

Neurofibromatosis 1
The neurofibromatosis disorder was named by Friedrich Daniel von Recklinghausen, who first described it in the medical literature. Neurofibromatosis 1 may affect many body organs as well as the central nervous system (CNS), where the lesions may affect the auditory and visual systems, and the intraspinal areas. (Mulvihill, 1990).

The diagnostic criteria for neurofibromatosis 1 are as follows: (1) six or more cafe-au-lait spots larger than 5 mm in diameter on prepubescent people and larger than 15 mm in diameter on postpubescent people; (2) two or more neurofibromas; (3) freckling in the axilla (associated with freckling of an area such as the nose) or inguinal (related to the groin) regions; (4) optic glioma (tumor from one of various cells that form interstitial tissue); (5) two or more Lisvch nodules; (6) distinctive bony lesion with or without pseudarthrosis (false joint); (7) a first-degree relative with neurofibromatosis 1 (Mulvihill, 1990; Miyamoto et al, 1991; NIH, 1991).

Neurofibromatosis 2

The less common genetic neurofibromatosis (only a few thousand in the United States according to Miyamoto et al [1991]), previously referred to as bilateral acoustic neurofibromatosis is now known as neurofibromatosis 2. This disorder has an autosomal dominant inheritance and is genetically distinct from neurofibromatosis 1. In addition, two forms of vestibular schwannomas occur with neurofibromatosis 2 (Parry, 1990). In the sporadic form, the vestibular tumor is usually unilateral. This is the more common form and accounts for about 95 percent of diagnosed vestibular schwannomas. With this form there is no history of close relatives who have the disorder. People with the sporadic form of neurofibromatosis 2 usually are older than 40 years and have no other tumors. In the familial form, 5 percent of the diagnosed vestibular schwannomas are bilateral (Parry, 1990). Furthermore, there is a history of relatives who have the disorder. People with familial neurofibromatosis 2 usually receive the diagnosis during adolescence and may have other CNS tumors as well. Meningiomas (tumors of the covering or lining of the brain) are commonly present with this form of neurofibromatosis 2.

Diagnostic criteria for neurofibromatosis 2 are as follows: (1) bilateral eighth nerve masses which can be viewed with magnetic resonance imaging (MRI) or computed tomography (CT); (2) a first-degree relative with neurofibromatosis 2 and unilateral eighth nerve mass or two other masses (neurofibroma, meningioma, glioma, schwannoma or juvenile posterior subcapsular cataract) (Mulvihill, 1990; Miyamoto et al, 1991; NIH, 1991)

Detection and Treatment

Early detection of a small vestibular schwannoma can mean preservation of both the facial and acoustic nerves. In some cases, hearing is preserved and useful; in others, the eighth cranial nerve is preserved but the hearing may be poor; and in still others the eighth cranial nerve cannot be preserved (Smith et al, 1990). Preoperative planning based on tests described in the next paragraph provides the basis for the decision regarding hearing preservation and surgical approach. Hearing preservation and thus the choice of surgical approach, according to some surgeons (Frerebeau et al, 1987) depends on the likelihood of serviceable hearing after the operation; the size of the tumor, those less than 20 mm in diameter being operable; whether nerve function would be jeopardized or there would be unnecessary risk to life; and the likelihood of complete tumor removal.

Although tests such as MRI are frequently utilized to monitor tumor growth and to determine where the growth has extended, the decision to use MRI, CT, or auditory brainstem response (ABR) depends on the clinical judgment of the physician. Gadolinium-enhanced MRI, while particularly useful and regarded as the most definitive for revealing tumors only a few millimeters in diameter, is extremely expensive, which hinders its use as a screening test unless there is a high probability that a tumor is present (Welling et al, 1990). If MRI produces normal findings, ABR is used to monitor and confirm the MRI results. Computed tomography is another approach used for tumor screening and for preoperative planning, particularly when MRI is not available. ABR, according to Welling et al (1990), is the preferred screening method when there is a low probability a tumor is present.

Surgical Procedures

Several surgical approaches may be used to treat vestibular schwannoma. The choice of approach depends on many factors. The ideal treatment is total removal of the tumor in a single-stage operation. Before a procedure is selected, consideration is given to the preoperative hearing status, facial nerve function, and the size and location of the tumor. When the preoperative audiometric results indicate a mild hearing loss and well-formed ABR waveforms, the prognosis for preserving hearing is fairly good (NIH, 1991). Conversely, if MRI indicates that the tumor is large and fills the internal auditory canal, the likelihood of preserving hearing during the operation is greatly reduced. Of course, hearing is not the only consideration, as good facial nerve function is a desired outcome and may influence the surgical approach as well.

The three major surgical techniques include the translabyrinthine, the middle fossa, and the retrosigmoid or suboccipital approaches. Each of these approaches has advantages and disadvantages that must be weighed for each patient (NIH, 1991).

Alternative Approaches

Other treatment options may include subtotal removal of the tumor, radiation treatment, or simple observation of the patient over time. Observation may be the management of choice for an elderly person who does not have neurologic symptoms and who has no evidence of tumor growth. Observation may be preferable in selected situations because most tumors progress very slowly and therefore leave intact a stable neurologic function for many years. Of course, elderly people need to be made aware of the potential for neurologic deterioration over time (NIH, 1991).

Follow-up Care

Regardless of the treatment approach, ongoing follow-up care is important. Monitoring the patient for new symptoms or progression of the disorder is important. Professional monitoring should include a neurologic examination, audiologic assessment, and radiographic imaging. Each of the professionals on the monitoring team may have an accepted monitoring interval, which can range from 3 months to 1 year (NIH, 1991). Intervals may change as time passes, and the duration of the follow-up period may vary. Certainly for patients with neurofibromatosis 2, the monitoring may be lifelong.

Information regarding the increased risk of hearing impairment in both ears should be included in management counseling regarding bilateral vestibular schwannoma. The disabling consequences of a bilateral hearing loss raises concerns such as the choice of ear for surgical treatment or the possibility of subtotal removal of the tumor on one side to preserve some hearing.

Loss of hearing is the most adverse consequence of a surgical approach (NIH, 1991). Noisy environments and situations in which sound location is needed provide a very difficult listening situation for people with unilateral hearing. Assistive listening devices (see Chapter 8) may be appropriate for these patients, particularly if the person is a student in an educational setting where communication is critical. Patients who experience a total loss of hearing may be able to undergo rehabilitation (see Chapters 9 and 10). Visual communication systems such as speech reading, communication boards, captioning, and sign language can be initiated. However, visual communication systems may not be appropriate for people with limited vision, which may be associated with neurofibromatosis 2, and consideration should be given to tactile systems (NIH, 1991) (see Chapter 9).

Most patients have abnormal vestibular function postoperatively (NIH, 1991). If surgical treatment was for unilateral tumor removal, the vestibular function of the other ear can compensate. Bilateral dysfunction, particularly when associated with other CNS or sensory impairments, may mean the patient should take precautions when swimming or bathing (NIH, 1991).

Other consequences of the operation may be compromise of functions such as eye closure, facial weakness, facial paralysis, or potential problems, such as headaches, tumor recurrence, and delayed radiation complications. The social and psychological factors associated with these compromised functions may have considerable impact on the patient and the family. The abnormal appearance of a person with facial nerve paralysis may be an unexpected consequence for family members. The health team, family members, and support groups need to be informed and supportive of the patient. The more knowledge the client and the family have, the easier it will be for them to cope with the consequences after surgical intervention (NIH, 1991).

Meningiomas

Meningiomas develop from the meningothelial arachnoid cells. They may develop in a variety of locations within the intracranial regions. Women are more frequently affected than are men (Hawke & Jahn, 1987). These tumors are slow growing and may not produce symptoms during the early stages; however, if a meningioma is within the cerebellopontine angle, it may produce subtle audiometric signs. Pure-tone thresholds may be symmetric and only when special auditory tests (ABR) are used will the abnormality be detected.

Audiometric Evaluation of Tumors

Early detection of vestibular schwannomas is vital and may require results of more than one test (Smith et al, 1990). A test that detects eighth-nerve involvement should be sensitive, specific, and noninvasive (Smith et al, 1990). Unfortunately, no single test fulfills these requirements.

The presence of a unilateral, asymmetric sensorineural hearing impairment (Monsell & Rock, 1990; Weaver & Staller, 1984; Pikus, 1990) should always be investigated. The hearing loss, when present, is usually slowly progressive, but it may be sudden in a small (10 percent) proportion of patients (Benecke, 1989; NIH, 1991). Many times the lesion is asymptomatic, but if symptoms are present, the first and most common auditory symptom may be tinnitus (75 percent of patients with vestibular schwannomas have tinnitus) with or without the unilateral sensorineural hearing loss (NIH, 1991).

The initial audiologic evaluation should include pure-tone air- and bone-conduction thresholds, word recognition thresholds, word discrimination scores, acoustic reflex thresholds, and acoustic reflex decay (NIH, 1991). Because the auditory pathways are so complex, the pure-tone test alone cannot detect an eighth nerve tumor. There is no one pure-tone configuration that is regularly associated with tumors. For example, a pure-tone audiogram may be flat with only a mild hearing loss or rising from slight impairment in the low frequencies to normal in the high frequencies, or both low and high frequencies may be normal with the greatest loss appearing in the mid-frequency range. However, approximately 70 percent of audiograms associated with vestibular schwannomas have a sloping high-frequency hearing impairment (NIH, 1991).

Speech tests are routinely performed as part of a basic test battery and it is not uncommon for the word discrimination test results to be relatively poor and out of proportion to expectations based on pure-tone thresholds (Welling et al, 1990). A common complaint from patients with symptoms associated with eighth nerve tumors is that there is a greater difficulty understanding speech in one ear than in the other ear when using a telephone.

The acoustic reflex threshold test is a good test for audiologists to include as part of the evaluation but it is not the most sensitive test for identification of schwannomas even though it has been reported to have a sensitivity of 88 percent and a specificity of 89 percent (McFarland et al, 1989) for eighth-nerve involvement. The auditory test most sensitive to eighth nerve tumor detection is the ABR. Selters and Brackmann (1977) reported a sensitivity of 98 percent and specificity of 92 percent for ABR for a group of patients with tumors. Use of the ABR in the medical setting is either as a diagnostic screen for possible referral for imaging techniques or as a cross check of the findings of MRI. The advantage of ABR is the ability of the test to measure the functional status of the system at a lower cost than MRI. Consequently, ABR is an excellent screening test. The specifics of ABR testing and results are described in Chapter 6.

Traumatic Fractures

Hearing loss that occurs with closed head injury is commonly associated with fractures of the temporal bone. Auditory abnormalities are a common occurrence with head injury, and the auditory system has been reported to be the sensory system most commonly impaired (Hough, 1973). Sakai and Mateer (1984) reported in a summary of several studies that the incidence of head injury and associated neurologic injury is estimated to be 400 injuries per 100,000 population with an increase in incidence as high as 700 injuries per 100,000 population each year among young men.

The two temporal bone fractures associated with head trauma and possible auditory abnormalities are longitudinal fractures and transverse fractures. A longitudinal fracture of the petrous bone is the most common fracture and is estimated to have an incidence of 70 to 90 percent (Parisier, 1983). A blow to the temporal or parietal region of the head produces a sideways tearing of structures and results in a longitudinal fracture (Hawke & Jahn, 1987) that runs parallel to the petrous portion of the temporal bone (Sakai & Mateer, 1984). Abnormalities associated with longitudinal fractures include a conductive hearing loss, which may result from damage to the ossicular chain or other structures in the middle ear, and bloody otorrhea in the middle ear space. The bleeding (hematoma or bloody otorrhea) may be a result of a fracture to the wall of the external bony canal and associated lacerations of the tympanic membrane (Hough, 1973). It is also possible that the temporomandibular joint becomes dislocated with the mandible portion of the joint forced into the external canal as a result of a blow to the head. Lacerations of the dura mater of the middle fossa may allow cerebrospinal fluid to leak into the ear or nose on the side of the injury (Hough, 1973). As the fracture heals with a fibrous seal, the fluid may dissipate. Complications for which one must be alert include meningitis, hemorrhage in the perilymphatic and or endolymphatic space, and purulent otorrhea.

The other less common fracture associated with auditory abnormalities (sensorineural hearing loss) is a transverse fracture. When a temporal bone fracture is transverse, the fracture is, most likely, the result of a blow to the occipital or frontal region of the head, which in turn produces a back-to-front shearing force on the internal structures. It is estimated that the incidence of transverse fractures from head injury accounts for 10 to 20 percent of temporal bone fractures (Sakai & Mateer, 1984). The transverse fracture line is vertical to the long axis of the petrous portion of the temporal bone and may be an extension of other fractures (Sakai & Mateer, 1984). Damage may involve the external and middle ear, but many of these abnormalities are transient in nature (Hall & Mackey-Hargadine, 1984) and do not occur frequently with transverse fractures. It is common, however, for the facial nerve to be involved with a transverse fracture because of the closeness of the fracture line to the facial nerve (Sakai & Mateer, 1984).

Concussion

A concussion, which results from a blow to the head, is a "temporary paralysis of nerve function" (Sakai & Mateer, 1984, p. 164). The reduced nerve function may compromise auditory function, resulting in a sensorineural hearing loss that could resolve within 6 months. If, however, the sensorineural loss persists, it is likely that the presence of microfractures or contusions have produced a permanent sensorineural hearing loss. As cited by Sakai and Mateer (1984), Schuknecht suggested the mechanism of damage is the vibratory energy transmitted to the inner ear structures. This violent vibratory motion within the cochlea injures the structures of the organ of Corti.

Electroacoustic measures (ABR and acoustic reflex threshold) have become common assessment and monitoring instruments. A working knowledge of the results is desirable for speech-language pathologists and health care professionals working with head trauma clients during long-term follow-up care. Auditory abnormalities and hearing sensitivity are described herein relative to the type of temporal bone fracture encountered. The relationship between the fracture and the hearing impairment is described in the next section. Either a conductive or sensorineural hearing impairment may result from a temporal bone fracture.

AUDIOLOGIC TEST RESULTS

Fractures

If a fracture is longitudinal, the auditory abnormalities are usually unilateral and the hearing loss is conductive. The degree of the hearing impairment may vary from mild to moderate (maximum) depending on the severity of the injury. A tympanogram may indicate reduced middle ear mobility (fluid- or blood-filled middle ear space) or increased middle ear mobility (disarticulation of the ossicular chain). Speech understanding in either case should be good when the stimulus presentation level is well above threshold. The conductive auditory abnormality commonly is transient, but if a sensorineural auditory component is present it will probably be permanent.

A transverse fracture of the temporal bone usually produces injury to the inner ear and possibly the central auditory system. Consequently, the audiometric results are consistent with a sensorineural hearing impairment. Accordingly, the tympanograms indicate normal middle ear function if no conductive component is present. Hearing status should be monitored for several months.

Concussion

In head trauma, it is possible for a patient to have a cochlear injury and to sustain a sensorineural hearing loss and to have an injury to the central auditory system without sustaining a temporal bone fracture. The hearing loss is sensorineural with the possibility of central auditory dysfunction (Sakai & Mateer, 1984).

Follow-up Care

Patients who have sustained a fracture of the temporal bone should be monitored for several months after the incident. The speech-language pathologist or possibly the health care professional may encounter a patient with a head injury during the monitoring months following the trauma and after the auditory symptoms have stabilized. If the hearing impairment appears to be stable and if the loss is unilateral, counseling regarding noise exposure and ear protectors as well as amplification options should be instituted. However, the hearing impairment may not be stable for several months following the injury. Consequently, the speech-language pathologist or health care professional should be alert to any complaints of fluctuating hearing loss, any remaining conductive hearing impairment or change in hearing status, any effects from noise exposure, and the need for amplification (Sakai & Mateer, 1984). If a patient describes problems that indicate a hearing loss, a referral should be made to an audiologist. If complaints of dizziness persist, a medical referral should be made.

Ménière's Disease

The incidence of Ménière's disease in the United States is not known. Arenberg reported that the incidence is between 97,000 and 300,000 cases per year and the prevalence is 2,425,000 to 7,500,000 (Dickins & Graham, 1983). These figures are speculative and unfortunately are taken from population data that was gathered in 1973. The derived prevalence does suggest, however, according to Dickins and Graham (1983) that Ménière's disease is a more common hearing disorder than otosclerosis. The difficulty in reporting prevalence and incidence rates for Ménière's disease is caused in part by its diagnostic classification.

It is known that Ménière's disease involves the inner ear, but the pathologic nature is still not well understood. Typically a person who has Ménière's disease, also known as endolymphatic hydrops, experiences a triad of symptoms during an episode. The typical triad of symptoms associated with Ménière's disease includes vertigo and possible nausea, sensorineural hearing loss, and tinnitus. Not all of the symptoms may be present at the same time. For example, the feeling of fullness or the change in hearing accompanied by tinnitus may precede an attack of vertigo. These symptoms may occur periodically over time, increasing and decreasing in occurrence. The onset of symptoms may be sudden and may last anywhere from a few minutes to several hours. Ménière's disease is difficult to diagnose; other disorders with similar symptoms must be ruled out before a firm diagnosis can be made on the basis of the history and auditory and vestibular tests (Hawke & Jahn, 1987; Pulec, 1984).

Varieties of Ménière's disease have different symptomatic patterns; in fact: the following four distinct subvarieties of Ménière's disease can be determined: Lermouyez syndrome, which includes improved hearing during and immediately after the attack; Tumarcinn syndrome, which includes sudden attacks of falling down and has a short duration of involvement; cochlear hydrops, which involves a low-frequency hearing loss and does not include dizziness; and vestibular hydrops, which includes dizziness and no hearing loss (American Speech-Language-Hearing Association, 1991).

In the normal inner ear, the vestibular and cochlear aqueducts allow for regulation of endolymph through the endolymphatic sac and perilymph through the cerebrospinal fluid (Horner & Cazals, 1990). If there is a malfunction in the resorption mechanism of the endolymphatic system, fluid pressure and volume increase, and Reissner's membrane may be distended (Hawke & Jahn, 1987). The membrane is elastic and may remain so through several increases and decreases in endolymphatic fluid, but the membrane loses its elasticity over time. Rupture of the membrane allows the perilymph and endolymph to mix and may thus be responsible for the fluctuating changes in hearing and vestibular function (Hawke & Jahn, 1987).

Ménière's disease generally refers to an increase in the amount of inner ear fluid, specifically an increase in endolymphatic fluid. Approximately one-half of people who describe symptoms of Ménière's disease have no known cause for the symptoms. For the other half, Ménière's disease is associated with allergy; a deficient adrenal gland, pituitary gland or thyroid gland; fracture of the temporal bone; viral infection; acoustic trauma; or a congenital abnormality (ASHA, 1991). Khetarpal and Schuknecht (1990) suggest that a small endolymphatic sac, a result of a congenital abnormality, reduces the resorption of endolymphatic fluid, which results in endolymphatic hydrops. The increased fluid pressure in the cochlea distorts the labyrinthine membranes and destroys the structures of hearing and balance.

Many treatments provide relief from the tinnitus and dizziness. Relief from the tinnitus may be obtained with a masking device. These devices resemble a hearing aid and produce a continuous noise that covers the internal tinnitus. Many people with Ménière's disease find that a hearing aid is useful on a full-time basis; hearing aids for patients with Ménière's disease need to have considerable flexibility in gain and frequency response.

Medical treatment of Ménière's disease ranges from reduction of sodium in the diet, administration of histamines or nicotinic acid, provision of an endolymphatic shunt, surgical destruction of the vestibular function, or denervation of the inner ear to the use of diuretics. Surgical intervention is usually required only if the episodes of vertigo are debilitating (Hawke & Jahn, 1987; Pulec, 1984). Patients who choose surgical treatment to relieve the excess fluid may have some hearing preserved. People with a more disabling form of Ménière's disease may find that surgical intervention destroys hearing and balance in the impaired ear (ASHA, 1991).

Audiologic Test Results

The fluctuating sensorineural hearing impairment associated with Ménière's disease may begin with greater impairment in the lower frequencies (generally normal above 2000 Hz) and progress to greater impairment in the higher frequencies with recurrent episodes. Some recovery of hearing thresholds to near normal may occur between episodes, thus the hearing loss is characterized by fluctuating hearing abilities. Continued fluctuation of hearing sensitivity is expected with Ménière's disease, and hearing thresholds gradually worsen and become a permanent impairment for most frequencies. Certainly, hearing should be monitored on a regular basis because of the fluctuating hearing loss. Furthermore, as hearing thresholds change and progress, hearing aid adjustments may be necessary to compensate for the fluctuations.

The hearing loss is generally unilateral. It has been reported, however, that 10 to 20 percent of patients have evidence of bilateral hearing impairment (Hawke & Jahn, 1987). The bilateral involvement may be a later development for patients who initially present with a unilateral hearing impairment.

As the hearing impairment increases, decreased sensation levels for the acoustic reflexes are expected. Speech discrimination is usually impaired during and after an episode, but good discrimination of speech is usually present in the early stages.

Multiple Sclerosis

Lesions in the white matter of the CNS were first described by Jean-Martin Charcot in 1868 when he stated there were "islands of scars" (Rivera, 1990). Multiple sclerosis (MS), a degenerative, demyelinating disease of the CNS (Cranford et al, 1990), is characterized by lesions that may affect the spinal cord, brainstem, optic nerve, and brain (Schweitzer & Shepard, 1989). The onset of symptoms usually occurs at about 30 years of age, and the symptoms are episodic; the disease progresses through active and inactive states. Recurrence of symptoms is likely during the first 3 to 4 years of the disease but can be followed by periods of remission over 20 to 30 years (Rivera, 1990). "The disease occurs most frequently in Caucasians living between latitude 40 degrees and 60 degrees north in both hemispheres . . . and is more common in the cold temperate areas" (Rivera, 1990, p. 210). The prevalence in the United States (58 per 100,000 population) varies depending on location; the prevalence in the Seattle area is 90 per 100,000, in the Denver area is 80 per 100,000, and in the Houston area is 14 per 100,000 (Riviera, 1990).

Exactly why MS develops is unclear, but it is probably due to many influences, chief among them is an altered immune-regulating system. According to Rivera (1990, p. 207), ". . . there is a continuous immunological alteration triggered possibly by a virus in genetically susceptible individuals." Since there are regions of the country where high numbers of cases occur, epidemiologic research has suggested that some environmental factor to which children are exposed may be responsible for MS later in life in certain susceptible individuals (Rivera, 1990).

Clinical symptoms of MS are highly variable and may develop over a period of days or weeks. Furthermore, the symptoms may improve but may just as likely plateau or worsen. Clinical symptoms of MS may include any of the following: "weakness, paralysis, brainstem deficits, cranial nerve deficits, abnormal reflexes, neurogenic bowel and bladder problems, impotence or frigidity and cerebellar dysfunction" (Rivera, 1990, p. 212).

MRI and CT are valuable imaging techniques for identifying MS. Imaging of two or more lesions in the white matter in the CNS with either procedure provides the diagnosis of MS (Rivera, 1990). Treatment of the disease and its symptoms may include any or all of the following: rehabilitative techniques, vocational training, psychological intervention, or pharmacological agents.

Audiologic Test Results

Acutely ill people with overt disabling symptoms of MS may be unconcerned with hearing status when reporting initial symptoms; thus the incidence of hearing loss with MS may be underreported. Furthermore, there is no typical audiologic pattern associated with MS (Franklin et al, 1989; Furman et al, 1989). If a loss is present, it is a sensorineural hearing impairment which can be unilateral, bilateral, transient, or permanent. Although unusual, hearing loss can be acute and rapidly progressive as a result of MS (Stach et al, 1990), but more commonly it is unilateral and transient (Barratt et al, 1988). Attempts to define the chronic hearing loss associated with MS have shown that the hearing impairment is highly variable. Even though no single audiometric pattern can be described that is typical of MS, pure-tone thresholds should be monitored for any changes in hearing status.

Speech discrimination measures have been somewhat more valuable. These measures are frequently abnormal when speech is presented in a background of noise to one or both ears at the same time (Stach et al, 1990). Although ABR is a useful clinical tool for determining and monitoring abnormal neural function (Schweitzer & Shepard, 1989), it cannot be used to specifically identify MS as the pathologic condition, nor can it be used to identify a specific location of a lesion (Jacobson & Jacobson, 1990).

Noise-Induced Hearing Loss

An important cause of hearing loss in the adult population is trauma, specifically noise trauma. According to Boettcher et al (1987), noise-induced hearing loss is a serious health problem in spite of increased public awareness and federal legislation. It is difficult to avoid noise exposure. Noise-induced hearing loss depends on the intensity, type, duration, and frequency of the noise exposure

(Chapter 12). Furthermore, individual susceptibility seems to play an important role. Exactly why large individual differences in susceptibility occur is not clear. However, it is possible that other factors such as aging and ototoxic drugs are involved. Certainly special precaution and counseling should be given to patients who take ototoxic drugs such as aminoglycoside antibiotics or cisplatin treatments. There is some evidence to support the concept that patients who take these drugs may have increased susceptibility to damage from noise (Boettcher et al, 1987).

Noise exposure alone, however, appears to have an impact on most auditory structures. The effects of the noise may cause alterations in the stereocilia, destruction of the support structures, or damage to the sensory hair cells. Over time, degeneration of the neurons associated with the damaged hair cells occurs (Boettcher et al, 1987; Hawke & Jahn, 1987). The exact relationship between various levels of noise and the damage that occurs within the system is unclear. Boettcher et al (1987) summarized several studies which suggested that low levels of noise exposure cause excessively high metabolic rates, which seem to be responsible for damage to hair cells and afferent nerves. At even higher sound levels, cells may rupture and allow for the mixing of endolymphatic and perilymphatic fluids which is destructive to hair cells in the ear. At the highest sound pressure levels, structures are damaged as the mechanical function of the system is exceeded. The result is that membranes may be torn and structures destroyed.

Continuous noise is not the only type of noise that is hazardous to the auditory system. Unfortunately, impulse noise in combination with continuous noise may have an even greater impact on the auditory structures than either continuous or impulse noise alone (Boettcher et al, 1987). Noise and hearing loss are discussed in Chapter 12.

Audiologic Test Results

Hearing loss that results from noise exposure can be permanent or temporary. Temporary hearing loss is a loss of hearing sensitivity in the high-frequency range that recovers over time. Permanent hearing loss is usually a result of chronic noise exposure to high-intensity noise or a combination of continuous and impulse noise. The audiometric configuration from noise-induced hearing loss is easily recognized during the initial stages. The sensorineural hearing loss is usually bilateral and symmetric with a characteristic notch at about 4000 Hz. This decrease in auditory sensitivity at 4000 Hz is present for both air- and bone-conduction thresholds but at 8000 Hz returns to a range that is closer to normal. It is possible for all frequencies below 4000 Hz to be within a normal range (less than 25 dB HL). Typically the sensorineural hearing impairment increases and the notch widens as noise exposure continues. In other words, the hearing impairment may extend into the higher frequencies (6000 Hz and 8000 Hz) and into the lower frequencies (2000 Hz and 3000 Hz). Protection from noise exposure is advocated for people exposed to noise on an infrequent basis as well as those exposed continuously.

Ototoxicity

The inner ear is susceptible to damage from therapeutic drugs. Of course, the risk of side effects from therapeutic, but ototoxic, drugs must be balanced with the potential benefit to the patient (Bergstrom & Thompson, 1984). Drug dosage must be monitored carefully as a therapeutic drug that may become ototoxic in some susceptible individuals. The amount of a therapeutic drug that can be administered with minimal ototoxic side effects depends on several risk factors which range from the concentration of drugs in the blood serum to individual susceptibility. Specifically, risk factors include drug dosage, renal function, state of hydration, and duration of drug administration (Bergstrom & Thompson, 1984; Hawke & Jahn, 1987). People most susceptible to ototoxicity are infants, elderly people, and possibly people who already have a hearing loss.

The incidence of hearing loss from ototoxicity varies depending on the risk factors already mentioned. Furthermore, the incidence of hearing loss within drug categories varies and is not well documented for any specific drug. Ototoxicity is thought to be an acquired adult disorder; however, a congenital hearing loss can occur as a result of damage to fetal ear structures when ototoxic drugs are ingested during pregnancy (Bergstrom & Thompson, 1984).

Mechanism of Toxicity

The inner ear maintains a functional filtering mechanism within the stria vascularis. As a result, most drugs cannot cross this barrier except in very small quantities. If, however, the barrier is crossed and drugs are introduced into the endolymph and allowed to accumulate, permanent hair-cell damage and a hearing loss are possible. Damage from drugs occurs within the cochlea and primarily results in damage to the hair cells, basal outer hair cells first (Hawke & Jahn, 1987), but also may damage the neurons associated with the vestibular portions of the eighth cranial nerve.

Bergstrom and Thompson (1984) suggest that aminoglycosides inhibit oxidative and metabolic enzymes and thus impair metabolic activities in the inner ear or that ionic transport in the inner ear is impaired by the change in membrane permeability, which is altered as a result of the drug and thus results in an imbalance of the inner ear fluids.

Ototoxic Drugs

There are five major categories of drugs (aminoglycosides, quinine and chloroquine, salicylates, loop-inhibiting diuretics, and chemotherapeutic agents) that can produce either temporary or permanent hearing impairment (Bergstrom & Thompson, 1984; Hawke & Jahn, 1987). The effects of hearing impairment due to drugs may be increased with exposure to noise or with administration of a second ototoxic drug.

Aminoglycoside Antibiotics

Aminoglycosides are drugs with similar chemical structure and therapeutic use (Bergstrom & Thompson, 1984). These drugs are administered to combat bacterial infections by inhibiting protein synthesis. Examples of aminoglycosides are kanamycin, neomycin, and amikacin, which are more toxic to the cochlea; other mycins (eg, tobramycin, gentamicin) may be more toxic to the vestibular system. In some cases, the cochleotoxic effect of the drugs may not be evident until weeks or months after administration (Bergstrom & Thompson, 1984; Hawke & Jahn, 1987).

The ototoxic effects of aminoglycoside antibiotics have been known for approximately 50 years, and yet the incidence of ototoxic effects is still controversial. Brummet and Morrison in 1990 reported that the incidence of hearing impairment from aminoglycoside antibiotics may be exaggerated. Some of the controversy surrounds clinical studies that use different criteria to determine hearing loss associated with ototoxic drugs. Many times it is difficult to test the patient receiving the ototoxic drugs either because of the ambient noise in the hospital room or because of the condition of the patient.

Quinine and Chloroquine

Both quinine and chloroquine have a toxic effect on the cochlea that can be temporary or permanent (Hawke & Jahn, 1987; Nielsen-Abbring et al, 1990). Quinine, which comes from the bark of the *Cinchona* tree, and chloroquine, which is the synthetic drug, are used as antimalarial drugs. Chloroquine, which is used in lieu of quinine, is less expensive and has fewer side effects (Nielsen-Abbring et al, 1990). However, some resistant malarial infections necessitate the use of quinine.

The embryonic inner ear changes caused by quinine range from destruction of the outer hair cells to changes in the stria vascularis to complete destruction of the organ of Corti (Hawke & Jahn, 1987). These drugs, like antibiotics, vary in the effect on each patient. Any woman who believes she is pregnant should not take these drugs because the inner ear of a developing fetus would be vulnerable to the effects of the drug. One of the more serious symptoms of quinine ototoxicity in the adult is tinnitus, which may be accompanied by a high-frequency temporary hearing impairment that can become permanent.

Salicylates

Aspirin (acetylsalicylic acid) is commonly used by older people with diseases such as arthritis. On occasion, a temporary hearing impairment may result from high dosages. However, about 1 week after the aspirin is discontinued hearing should return to normal (Bergstrom & Thompson, 1984; Hawke & Jahn, 1987). The mechanism thought to be responsible for the temporary threshold change is interruption of the enzyme activity of the hair cell.

Loop-Inhibiting Diuretics

Loop-inhibiting diuretics are commonly reported to cause temporary hearing impairment (Bergstrom & Thompson, 1984). However, there have been infrequent reports of permanent hearing impairment occurring with loop-inhibiting diuretics (Hawke & Jahn, 1987). In general, when diuretics have been given in isolation, the effect of impairment is initially in the cell structure of the stria vascularis followed by possible damage to the hair-cell population in later stages. Compounding effects have been seen in instances in which diuretics have been given in conjunction with aminoglycoside antibiotics (Boettcher et al, 1987; Hawke & Jahn, 1987). In these instances, extensive destruction can be found throughout the hair cell population, resulting in permanent impairment.

Cisplatin

Many drugs (nitrogen mustard and *cis*-diamminedichloroplatinum) may be given as part of chemotherapy for malignant tumors and may unavoidably place normal hearing at risk (Hawke & Jahn, 1987; Kopelman et al, 1988). Cisplatin is a new class of drug used to treat malignant neoplasms and has been directly related to damage within the organ of Corti, particularly the outer hair cells in the basal end of the cochlea (Kopelman et al, 1988). Kopelman et al followed nine patients who underwent cisplatin treatment and found that none of the patients responded to frequencies of 9000 Hz and above at ultra high-frequency audiometry after only one or two doses of cisplatin. Tests with more conventional frequencies (4000 Hz to 8000 Hz) showed impairment with repeated drug administration. The impairment appeared to plateau within the moderate hearing-loss range for the higher frequencies. All patients experienced tinnitus and poor speech discrimination in the presence of background noise regardless of dosage or method of administration of cisplatin. Waters et al (1991) studied 60 patients and compared serial audiograms. Patients in the study received different drug dosages under different schedules. Their results indicated that the most severe ototoxic effects were associated with administration of high doses over a short period of time. The greatest effect from cisplatin was between 4000 Hz and 8000 Hz. Tinnitus occurred primarily in the group that received the high doses at the onset of treatment. It is not clearly established whether the presence of pre-existing hearing loss places a person at greater risk for further hearing impairment after cisplatin treatment. Results of a preliminary study with a small number of subjects (Durrant et al, 1990) suggested that there is no greater risk for hearing impairment in people who already have a hearing loss.

Audiologic Test Results

The audiometric pattern that results from ototoxicity is usually a bilateral, moderate to severe sensorineural hearing impairment that primarily affects the high-frequency range. The toxic effect on hearing may not occur immediately but may be delayed in onset. The amount of the impairment may continue to increase for some time after termination of the drug. In a few cases, the hearing impairment may be temporary. Frequently a high-pitched, ringing tinnitus precedes the hearing impairment. Establishing a baseline audiogram is desirable followed by periodic monitoring of the hearing sensitivity. It is recommended that (Bergstrom & Thompson, 1984) air-conduction thresholds at 500 Hz, 1000 Hz, 2000 Hz, 4000 Hz, and 8000 Hz be monitored regularly. If possible, thresholds in the high-frequency range from 8000 Hz to 20,000 Hz should be obtained to determine hearing loss at an early stage. Any patient who takes ototoxic drugs and exhibits symptoms such as tinnitus, hearing loss, or dizziness should be referred to an audiologist. Any patient with a change of 15 dB HL at any test frequency threshold should be referred for a complete audiologic evaluation. Because individual variability has a great effect in determining susceptibility to a drug, hearing should be systematically monitored once a week during therapy and 1 month and 3 months after therapy (Bergstrom & Thompson, 1984). Diuretic-induced hearing impairment typically does not produce the high-frequency hearing impairment seen with other ototoxic drugs. Rather, the impairment may be concentrated in the middle to low frequency range and usually reverses itself within 24 hours after discontinuation of the drug (Bergstrom & Thompson, 1984).

Speech-language pathologists who are part of a health care team monitoring a patient in a nursing home or hospital should assume that part of their responsibility is to assure that patients who fit the following criteria receive audiometric monitoring. Patients at risk for hearing loss are those who have decreased renal function; are taking drugs in high dosages; have high serum levels of a drug; have tinnitus, hearing loss, or dizziness; have taken multiple ototoxic drugs; or have a pre-existing hearing loss or other sensory impairment (Bergstrom & Thompson, 1984). Patients who begin to experience a hearing loss in the frequency range from 2000 Hz through 8000 Hz should begin aural rehabilitation to make use of the residual hearing (Kopelman et al, 1988). A hearing threshold change of greater than 20 dB at one frequency or greater than 15 dB for two frequencies is among the criteria used to determine ototoxic effects in clinical studies.

Presbycusis

The term *presbycusis*, "old age hearing," applies to the degenerative changes that occur in the aging auditory system (Mangham & Yarington, 1984; Hawke & Jahn, 1987). It is a common term related to all aspects of the decline of age-related auditory performance (Gates et al, 1989). This type of hearing loss affects people older than 50 years who do not have a history of noise exposure or ototoxicity (Hawke & Jahn, 1987). Gates et al (1989, p. 268) reported that "23% of the population between 65 and 75 years of age and 40% of the population above 75 years is affected," which certainly suggests that presbycusis is one of the most common chronic conditions that affect the elderly (Bess et al, 1989). Brown (1990) reported that although overall prevalence data for aging and hearing loss are updated by the National Health Interview Survey, there are not reliable data about the prevalence of the various degrees of hearing impairment. Further, it is difficult to separate hearing loss due to aging from hearing loss due to other factors, such as noise, ototoxicity, and infections (Rosenhall et al, 1990). The diagnosis of hearing loss due to aging is now made primarily on the basis of exclusion of other causes (Mangham & Yarington, 1984). As the population ages and this health problem increases, the need for more specific data will become even more important than it is now.

The pathologic changes that occur in the auditory system (Chapter 11) range from arthritic alterations, primarily within the ossicular chain joints (Mangham & Yarington, 1984), to devascularization of the cochlea from the basal to the apical end coupled with a corresponding loss of sensory hair cells in the organ of Corti (Hawke & Jahn, 1987). Secondary to the hair-cell loss is a loss of neurons from the cochlea through the brainstem and, in fact, throughout the central auditory system (Hawke & Jahn, 1987).

The most common measure of the impairment is the pure-tone audiogram. Unfortunately, the hearing loss visualized on the audiogram cannot always be equated with the communication difficulty experienced. Moreover, it has been suggested (Bess et al, 1989) that hearing impairment has a serious psychosocial impact on older people. Thus as the hearing loss increases in an older adult, a similar increase in physical and social dysfunction occurs. Presbycusis is a complex state and is an important health concern in need of further research. Information about older adults and hearing is contained in Chapter 11.

Audiologic Test Results

The hearing loss associated with aging is a bilateral, sensorineural hearing impairment with greater hearing loss in the high frequencies than the low frequencies. Initially the hearing loss may be mild with a loss of sensitivity in the high frequencies that continues to increase with increasing age. Word discrimination scores vary depending on the degree and configuration of the hearing impairment. However, as indicated previously, it is difficult to predict speech discrimination ability on the basis of audiometric thresholds. It is possible for a person who has only a mild hearing impairment to experience considerable difficulty communicating in a noisy atmosphere, and older people may have particular difficulty understanding speech in a noisy atmosphere. Gaeth, according to Marshall (1985), called the poor speech understanding phonemic regression. In other words, the ability to understand speech is much poorer than might be expected when compared with the pure-tone thresholds. This phenomenon is associated with central auditory dysfunction. Special auditory tests may be used to determine if there is a disruption in the central auditory function (Chapter 13). If results from the special tests indicate the presence of central auditory dysfunction, the speech-language pathologist and health care professional should be aware that adjustments to the environment can be made to assist the person. These modifications and others are described in Chapter 11.

Sudden Hearing Loss

Sudden hearing loss, approximately 1 percent of all sensorineural hearing losses (Hawke & Jahn, 1987), is a hearing loss that occurs immediately or over a very short time span. For example, a person may have normal hearing on retiring at night but on arising in the morning may notice a loss of hearing (Mattox & Lyles, 1989). Fortunately, though it is not clear why it happens, in approximately 65 percent of cases of sudden hearing loss, spontaneous recovery occurs within 2 to 4 weeks of onset regardless of treatment (Mattox & Simmons, 1977). Mattox and Lyles (1989) wrote that recovery from the loss is inversely related to the degree of the hearing loss and that the prognosis is related to the frequency of the hearing impairment. In other words, if the damage from the sudden loss occurs in the middle and apical ends of the cochlea (rising audiogram), the prognosis for improvement is greater than if the damage is elsewhere in the cochlea.

Even though the cause of the sudden hearing loss is frequently unknown, several possible causes have been suggested. Two important causes of sudden hearing loss (Hawke & Jahn, 1987) are viral infection and vascular occlusion. The first of these conditions, acute viral infection, includes diseases such as rubella, mumps, influenza B and A3, and cytomegalovirus infection. The second proposed cause of sudden hearing loss is acute vascular occlusion of the inner ear. If the hearing loss is vascular in origin, it is believed that the most likely site of involvement is the stria vascularis. Examinations of temporal bones have confirmed that approximately 50 percent of people with a sudden hearing loss ". . . show evidence of degeneration of the stria. Other conditions associated with sudden hearing loss include trauma, congenital syphilis, measles, meningitis, otitis media, leukemia, spontaneous rupture of the round window, and spontaneous hemorrhage of the perilymphatic spaces" (Hawke and Jahn, 1987, p. 5.33).

Audiologic Test Results

The pure-tone audiogram of a person suffering a sudden, unilateral hearing loss may vary from a mild to profound sensorineural impairment. The effect may be evident at all frequencies or only at one or two selected frequencies. The audiogram configuration may be flat, upward or downward sloping, or notched. Word discrimination associated with the loss varies depending on the degree of the hearing loss and the frequencies involved. Speech understanding improves as the pure-tone thresholds improve. Improvement does not occur in all cases. People who experience a sudden hearing impairment should seek an audiometric evaluation and medical attention immediately.

Sickle Cell Anemia

Sickle cell disease has many variants (HbSS or sickle cell anemia, HbSC or sickle cell C disease, and HbSS-thal or sickle cell thalassemia), but the term *sickle cell anemia* refers to all variants (Crawford et al, 1991). The disease is described as an abnormal blood condition with sickle-shaped cells. People who have sickle cell anemia suffer from the destruction of blood cells that assist with the concentration of oxygen transporting material in the blood; this is known as hemolytic anemia (Crawford et al, 1991). As a result of the anemia, other relatively unimportant infections may become life-threatening. The most serious problem, however, occurs during crises. Crises, which occur periodically, involve the closing or narrowing of blood vessels. A long-standing problem due to mechanical obstruction may produce a localized narrowing of the arterial blood supply. Because sickle cell anemia is a chronic condition, cells, or portions of tissue or vital organs, may die with the repeated obstruction of the blood supply.

The incidence of communication disorders associated with sickle cell anemia is unknown. Even though the hearing status is unclear, it is known that sickle cell anemia involves the vascular and neurologic systems, which means there is the potential for involvement of the auditory system. Crawford et al (1991) suggested, on the basis of their study of patients with sickle cell anemia, that the prevalence of a hearing loss in a population of people with sickle cell disease is 41 percent. This proportion is higher than expected in the general population. It appears as if people who have sickle cell anemia are at greater risk than the general population for acquiring a hearing loss. Crawford et al (1991) also reported that people who have the HbSC variant are at greater risk for hearing loss than people with other variants of sickle cell anemia.

Gould et al (1991) evaluated a group of African American adults who had sickle cell anemia and was unable to find any consistent auditory patterns but did report that the group studied was at greater risk for a peripheral hearing loss and central auditory dysfunction than the general population. Because the cochlea is highly vascular and in need of a continuous oxygen supply to continue to function properly, disruption of the oxygen and blood supply places the cochlea and central auditory system at risk for hearing impairment.

Audiologic Test Results

There is no identifiable type of hearing loss associated with sickle cell disease. Gould et al (1991) found that 63 of 68 people tested had normal hearing as defined by the pure-tone average. Speech reception thresholds were similar to the results of the pure-tone average and were predominately normal. Word recognition scores were usually normal. The Synthetic Sentence Identification with Ipsilateral Competing Message test, a test sensitive to intra-axial brainstem involvement, demonstrated the highest abnormality rate (only 10 ears). Auditory brainstem responses, which are generally considered to be the most sensitive and specific tests for neural function, were also predominately normal. Only six ears were found to have abnormal function, but this was higher than the expected fail rate in the general population. Overall, no consistent pattern exists that can be associated with sickle cell anemia, but awareness of the potential for cochlear and central auditory dysfunction within this population is warranted.

REFERENCES

Alford, B. R., & Guilford, F. R. (1962). A comprehensive study of tumors of the glomus jugulare. *Laryngoscope, 72,* 765-787.

American Speech-Language-Hearing Association (1991). Let's talk: Ménière's disease. *Asha, 30,* 61-62.

Barratt, J. J., Miller, D., & Rudge, P. (1988). The site of lesion causing deafness in multiple sclerosis. *Scandinavian Audiology, 17,* 67-71.

Benecke, J. E. (1989). Diagnosis and management of acoustic tumors: An overview. *Seminars in Hearing, 10,* 307-312.

Bergstrom, L., & Thompson, P. L. (1984). Ototoxicity. In J. L. Northern (Ed.), *Hearing Disorders* (pp. 119-139). Boston: Little, Brown.

Bess, F. H., Lichtenstein, M., Logan, S. A., Burger, C., & Nelson, E. (1989). Hearing impairment as a determinant of function in the elderly. *Journal of the American Geriatric Society, 37,* 123-128.

Boettcher, F. A., Henderson, D., Gratton, M. A., Danielson, R. W., & Byrne, C. D. (1987). Synergistic interactions of noise and other ototraumatic agents. *Ear and Hearing, 8,* 192-212.

Bratt, G. W., Bess, F. H., Miller, G. W., & Glasscock, M. E. (1979). Glomus tumor of the middle ear: Origin, symptomatology, and treatment. *Journal of Speech and Hearing Disorders, 44,* 121-137.

Brown, S. C. (1990). The prevalence of communicative disorders in the aging population. *Asha, 19,* 14-25.

Brummet, R. E., & Morrison, R. B. (1990). The incidence of aminoglycoside antibiotic-induced hearing loss. *Archives of Otolaryngology: Head & Neck Surgery, 116,* 406-410.

Cohn, A. M. (1981). Etiology and pathology of disorders affecting hearing. In F. Martin (Ed.), *Medical audiology: Disorders of hearing* (pp. 123-144). Englewood Cliffs: Prentice Hall.

Cranford, J. L., Boose, M., & Moore, C. A. (1990). Tests of the precedence effect in sound localization reveal abnormalities in multiple sclerosis. *Ear and Hearing, 11,* 282-288.

Crawford, M. R., Gould, H. J., Smith, W. R., Beckford, N., Gibson, W. R., Bobo, L. (1991). Prevalence of hearing loss in adults with sickle cell disease. *Ear and Hearing, 12,* 349-351.

Derlacki, E. L. (1984). Otosclerosis. In J. L. Northern (Ed.), *Hearing disorders* (pp. 111-118). Boston: Little, Brown.

Dickins, J. R. F., & Graham, S. S. (1983). Ménière's disease: 1978-1982. *The American Journal of Otology, 5,* 137-154.

Durrant, J. D., Rodgers, M. D., Myers, E. N., & Johnson, J. T. (1990). Hearing loss-risk factor for cisplatin ototoxicity? Observations. *The American Journal of Otology, 11,* 375-377.

Franklin, D. J., Coker, N. J., & Jenkins, H. A. (1989). Sudden sensorineural hearing loss as a presentation of multiple sclerosis. *Archives of Otolaryngology: Head & Neck Surgery, 115,* 41-47.

Frerebeau, P., Benezech, J., Uziel, A., Coubes, P., Segnarbieux, F., & Malonga, M. (1987). Hearing preservation after acoustic neurinoma operation. *Neurosurgery, 21,* 197-120.

Frolsch, M., & Sommer, A. (1991). *Handbook of congenital and early onset hearing loss.* New York: Igaku-Shoin.

Furman, J. M. R., Durrant, J. D., & Hirsch, W. (1989). Eighth nerve signs in a case of multiple sclerosis. *American Journal of Otolaryngology, 10,* 376-381.

Gates, G., Caspary, D., Clark, W., Pillsbury, H., Brown, S. C., & Dobie, R. (1989). Presbycusis. *Invitational Geriatric Otorhinolaryngology Workshop, 100,* 266-271.

Glasscock, M. E., Harris, P. F., & Newsome, G. (1974). Glomus tumors: Diagnosis and treatment. *Laryngoscope, 84,* 2006-2032.

Glasscock, M. E., Miller, O. W., Drake, F. D., & Kanok, M. M. (1978). Surgery of the skull base. *Laryngoscope, 88,* 905-923.

Gould, H. J., Crawford, M. R., Smith, W. R., et al. (1991). Hearing disorders in sickle cell disease: Cochlear and retrocochlear findings. *Ear and Hearing, 12,* 352-354.

Hall, J. W., & Mackey-Hargadine, J. (1984). Auditory evoked responses in severe head injury. *Seminars in Hearing, 5,* 313-336.

Hawke, M., & Jahn, A. F. (1987). *Diseases of the ear.* Philadelphia: Lea & Febiger.

Horner, K. C., & Cazals, Y. (1990). Alterations of CAP audiogram by increased endolymphatic pressure and its relation to hydrops. *Hearing Research, 45,* 145-150.

Hough, J. V. D. (1973). Otologic trauma. In M. M. Paparella & D. A. Sumric (Eds.), *Otolaryngology: The ear* (Vol. 2) (pp. 241-262). Philadelphia: Saunders.

Jacobson, J. T., & Jacobson, G. P. (1990). The auditory brainstem response in multiple sclerosis. *Seminars in Hearing, 11,* 248-264.

Khetarpal, V., & Schuknecht, H. F. (1990). Temporal bone findings in a case of bilateral Meniere's disease treated by parenteral streptomycin and endolymphatic shunt. *Laryngoscope, 100,* 407-414.

Kopelman, J., Budnick, A., Sessions, R. B., Kramer, M., & Wong, G. (1988). Ototoxicity of high-dose cisplatin by bolus administration in patients with advanced cancers and normal hearing. *Laryngoscope, 98,* 858-864.

Kristensen, S., Juul, A., Gammelgaard, N. P., & Rasmussen, O. R. (1989). Traumatic tympanic membrane perforations: Complications and management. *Ear, Nose and Throat Journal, 68,* 503-515.

Mangham, C. A., & Yarington, C. T., Jr. (1984). Presbycusis. In J. L. Northern (Ed.), *Hearing disorders* (pp. 161-169). Boston: Little, Brown.

Marshall, L. (1985). Audiological assessment of older adults. *Seminars in Hearing, 6*(2), 161-180.

Mattox, D. E., & Lyles, A. C. (1989). Idiopathic sudden sensorineural hearing loss. *The American Journal of Otology, 10,* 242-247.

Mattox, D. E., & Simmons, F. B. (1977). Natural history of sudden sensorineural hearing loss. *Annals of Otology, 86,* 463-480.

McFarland, W. H., Inthicum, F. H., & Waldorf, R. (1989). Auditory and vestibular tests. *Seminars in Hearing, 10,* 313-326.

Monsell, E. M., & Rock, J. P. (1990). Sensorineural hearing loss and the diagnosis of acoustic neuroma. *Henry Ford Hospital Medical Journal, 38,* 9-12.

Miyamoto, R. T., Roos, K. L., Campbell, R. L., & Worth, R. M. (1991). Contemporary management of neurofibromatosis. *Annals of Otology Rhinology and Laryngology, 100,* 38-43.

Mulvihill, J. J. (Moderator); Parry, D. M., Sherman, J. L., Pikus, A., Kaiser-Kupfer, M., & Eldridge, R. (Discussants) (1990). Neurofibromatosis 1 (Recklinghausen disease) and neurofibromatosis 2 (bilateral acoustic neurofibromatosis): An update (NIH Clinical Staff Conference Summary, April 1989; © 1990 American College of Physicians). *Annals of Internal Medicine, 113,* 39-52.

National Institutes of Health (1991). Acoustic neuroma. (Reprinted from NIH Consensus Development Conference Consensus Statement, December 11-13, 9(4).)

Nielsen-Abbring, F. W., Perenboom, R. M., & van der Hulst R. J. A. M. (1990). Quinine-induced hearing loss. *Otorhinolaryngology, 52,* 65-68.

Pahor, A.L. (1981). The ENT problems following the Birmingham bombings. *Journal of Laryngology and Otology, 95,* 399-406.

Parisier, S. C. (1983). Injuries of the ear and temporal bone. In C. D. Bluestone & S. E. Stool (Eds.). *Pediatric otolaryngology* (Vol. 1) (pp. 614-636). Philadelphia: Saunders.

Parry, D. M. (1990). Gene mapping and tumor genetics (pp. 41-42). In J. J. Mulvihill (Moderator). Neurofibromatosis 1 (Recklinghausen disease) and neurofibromatosis 2 (bilateral acoustic neurofibromatosis): An update (NIH Clinical Staff Conference Summary, April 1989; © 1990 American College of Physicians). *Annals of Internal Medicine, 113,* 39-52.

Pikus, A. (1990). Audiological manifestations (pp. 44-46). In J. J. Mulvihill (Moderator). Neurofibromatosis 1 (Recklinghausen disease) and neurofibromatosis 2 (bilateral acoustic neurofibromatosis): An update (NIH Clinical Staff Conference Summary, April 1989; © 1990 American College of Physicians). *Annals of Internal Medicine, 113,* 39-52.

Pulec, J. L. (1984). Ménière's disease. In J. L. Northern (Ed.), *Hearing disorders* (pp. 135-143). Boston: Little, Brown.

Rivera, V. M. (1990). The nature of multiple sclerosis. *Seminars in Hearing, 11,* 207-220.

Rosenhall, U., Pedersen, K., & Svanborg, A. (1990). Presbycusis and noise-induced hearing loss. *Ear and Hearing, 11,* 257-262.

Rosenwasser, H. (1945). Carotid body tumor of the middle ear and mastoid. *Archives of Otolaryngology, 41,* 64-67.

Sakai, C. S., & Mateer, C. A. (1984). Otological and audiological sequelae of closed head trauma. *Seminars in Hearing, 5,* 157-173.

Schweitzer, V. G., & Shepard, N. (1989). Sudden hearing loss: An uncommon manifestation of multiple sclerosis. *Archives of Otolaryngology: Head & Neck Surgery, 100,* 327-332.

Selters, N. A., & Brackman, D. E. (1977). Acoustic tumor detection with brainstem electric response audiometry. *Archives of Otolaryngology, 103,* 181-187.

Smith, I. M., Turnbull, L. W., Sellar, R. J., Murray, J. A. M., & Best, J. J. K. (1990). A modified screening protocol for the diagnosis of acoustic neuromas. *Clinical Otolaryngology, 15,* 167-171.

Stach, B. A., Delgado-Vilches, G., & Smith-Farach, S. (1990). Hearing loss in multiple sclerosis. *Seminars in Hearing, 11,* 221-230.

Waters, G. S., Ahmad, M., Katsarkas, A., Stanimer, G., & McKay, J. (1991). Ototoxicity due to cis-diamminedichloro-platinum in the treatment of ovarian cancer: Influence of dosage and schedule of administration. *Ear and Hearing, 12,* 91-102.

Weaver, M., & Staller, S. J. (1984). The acoustic nerve tumor. In J. L. Northern (Ed.), *Hearing disorders* (pp. 171-177). Boston: Little, Brown.

Welling, D. B., Glasscock, M. E., III, Woods, C. I., & Jackson, C. G. (1990). Acoustic neuroma: A cost-effective approach. *Archives of Otolaryngology: Head and Neck Surgery, 103,* 364-370.

SUGGESTED READING

Gerber, S. E., & Mencher, G. T. (1980). *Auditory dysfunction.* Houston: College-Hill Press.

Jerger, S., & Jerger, J. (1981). *Auditory disorders: A manual for clinical evaluation.* Boston: Little, Brown.

McFarland, W. H. (1989). The acoustic tumor. *Seminars in Hearing, 10*(4). New York: Thieme Medical Publishers, Inc.

Northern, J. L. (1984). *Hearing disorders* (2nd ed.). Boston: Little, Brown.

4

Identification and Evaluation of Hearing Loss in Infants and Preschool Children

Susan D. Dalebout

It commonly is stated that severe or profound bilateral sensorineural hearing impairment is present in approximately one infant in every 1000 live births (Mauk & Behrens, 1993; Welsh & Slater, 1993) and that less severe bilateral sensorineural hearing loss or unilateral hearing loss is present in approximately 6 in every 1000 live births (Goldberg, 1993). However, the incidence of hearing loss in newborns varies according to infant condition and nursery placement (Yellin, 1993). That is, for infants in a neonatal intensive care nursery (NICU), incidence estimates are as high as 20 to 40 infants per 1000 live births (American Speech-Language-Hearing Association [ASHA], 1989). In addition to those infants born with hearing loss, others will acquire hearing impairment during infancy and early childhood.

Speech-language pathologists, along with other health care professionals and educators, play a critical role in the development and implementation of early intervention programs for hearing-impaired children and their families. However, they also can assist in the identification of young children who have hearing losses by making appropriate referrals. In this chapter, the history of the neonatal hearing screening movement in the United States is reviewed, and the current guidelines for screening developed by both the national Joint Committee on Infant Hearing (1994) and the ASHA Committee on Infant Hearing (1989) are discussed. In addition, a model for the comprehensive, clinical assessment of infants and young children who are referred by screening programs, professionals, or parents is presented, and practical guidelines for making audiologic referrals are suggested. Federal mandates regarding early identification and intervention are highlighted, and, finally, information relevant to the interpretation of pediatric audiologic assessment reports is offered.

THE IMPORTANCE OF EARLY IDENTIFICATION OF HEARING LOSS

In 1986, Downs asserted that the age at which a hearing loss is identified and habilitation is initiated may have an even greater impact on a deaf child's future language abilities than the severity of the hearing loss itself. This assertion was borne out in a study by Levitt, McGarr, and Geffner (1987), in which language and educational achievement skills were *not* related to the degree of hearing loss. In fact, the only major variable affecting language was the age at which intervention was initiated. Downs' (1987) observation is consistent with the concept that critical periods in development exist, during which certain types of input are used to their maximum potential. After these periods have passed, the input never again is as effective for learning or skill development. For example, prominent linguists, among them Chomsky (1966) and Lenneberg (1967) have theorized that language is an innate function, time-locked to early periods in development when the brain is in its most plastic state and can use the language input it receives to the greatest benefit.

There is a similar critical period for auditory stimulation. For example, Ruben and Rapin (1980) presented evidence for the early plasticity of the brain and stated that input from the peripheral auditory system is critical to the maturation and innervation of portions of the central auditory system. They suggested that auditory stimulation has the greatest effect in shaping auditory abilities during the first three years of life. Extrapolating from animal studies (eg, Webster & Webster, 1977; 1979; 1980), it has been suggested that irreversible deterioration of central auditory pathway nuclei secondary to a lack of sound stimulation imposed at birth might occur in humans as it does in some experimental animals (eg, mice). However, findings from a more recent study (Doyle & Webster, 1991) suggested that in animals for whom hearing begins in utero, changes in the central auditory nervous system do *not* result from conductive hearing losses imposed at birth. This includes the human fetus, in whom the auditory system is functional by five months gestation. Downs (1994) suggested that the more recent findings do not refute earlier assumptions about the plasticity of the central nervous system and its ability to be shaped through experiential deprivation of auditory stimuli; rather, the results of the latter study serve to confirm the power of early auditory stimulation—even in utero. It appears that the most critical period for language and auditory input may be very early in life.

The importance of the early identification of hearing loss cannot be overemphasized. The prognosis of the hearing impaired child in areas ranging from speech, language, cognition, and psychosocial development to academic achievement depends on early identification. Moreover, although it has long been recognized that severe or profound bilateral hearing loss has a pervasive effect on virtually all areas of development, more recent research has demonstrated that unilateral hearing loss and milder degrees of bilateral hearing loss also have negative effects. For example, Bess and Tharpe (1984) reported that the rate of grade failure was ten times higher in a sample of 60 children with unilateral hearing loss than it was in a local public school population.

A report issued by the U.S. Department of Health and Human Services (DHHS), entitled *Healthy People 2000* (1990), emphasized the importance of identifying hearing loss at the youngest possible age. In this report, a goal was set to "reduce the average age at which children with significant hearing impairment are identified to no more than 12 months" (p. 460). Unfortunately, despite the acknowledged importance of identifying hearing loss as early as possible, the average age at identification in this country is 24 to 30 months (Commission on Education of the Deaf, 1988; U.S. DHHS, 1990). Children with milder but nonetheless detrimental hearing losses frequently are not identified until they are 5 to 6 years of age (White & Behrens, 1993).

According to Downs (1986), the need to identify hearing disorders at birth was recognized as early as the 1950s, when a number of investigators throughout the world began to explore techniques for newborn screening. However, progress in the early identification of hearing loss has been painfully slow (Mauk & Behrens, 1993). In 1992, Bess and Hall reported that 95 to 97 percent of the 4 million infants born in the United States each year were not screened for hearing loss.

Before screening and clinical assessment practices are discussed, the techniques involved in each are described. These descriptions should give readers a common reference point for understanding the information that follows. Because some of the techniques described herein may be used both for screening and for clinical assessment (eg, auditory brainstem response [ABR] audiometry), it is important to emphasize the different purposes of screening and assessment procedures. A screening test is a measure that is used to differentiate apparently healthy people who probably have a disease from those who probably do not (Jacobson, 1990).

As described by Johnson et al (1993), hearing screening involves the use of a relatively quick, inexpensive, simple, reliable technique to reduce the size of the population that needs to be examined more closely for possible hearing loss. Infants who do not pass the screening are referred for more comprehensive, definitive procedures to determine if a hearing loss is present and, if so, to describe its degree and nature so that appropriate intervention can begin. By focusing diagnostic resources on a smaller group of children more likely to have a hearing loss, money, time, and unnecessary anxiety are saved. Thus, although ABR audiometry may be used to screen infants for hearing loss and also as part of the clinical assessment of an infant referred by a screening program, the purposes and protocols are quite different.

SCREENING AND ASSESSMENT OF HEARING IN INFANTS AND YOUNG CHILDREN

Screening Techniques and Practices

High-Risk Register

The high-risk register concept is based on the premise that a subgroup of the general population can be selected for further study on the basis of certain criteria that indicate an increased risk for the target disorder or illness (in this case, hearing loss). The risk criteria may involve history or physical findings or a combination of both. For example, a high-risk register may be used to identify a subpopulation of newborns who are at increased risk for hearing impairment and, therefore, will be screened further with a second technique. Use of a high-risk register for hearing loss reduces the focus to approximately 10 percent (Johnson et al, 1993) of the general neonatal population, 2 to 4 percent of whom will have moderate to profound hearing impairments (Welsh & Slater, 1993).

Unfortunately, a grave limitation of using a high-risk register to identify hearing loss is that a substantial percentage (ie, up to 50 percent) of children with hearing impairments manifest no identifiable risk factors and, therefore, are missed by screening programs (Jerger, 1993; Mauk & Behrens, 1993; White et al, 1993). For example, studies indicate that as many as 50 percent of congenital hearing losses with a known origin are due to hereditary factors. However, 80 to 90 percent of all genetic hearing losses are inherited recessively (Northern & Downs, 1991; Martin, 1994). Children with recessively inherited hearing loss typically have two parents with normal hearing who are carriers for the recessive gene. There is no history of familial hearing loss; thus, it is not possible to identify such families in the general population until they have produced an affected child.

Behavioral Observation Screening

Behavioral screening implies the observation of overt changes in behavior that occur in response to high-intensity stimuli presented with a handheld instrument positioned near the infant. The behavioral responses are reflexive and may include arousal from sleep, a startle, or an eyeblink. Some of the major limitations of behavioral observation techniques are as follows: the protocols must use stimuli that, at best, only identify infants with bilateral severe or profound hearing losses; determination of whether the observed change in behavior was indeed a response to the auditory stimulus relies on the subjective judgment of the observers; and the state (ie, activity level) of the infant has a substantial effect on responsiveness. Because of the high number of false-positive and false-negative results, behavioral observation is not widely accepted as an effective screening procedure.

Crib O-Gram

Use of the Crib-O-Gram device (Telesensory Systems, Inc., Palo Alto, Calif.) involves placement of a motion-sensitive transducer under a crib mattress to detect motor activity produced by the infant. The infant's activity level is monitored automatically for 10 to 15 seconds before and 2 to 5 seconds after the presentation of an auditory stimulus. The stimulus is a 2000- to 4000-Hz bandpass noise of 92 decibels sound pressure level (dB SPL) delivered from an earphone placed in the crib. The stimulus is presented 20 or more times. Responses in the form of motor movement are analyzed by a microprocessor until the unit can make a statistically valid decision as to whether the infant passed or failed the screening. In recent years, the sensitivity, specificity, and reliability of this screening method have been questioned (Durieux-Smith et al, 1985; Wright & Rybak, 1983). Also, because high stimulus intensities are needed to elicit a detectable behavioral response, the Crib O-Gram, like behavioral observation screening, is likely to miss mild and moderate hearing losses (Mauk & Behrens, 1993). Both techniques are insensitive to unilateral hearing losses.

Auditory Brainstem Response Audiometry

The ABR consists of seven components of the auditory evoked response that occur within the first 10 milliseconds (msec) after stimulus onset. The term *auditory evoked response* refers to changes in the ongoing electrical activity of the brain (indicated by electroencephalographic [EEG] recordings) that occur in response to auditory stimulation. These changes are extremely small relative to ongoing EEG activity and cannot be detected without the use of signal-averaging computers. These computers use a technique in which activity time-locked to the stimulus is added together and averaged over successive trials. In contrast, the background activity, which is random and not time-locked to the stimulus, theoretically consists of an equal number of positive and negative electrical voltages and cancels itself out over repeated trials. Thus, the changes that occur in response to auditory stimulation are enhanced relative to background brain activity.

The ABR is considered to reflect the electrical activity of cranial nerve VIII (the auditory nerve) and the auditory pathways of the brainstem. As such, ABR results reflect neural integrity but cannot be considered a perceptual response to sound or a reflection of *hearing*. Thus, the ABR should not be viewed as a substitute for behavioral assessment, but as an adjunct measure to be used when behavioral results are unavailable, inconclusive, or unreliable. The ABR seves a variety of clinical purposes; it is considered here only as a technique for screening the hearing of newborns and for estimating hearing sensitivity in difficult-to-test populations such as infants and young children.

ABR testing currently is the most popular technique for screening the hearing of neonates. Limitations associated with ABR screening include its relatively high cost, the time required for testing, the need for electrode placement on the scalp or forehead and ears, and the fact that the screening does not provide frequency-specific information. The screening ABR, typically evoked by click stimuli, provides an estimate of hearing sensitivity in the high-frequency range only.

Fortunately, this frequency range is the most critical for speech perception; however, to ascertain the status of hearing across the frequency range, protocols employing frequency-specific stimuli, such as tone pips, are necessary. Such protocols generally are performed only within the context of clinical assessment. Thus, it is conceivable that an infant with a hearing loss affecting only the mid or low frequencies could pass an ABR screening.

Despite these limitations, ABR testing holds several important advantages over the behavioral observation and Crib-O-Gram screening methods. For example, unilateral hearing losses and bilateral losses of mild to moderate degree can be identified with ABR screening. The use of a high-intensity stimulus that is presented to both ears precludes the identification of such losses with behavioral observation and Crib-O-Gram screening. Also, the ABR is a physiologic response that is not affected by sleep or by pharmacologic agents.

Automated ABR devices are commercially available for screening the hearing of newborns. Such devices deliver a pass–refer outcome after comparing an individual neonate's ABR with a normative template algorithm (Mauk & Behrens, 1993). The primary advantage of an automated ABR screener is that it does not require an audiologist for administration and interpretation, thereby resulting in a lower cost per test than conventional ABR screening.

Otoacoustic Emissions

Otoacoustic emissions (OAEs) are acoustic responses associated with the normal hearing process that can be measured in the external ear canal. They represent physiologic activity from within the cochlea, specifically, from normally functioning outer hair cells. In a normal ear, OAEs can be elicited with brief acoustic stimuli, such as clicks. Sound enters the ear canal and moves through the middle ear into the cochlea, where hundreds of thousands of frequency-specific hair cells vibrate to transmit the signal through cranial nerve VIII to the brain (White et al, 1993). If the cochlea is functioning normally, the hair cells emit sound as they vibrate, or send an echo back through the middle ear (White et al, 1993). This echo can be recorded in the ear canal by a small, sensitive microphone connected to a specially equipped computer (White et al, 1993). These responses are known as OAEs. A strong OAE cannot be obtained without a normally functioning cochlea (Vohr et al, 1993).

Because OAE screening has been shown to be simple, fast, economical, noninvasive, and accurate (White et al, 1993), it recently has been proposed as a standard screening technique for *all* infants born in the United States (National Institutes of Health [NIH], 1993; Joint Committee on Infant Hearing, 1994). This may represent the first step toward achieving the goal of universal screening. White et al (1993) reported results from the Rhode Island Hearing Assessment Project, a large-scale program in which OAEs were used to screen the hearing of 1850 infants born during a 6-month period in 1990–1991. In this project, if only those infants identified as at-risk by the high-risk register or only infants in the NICU had been screened, approximately one-half of the infants identified with OAEs as having a hearing impairment would have been missed. Moreover, if only high-risk infants had been screened, 30 of the 37 infants with fluctuating, conductive hearing loss would have been missed.

A limitation of using OAEs as a hearing screening technique involves its sensitivity to background noise. It is sometimes difficult to obtain reliable responses in the nursery. It also should be noted that OAEs are thought to reflect outer hair cell activity. As such, an infant with normal cochlear function and a lesion of the auditory system beyond the cochlea could pass an OAE screening. Also, as with ABR, OAEs represent a physiologic response and do not reflect hearing in the perceptual sense. Other limitations include the presence of vernix caseous and other debris in the external ear canal and canal collapse (Norton, 1993). Vernix is a sebaceous deposit that covers the skin of the fetus in utero. It can accumulate in creases and crevices, such as the ear canal, and block both the microphone and the sound delivery ports of the OAE probe. In addition, the walls of the neonatal ear canal are very pliable and collapse easily, which also may result in blockage of the probe.

Universal Screening

It has become apparent that high-risk screening misses approximately 50 percent of infants with congenital hearing loss (Jerger, 1993). There is currently a national movement toward universal screening of all newborns which is supported by proposed congressional legislation, the most recent statement from the national Joint Committee on Infant Hearing (1994), and a report drafted by the NIH Consensus Development Conference on Early Identification of Hearing Impairment in Infants and Young Children (1993). The NIH panel recommended the screening of all neonates with OAEs, followed by ABR screening of infants who do not pass the initial OAE screening. The panel noted that although ABR has been the hearing screening method of choice for infants identified by the high-risk register for nearly 15 years (Goldberg, 1993), factors such as its high cost, the time required for testing, and the need for electrode placement have discouraged its use as a universal screening tool. The development of techniques involving OAEs prompted the panel to recommend, for the first time, universal screening of all newborns. In 1994, the Joint Committee on Infant Hearing also endorsed the goal of universal detection of infants with hearing loss. Like the NIH panel, the Joint Committee suggested the use of ABR and OAEs to accomplish this goal. The 1994 position statement of the Joint Committee will be discussed in more detail in this chapter.

Clinical Assessment Techniques and Practices

Behavioral Observation Audiometry

In behavioral observation audiometry (BOA), similar to behavioral observation screening, a baby's behavior is observed in the presence and absence of sound stimuli. The audiologist looks for a change in behavior that implies the baby has heard the sound presented. In contrast to behavioral observation screening, in which stimuli are presented to infants in the nursery from a handheld instrument,

BOA involves the presentation of calibrated, frequency-specific stimuli from loudspeakers in a sound-controlled environment. However, not unlike behavioral observation screening, BOA has a number of serious limitations.

BOA may be confounded by factors such as the expectations of the observer; the nonspecific responses given by infants to sound stimuli; and the fact that reflexive responses vary as a function of the nature of the stimulus, the state (ie, sleep state or activity level) of the infant, and the infant's age (Widen, 1993). Moreover, habituation to the test stimulus in BOA results in large intrasubject variability. Research has shown (Thompson & Weber, 1974) that the dispersion of results among normally hearing, normally developing infants is so great that it is difficult to define hearing loss as a deviation from the norm.

Visual Reinforcement Audiometry

The most commonly used audiologic procedure for screening or assessing the hearing of infants who are 6 months through 2 years of age is visual reinforcement audiometry (VRA) (Moore et al, 1992; Gravel, 1994). Research has demonstrated that it is possible to elicit reliable, behavioral responses from children using operant conditioning and visual reinforcement. Normally developing children as young as 5 months of age can be conditioned to produce a specific motor response contingent on the presence of an auditory stimulus (ASHA, 1991). Frequency-specific thresholds may be obtained from infants, allowing the accurate evaluation of hearing sensitivity regardless of the type, degree, or configuration of hearing impairment (ASHA, 1991). Test reliability and validity have been documented; VRA threshold estimates obtained from infants with sensorineural hearing loss are comparable to thresholds obtained from the same children at older ages using conditioned play audiometry (Gravel, 1994).

In the VRA operant conditioning paradigm unidirectional head turns are conditioned and maintained with visual reinforcement such as the activation of a lighted, animated toy. Several different toys may be used, each of which is housed in a smoked Plexiglas case. Thus, the infant can see the toy only when it is lighted and activated as a reinforcer. Head turns toward the reinforcer in the absence of a stimulus are minimized by a test assistant who sits in front of the infant and directs attention toward the midline. Both the test assistant and the mother may wear masking earphones during the evaluation so that they do not provide cues to the infant regarding the presence of test sounds. The infant initially is conditioned to the task by pairing the presentation of a sound stimulus with the visual stimulus (reinforcer). Once conditioning has been established, hearing thresholds can be determined by varying the intensity level of the auditory stimulus and using the visual stimulus only to reinforce an appropriate head-turn response. If a child does not condition readily, it is possible that he or she is unable to hear the auditory signal; however, it is also possible that the child is slow to learn the task. To resolve this question, a vibrotactile signal from the bone-conduction vibrator may be used for conditioning. In this case, the clinician can be certain that the infant is able to perceive the signal. The bone-conducted signal is paired with the visual stimulus for several trials until the infant learns the response contingency. If the infant is conditioned readily using a vibrotactile signal, a severe or profound hearing loss is suspected. On the other hand, if the child continues to demonstrate difficulty learning the task, the possibility of developmental delay should be investigated (Gravel, 1994).

Use of a VRA paradigm eliminates some of the subjectivity inherent in BOA. For example, both examiners, one of whom is naive to the presentation of stimuli, may vote independently about whether a head-turn response has occurred. Only if both examiners vote affirmatively after a stimulus indeed has been presented is the reinforcer activated. In addition, once conditioning has been established, the nature of the stimulus no longer affects the type or the level of the response, and responses do not vary as a function of age (over a range of 6 to 24 months). The use of a visual reward also reduces the habituation problem, dramatically decreasing intrasubject variability. Studies have shown that infant VRA thresholds differ only slightly (10–15 dB) from those of adults and that the dispersion of normal responses is small, allowing even mild hearing losses to be accurately defined (Widen, 1993). This procedure has been found to be effective for infants between 5 and 24 months of age.

Tangible Reinforcement Operant Conditioning Audiometry

Tangible reinforcement operant conditioning audiometry (TROCA) involves the use of specially designed audiometric equipment from which a tangible reinforcer such as candy, cereal, or a token can be dispensed. The child is conditioned to push a button whenever a test sound is heard. Depending on the age of the child, variations could include, for example, the dispensation of pegs with which the child can complete a design on a pegboard. Correct responses, time-locked to the stimulus, are reinforced; false responses are followed by silent periods during which testing stops and the possibility of reinforcement is taken away. Although effective, these procedures tend to be time-consuming.

Visual Reinforcement Operant Conditioning Audiometry

Visual reinforcement operant conditioning audiometry (VROCA) is a variation of TROCA in which a correct response (eg, a button press upon hearing a sound) is visually reinforced. Visual reinforcement may be in the form of videotapes or the activation of mechanical toys and puppets.

Conditioned Play Audiometry

For this procedure, the child is conditioned to insert a peg in a pegboard, place a ring on a stick, toss blocks in a bucket, or to perform another activity upon hearing the test stimulus.

Immittance Audiometry

Immittance audiometry is the term used to encompass a battery of three tests: tympanometry, compensated static acoustic immittance, and acoustic reflex testing. Because compensated static acoustic immittance measurements are not discussed within the recommended protocols to be presented later in this chapter, only tympanometry and acoustic reflex testing are discussed here.

Tympanometry

Tympanometry is a technique for measuring relative changes in the compliance of the tympanic membrane as air pressure is mechanically varied in the external auditory canal. The compliance of the tympanic membrane at specific air pressures is plotted on a graph known as a tympanogram. The tympanometric pattern obtained provides information regarding the status of the middle ear. For example, a tympanogram may suggest normal middle ear function, the presence of middle ear effusion ("fluid"), eustachian tube dysfunction, ossicular fixation, or ossicular discontinuity. Tympanometry also can be used to follow the progression and resolution of otitis media in children, to determine the patency of tympanostomy tubes, and to detect perforations in the tympanic membrane not readily seen with the aid of an otoscope. Tympanometry should be a component of every pediatric hearing assessment.

Acoustic Reflex Testing

The acoustic reflex threshold represents the lowest stimulus intensity level at which a contraction of the stapedius muscle in the middle ear is detectable as a change in tympanic membrane compliance. In general, thresholds are obtained for the octave frequencies of 500 to 4000 Hz. Because the stapedius muscles contract bilaterally in response to an appropriate stimulus presented to either ear, both ipsilateral (uncrossed) and contralateral (crossed) reflexes may be obtained. Acoustic reflex thresholds can provide considerable information regarding the presence or absence of middle ear pathology in the ear where the reflex is measured and the type of hearing loss (conductive or sensorineural) in the ear receiving the stimulus (ie, the stimulus used to elicit the acoustic reflex). Acoustic reflex thresholds also can be used to infer information regarding the degree of hearing loss in the stimulated ear. Along with tympanometry, acoustic reflex testing should be a part of every pediatric hearing assessment.

Early Intervention

The early identification of a hearing loss is of benefit only if early intervention services are available (Johnson et al, 1993). In fact, without aggressive follow-up, the initiation of a hearing screening program is indefensible (Jacobson, 1990). A comprehensive program should include a neonatal screening program, parent education and involvement, appropriate diagnostic testing, audiologic management, and intervention designed to optimize parent–child interaction for language growth (Brackett et al, 1993).

Although it is widely acknowledged that early intervention is essential for children with moderate, severe, or profound bilateral sensorineural hearing losses, it is important to recognize that even a mild hearing loss can interfere with a child's ability to perceive and categorize speech sounds, internalize acoustic cues, discriminate words, and distinguish the characteristics of speech (Yellin, 1993). This may be particularly true if the hearing loss fluctuates, as is often the case in hearing loss associated with recurrent otitis media and other conductive pathologies. When the hearing loss is identified early, systematic intervention programs can prevent the developmental sequelae of mild bilateral, unilateral, or fluctuating conductive hearing loss and can reduce the amount of special education required over the long term (Brackett et al, 1993).

NEONATAL HEARING SCREENING
Background

Downs and Sterritt (1964) and Downs and Hemenway (1969) developed and described protocols for infant hearing screening that were based on the observation of reflexive responses to sound (eg, the auropalpebral [eyeblink] response, the startle response, and a variety of subtle head and limb movements). These protocols involved the mass behavioral screening of newborns using a 3000-Hz narrow-band noise stimulus of approximately 90 dB SPL. The goals of these early efforts were to identify newborn infants with bilateral severe or profound congenital hearing loss and to develop screening techniques that could be expanded to other newborn nurseries at a modest cost (Weber, 1987).

The reports of Downs and associates prompted considerable enthusiasm for the development of neonatal screening programs (Dennis, 1987). However, it soon became apparent that such programs were neither cost-effective nor adequate in terms of sensitivity and specificity. That is, tests that relied on the behavioral responses of neonates, the subjective judgments of volunteers, and that were applied to all infants resulted in unacceptable rates of overreferral and underreferral. Moreover, a protocol in which a stimulus was presented to both ears at a level of 90 dB SPL could not identify unilateral, mild, or moderate hearing losses. Still, these pioneering efforts can be credited with the generation of substantial research and development in the area of newborn hearing screening (Dennis, 1987).

In response to the proliferation of "unstructured and nondirected attempts" (Gerkin & Downs, 1984, p. 9) at behavioral screening that followed the reports of Downs et al, professionals called for standards. The idea of newborn screening was embraced, but the techniques for accomplishing it were in question (Gerkin & Downs, 1984). In 1970, Downs approached ASHA requesting that a joint committee, composed of representatives from the American Academy of Ophthalmology and

Table 4.1 Risk Criteria—1982 Position Statement of the Joint Committee
on Infant Hearing

Factors that identify infants who are AT RISK for having hearing impairment:

1. A family history of childhood hearing impairment.
2. Congenital perinatal infection (eg, cytomegalovirus, rubella, herpes, toxoplasmosis, syphilis).
3. Anatomic malformations involving the head or neck (eg, dysmorphic appearance including syndromal and nonsyndromal abnormalities, overt or submucous cleft palate, morphologic abnormalities of the pinna).
4. Birthweight less than 1500 grams.
5. Hyperbilirubinemia at level exceeding indications for exchange transfusion.
6. Bacterial meningitis, especially *H. influenza.*
7. Severe asphyxia, which may include infants with Apgar scores of 0 to 3 who fail to institute spontaneous respiration by 10 minutes and those with hypotonia persisting to 2 hours of age.

Otolaryngology, the American Academy of Pediatrics, and ASHA be formed to evaluate the status of newborn screening and to make recommendations (Downs, 1986; Mahoney & Eichwald, 1987). The initial membership of the Joint Committee on Infant Hearing was composed of four ASHA members, two pediatricians, and one otolaryngologist. Downs was appointed chairperson by committee vote (Gerkin & Downs, 1984).

In 1970, the Joint Committee issued a statement that discouraged mass screening of all infants but highlighted the need for further research. In 1973, the committee published a high-risk register for deafness, which included five criteria that indicated a newborn infant was at increased risk for hearing impairment. The records of each infant were to be reviewed so that the presence of any of the five factors could be identified. The 1973 statement suggested in-depth audiologic evaluation of infants identified by the high-risk register within the first 2 months of life. The Joint Committee has continued to revise its statements periodically, publishing new position statements in 1982, 1990, and 1994. In 1982, the Joint Committee recommended identification of infants at risk for hearing loss in terms of seven specific risk factors and suggested follow-up audiologic evaluation until an accurate assessment of hearing could be made. In 1990, the position statement was modified to expand the list of risk factors and recommend a specific hearing screening protocol (ABR). The high-risk indicators included in position statements in 1982 and 1990 are shown in Tables 4.1 and 4.2, respectively. The 1994 position statement, including the current high-risk register, will be discussed later in this chapter.

Table 4.2 Risk Criteria for Neonates and Infants—1990 Position Statement
of the Joint Committee on Infant Hearing

A. **Neonates (birth to 28 days)**
1. Family history of congenital or delayed-onset childhood sensorineural impairment.
2. Congential infection known or suspected to be associated with sensorineural hearing impairment such as toxoplasmosis, syphilis, rubella, cytomegalovirus, and herpes.
3. Craniofacial anomalies including morphologic abnormalities of the pinna and ear canal, absent philtrum, low hairline, and so on.
4. Birth weight less than 1500 grams (3.3 lbs).
5. Hyperbilirubinemia at a level exceeding indication for exchange transfusion.
6. Ototoxic medications, including but not limited to the aminogycosides used for more than 5 days (eg, gentamycin, tobramycin, kanamycin, streptomycin) and loop diuretics used in conjunction with aminoglycosides.
7. Bacterial meningitis.
8. Severe depression at birth, which may include infants with Apgar scores of 0 to 3 at 5 minutes or those who fail to initiate spontaneous respiration by 10 minutes or those with hypotonia persisting to 2 hours of age.
9. Prolonged mechanical ventilation for a duration equal to or greater than 10 days (eg, persistent pulmonary hypertension).
10. Stigmata or other findings associated with a syndrome known to include sensorineural hearing loss (eg, Waardenburg or Usher's syndrome).

B. **Infants (29 days to 2 years)**
1. Parent/caregiver concern regarding hearing, speech, language, and/or developmental delay.
2. Bacterial meningitis.
3. Neonatal risk factors that may be associated with progressive sensorineural hearing loss (eg, cytomegalovirus, prolonged mechanical ventilation, and inherited disorders).
4. Head trauma especially with either longitudinal or transverse fracture of the temporal bone
5. Stigmata or other findings associated with syndromes known to include sensorineural hearing loss (eg, Waardenburg or Usher's syndrome).
6. Ototoxic medications, including but not limited to the aminoglycosides, used for more than 5 days (eg, gentamycin, tobramycin, kanamycin, streptomycin) and loop diuretics used in combination with aminoglycosides.
7. Children with neurodegenerative disorders such as neurofibromatosis, myoclonic epilepsy, Friedreich's ataxia, Huntington's chorea, Werdnig-Hoffman disease, Tay-Sach's disease, Niemann-Pick disease, Charcot-Marie-Tooth disease, any metachro-matic leukodystrophy, or any infantile demyelinating neuropathy.
8. Childhood infectious diseases known to be associated with sensorineural hearing loss (eg, mumps, measles).

Guidelines for Audiologic Screening of Newborn Infants at Risk for Hearing Impairment*

The ASHA Committee on Infant Hearing was established in 1984. The initial activity of the committee was to determine the procedures most appropriate for audiologic screening of infants at risk for hearing impairment. After consideration of the many issues related to infant hearing, the committee concluded that all newborn infants who are at risk for hearing impairment should be identified using the seven-item high-risk register included in the 1982 position statement of the Joint Committee. Infants identified as at-risk should be screened by an audiologist or under the supervision of an audiologist before being discharged from the hospital. The rationale for screening before discharge was, in part, the substantial loss-to-follow-up that can occur if screening is deferred (ASHA, 1989). It was recommended that hearing be screened using auditory evoked potentials (ABR); infants who do not pass the initial audiologic screening or who are not screened before hospital discharge should enter an audiologic evaluation, follow-up, and management program.

The guidelines called for the use of stimuli that contain energy in the frequency region important for speech recognition and a pass–fail criterion of 40 dB nHL or less for each ear. (Thresholds reported in dB nHL are referenced to average thresholds obtained from young, normally hearing adults with whom the same test stimuli and procedures are used.) Estimates of peripheral sensitivity based on electrophysiologic procedures should be confirmed by behavioral techniques as soon as possible. Thus, although the 1982 position statement of the Joint Committee had not recommended a particular method of screening, the guidelines developed by the ASHA Committee on Infant Hearing reflected a consensus among speech-language-hearing professionals that the ABR technique, in conjunction with the high-risk register, was the best available tool for infant screening. Thoughtful analysis and comments regarding potential limitations of the recommended protocol were provided by Turner (1990).

The early identification program outlined in the ASHA guidelines included two additional components: parent–caregiver education and evaluation, and follow-up and management. According to the guidelines, parents–caregivers of all newborns should receive information about normal auditory, speech, and language development and should be informed of the importance of early audiologic evaluation of suspected hearing problems. Definition of the third component of the identification program, a specific system for evaluation, follow-up, and management, was not included in this document. The committee did state, however, that habilitation should be initiated by the age of 6 months.

---

*ASHA Committee on Infant Hearing (1989).

1994 Position Statement*

In 1994, the Joint Committee on Infant Hearing represented the American Speech-Language-Hearing Association, the American Academy of Audiology, the American Academy of Otolaryngology–Head and Neck Surgery, the American Academy of Pediatrics, and the Directors of Speech and Hearing Programs in state health and welfare agencies. The 1994 position statement endorsed the goal of universal detection of infants with hearing loss as early as possible. All infants with hearing loss should be identified before 3 months of age, and receive intervention by 6 months of age. Establishment of this goal reflects concern that risk-factors screening identifies only 50 percent of infants with hearing loss (Pappas, 1983; Elssman et al, 1987; Mauk et al, 1991).

Additional considerations included evidence that normal hearing is critical for speech and oral language development as early as the first 6 months of life (Kuhl et al, 1992) and knowledge that hearing loss of 30 dB hearing level (HL) and greater in the frequency range important for speech recognition (approximately 500 through 4000 Hz) will interfere with the development of speech and oral language. Thus, it was necessary that the techniques suggested by the committee be capable of detecting hearing loss of this degree in infants by age 3 months and younger. Two physiologic approaches, ABR and OAEs, were recommended by the Joint Committee. The committee acknowledged that specific characteristics of test performance for ABR and OAEs had not yet been fully defined in universal hearing detection applications and recommended that each team of health care professionals responsible for the development and implementation of infant hearing programs evaluate and select the technique most suitable for their care practices. The committee noted that although each of the physiologic measures has advantages and disadvantages, both outperform behavioral and automated techniques in their ability to detect hearing loss of 30 dB HL in infants less than 6 months of age (Jacobson & Morehouse, 1984; Durieux-Smith et al, 1985; Hosford-Dunn et al, 1987).

It was recommended that specific timelines be established by each infant hearing program for moving toward the Joint Committee's goal of universal detection. Pending the development of universal screening programs, the Joint Committee recommended that programs based on high-risk indicators be continued. On implementation of universal programs, these indicators should be used to aid in the etiologic diagnosis of hearing loss and to identify infants who require ongoing hearing monitoring. Thus, the 1994 position statement maintained a role for the high-risk indicators described in the 1990 position statement.

The list of indicators associated with sensorineural and conductive hearing loss in newborns and infants is shown in Table 4-3. Indicators associated with late-onset hearing loss were identified for the first time in the 1994 position

---

*Joint Committee on Infant Hearing (1994).

statement and procedures for monitoring infants with those indicators were recommended. The adverse effects of fluctuating, conductive hearing loss from persistent or recurrent otitis media with effusion (OME) also were recognized for the first time, and the Joint Committee recommended monitoring infants with OME for hearing loss. In addition, the Joint Committee recommended that hearing assessment programs be supervised by audiologists.

When a hearing loss is identified, the Joint Committee recommended that evaluation and early intervention services be provided in accordance with the Individuals with Disabilities Education Act (IDEA)—Public Law 102-119 (formerly Public Law 99-457). In accordance with IDEA, a multidisciplinary evaluation must be completed to determine eligibility and to assist in the development of an Individualized Family Service Plan (IFSP) to describe the early intervention program. Because specific services and service eligibility are not uniform from state to state, the Joint Committee suggested that service users and providers contact their state Resource Access Projects (RAP) coordinators for information.

According to the IDEA, the full evaluation process should be completed within 45 days of referral. However, intervention services may commence before completion of the evaluation if parent–caregiver's consent is obtained and an interim IFSP is developed. Early intervention services that might be offered before completing the full evaluation of all developmental areas include the initiation of procedures related to the fitting of amplification and provision of support and information to parents regarding hearing loss and the range of intervention alternatives available. The interim IFSP should include the name of the service coordinator who will be responsible for both implementation of the interim IFSP and coordination of activities among other agencies and persons.

The multidisciplinary evaluation and assessment of an infant identified with a hearing loss should be performed by a team of professionals working in conjunction with the parent–caregiver. The professionals may include, depending on the needs of the individual:

1. A physician with expertise in the management of early childhood otologic disorders.
2. An audiologist with expertise in the assessment of infants and young children to determine the type, degree, symmetry, stability, and configuration of the hearing loss, and to recommend amplification devices appropriate to the child's needs (eg, hearing aids, personal frequency modulation [FM] systems, vibrotactile aids, and/or cochlear implants).
3. A speech-language pathologist, audiologist, sign language specialist, and/or teacher of children who are deaf or hard-of-hearing with expertise in the assessment of communication skills.
4. Other professionals as appropriate for the individual needs of the child and family.

This team will develop a program of early intervention services (an IFSP) based on the child's unique strengths and needs and consistent with the family's

Table 4.3 Risk Criteria—1994 Position Statement of the Joint Committee on Infant Hearing

INDICATORS ASSOCIATED WITH SENSORINEURAL AND/OR CONDUCTIVE HEARING LOSS

A. **For use with neonates (birth through age 28 days) when universal screening is not available:**

1. Family history of hereditary childhood sensorineural hearing loss.
2. In utero infection such as cytomegalovirus, rubella, syphilis, herpes, and toxoplasmosis.
3. Craniofacial anomalies, including those with morphological abnormalities of the pinna and ear canal.
4. Birth weight less than 1500 grams (3.3 lbs).
5. Hyperbilirubinemia at serum level requiring exchange transfusion.
6. Ototoxic medications, including but not limited to aminoglycosides, used in multiple courses or in combination with loop diuretics.
7. Bacterial meningitis.
8. Apgar scores of 0 to 4 at 1 minute or 0 to 6 at 5 minutes.
9. Mechanical ventilation lasting 5 days or longer.
10. Stigmata or other findings associated with a syndrome known to include sensorineural and/or conductive hearing loss.

B. **For use with infants (age 29 days through 2 years) when certain health conditions develop that require rescreening:**

1. Parent–caregiver concern regarding hearing, speech, language, and/or developmental delay.
2. Bacterial meningitis and other infections associated with sensorineural hearing loss.
3. Head trauma associated with loss of consciousness or skull fracture.
4. Stigmata or other findings associated with a syndrome known to include a sensorineural and/or conductive hearing loss.
5. Otoxic medications, including but not limited to chemotherapeutic agents or aminoglycosides, used in multiple courses or in combinatin with loop diuretics.
6. Recurrent or persistent otitis media with effusion for at least 3 months.

C. **For use with infants (age 29 days through 3 years) who require periodic monitoring of hearing:)**

Some newborns and infants may pass initial hearing screening but require periodic monitoring of hearing to detect delayed-onset sensorineural and/or conductive hearing loss. Infants with these indicators require hearing evaluation at least every 6 months until age 3 years and at appropriate intervals thereafter.

INDICATORS ASSOCIATED WITH DELAYED-ONSET SENSORINEURAL HEARING LOSS

1. Family history of hereditary childhood hearing loss.
2. In utero infection such as cytomegalovirus, rubella, syphilis, herpes, or toxoplasmosis.
3. Neurofibromatosis Type II and neurodegenerative disorders.

INDICATORS ASSOCIATED WITH CONDUCTIVE HEARING LOSS

1. Recurrent or persistent otitis media with effusion.
2. Anatomic deformities and other disorders that affect eustachian tube function.
3. Neurodegenerative disorders.

resources, priorities, and concerns related to enhancing the child's development. This multidisciplinary team must include the parent–caregiver. Team planning should be cognizant of and sensitive to the range of available communication and educational choices, and parents should be given sufficient information regarding all options to enable them to exercise informed consent when selecting their child's program. In accordance with the IDEA, the components of an early intervention program for children with hearing loss and their families should include:

1. Family support and information regarding hearing loss and the range of available communication and educational intervention options. Such information must be provided in an objective, nonbiased way to support family choice. It is recommended that consumer organizations and persons who are deaf or hard-of-hearing be used to provide such information. Professional, consumer, state- and community-based organizations should be accessed to provide ongoing information regarding legal rights, educational materials, support groups and/or networks, and other relevant resources for children and families.

2. Implementation of learning environments and services designed with attention to the family's preferences. Such services should be family-centered and consistent with the needs of the child, the family, and their culture.

3. Early intervention activities that promote the child's development in all areas, with particular attention to language acquisition and communication skills.

4. Early intervention services that provide ongoing monitoring of the child's medical and hearing status, amplification needs, and development of communication skills.

5. Curriculum planning that integrates and coordinates multidisciplinary personnel and resources so that intended outcomes of the IFSP are achieved.

Finally, the Joint Committee addressed several additional considerations in their 1994 position statement. These considerations are based on the belief that successful programs for identifying infants with hearing loss are characterized by commitment and support from health care administrators, physicians, audiologists, families and caregivers, and a community educated about the importance of hearing and infant development. Because of the dynamic changes in technology and in education and health care policy, the Joint Committee on Infant Hearing made the following recommendations to facilitate establishment and maintenance of infant hearing programs:

1. Development of a uniform state and national database incorporating standardized technique, methodology, reporting, and system evaluation. This database will enhance patient outcomes, program evaluation (including efficacy and cost/benefit analysis), continuous quality improvement, and public policy development.
2. Development of a tracking system to ensure that newborns and infants identified with or at risk for hearing loss have access to evaluation, follow-up, and intervention services.

3. Systematic evaluation of techniques for identification, assessment, and intervention for hearing loss in infants. Replication and ongoing assessment of current programs will assist in evaluating the efficacy of infant hearing programs and facilitate widespread acceptance of the benefits of early identification of infants with hearing loss.
4. Ongoing refinement of current indicators associated with sensorineural and/or conductive hearing loss.
5. Outcome studies to investigate the impact of early identification on the degree of literacy and communication competence achieved by children with hearing impairments and to establish factors that contribute to outcome.
6. Continued research into the prevention of hearing loss in newborns and infants.

PUBLIC LAW 102-119: INDIVIDUALS WITH DISABILITIES EDUCATION ACT

Federal law stipulates that every child in the United States is entitled to a free and appropriate public education. In 1975, Public Law 94-142 extended this right to all school-aged children with disabilities. The provisions of Public Law 94-142 include free and appropriate public education, nondiscriminatory assessment, an individualized educational program, due process mechanisms for monitoring and appealing decisions, and educational placement in the least restrictive environment (American Speech-Language-Hearing Foundation [ASHF], 1989). In addition to special education services, eligible students also may receive related services, which are supportive services that allow children with disabilities to benefit from special education (Power-deFur & Harvey, 1994). Related services include audiology and speech-language pathology.

In 1986, Public Law 99-457 (Education of the Handicapped Act Amendments) was enacted, reauthorizing Public Law 94-142 and amending it to include mandatory special education for children 3 to 5 years of age. Also provided were incentives for states to offer services to infants and toddlers (and their families) who have disabilities or are at developmental risk. In 1990, Public Law 99-457 was renamed the "Individuals with Disabilities Education Act" in response to persons with disabilities and advocacy groups who called for a change in language (Power-deFur & Harvey, 1994). The "Individuals with Disabilities Education Act Amendments of 1991" were signed into law on October 7 (Public Law 102-119).

Services for 3- and 4-Year-Old Children (Part B)

Public Law 102-119 requires the provision of special education services to all children between 3 and 21 years of age with disabilities. That is, it extends to preschool children all of the services, rights, and protections afforded to school-aged children under Public Law 94-142. States not serving all 3- and 4-year-old children with disabilities risk losing federal funds for all early-education services.

The services provided by audiologists and speech-language pathologists to 3- and 4-year-olds are similar to those provided to older children under Public Law 94-142.

Roush and McWilliam (1990) highlighted six principles originally contained within Public Law 94-142 that are extended to 3- and 4-year-old children by Public Law 102-119:

1. *Zero reject.* All children with disabilities must be provided with a free, appropriate public education; local school divisions are required to seek out all such children. That is, local school divisions must operate ongoing identification and referral programs. These programs involve informing the public of a person's right to a free, appropriate public education and the availability of special education services. The nature of disabilities, the early warning signs, and the need for early intervention must be included (Power-deFur & Harvey, 1994).

2. *Nondiscriminatory evaluation.* Every child referred to the school division must receive an individualized, culturally appropriate evaluation before placement in a special education program. A child suspected of having a hearing loss should receive a full audiologic evaluation and assessment of communicative skills. Eligibility for special education services is based upon the presence of a disability or a developmental delay. Use of "developmental delay" as an eligibility category is at each state's discretion, and will be reflected in each state's special education regulations (Power-deFur & Harvey, 1994). All evaluations are to be conducted by professionals who are recognized by the state as qualified to practice their specific profession.

3. *Individualized Education Plan* (IEP). If found eligible for special education or related services, a written document that directs the child's educational program must be developed with the parents as key participants. The IEP must include a statement of the present level of performance; a statement of annual goals, including short-term instructional objectives; a statement of the specific education and related services to be provided; the extent to which the child will participate in higher education programs; the projected date for initiation and the anticipated duration of services; and appropriate objective criteria, evaluation procedures, and schedules for determining, at least on an annual basis, whether instructional objectives are being achieved (Power-deFur & Harvey, 1994).

4. *Least restrictive environment.* To the maximum extent possible, a child with a disability must be educated with children who do not have disabilities. A full range of alternative placements must be available to every child with a disability. For preschool children, special education services may be delivered at home, in community-based preschool or child-care centers, in Head Start programs, in preschool classes for children with disabilities, and in other places based on the needs of the child (Power-deFur & Harvey, 1994).

5. *Due process.* A series of checks and balances must be included to provide parents with a mechanism for monitoring and appealing decisions regarding identification, placement, and provision of services.

6. *Parental participation.* Parents must be allowed substantial access to school records regarding their child's special education and have the right to be involved in decision making on the IEP.

Early Intervention Services for Children from Birth to 3 Years of Age (Part H)

This component of Public Law 102-119 provides states with funding designed to assist in the development of comprehensive, multidisciplinary, interagency programs for children from birth through 3 years of age who are in need of early intervention services. Children may be served because they are experiencing developmental delays in one or more of five developmental domains (physical, including hearing and vision; cognitive; communication; psychosocial; self-help and adaptive), as measured by appropriate diagnostic instruments and procedures; have a diagnosed physical or mental condition that has a high probability of resulting in developmental delay (eg, Down syndrome); or are considered to be at risk for having substantial developmental delays (to be defined at each state's discretion) if early intervention services are not provided (Houle & Hamilton, 1991; ASHF, 1989).

This program is discretionary; that is, states are not required to participate, but those that elect to do so are required to develop and implement a statewide plan for providing services to children between birth and age 3 years and their families. Within each state a lead agency is responsible for the general administration of the early intervention system. The governor of each state chooses the lead agency. State departments of education, of health, and of human resources frequently are designated as lead agencies (Power-deFur & Harvey, 1994). The early intervention program is intended to be developed primarily through the coordination of existing services and resources already functioning within a given state. The governor appoints a state Interagency Coordinating Council composed of parents of children with disabilities, providers of early intervention services, state agency representatives, at least one person involved in personnel preparation, at least one state legislator, and others at the governor's discretion.

A fundamental difference between Part B and Part H of the IDEA is the shift in focus of Part H from the child's educational needs to the child's developmental needs. This focus is based on the premise that early intervention can reduce the effects of a child's delay or disability, or even may prevent disabilities. Another difference is the focus of Part H on the family rather than on the child. This is consistent with the Congressional finding that there is an urgent and substantial need to enhance the capacity of families to meet the special needs of their infants and toddlers with disabilities (Power-deFur & Harvey, 1994).

Procedures related to screening, multidisciplinary evaluation, and development of an IFSP, as well as the necessary components of an early intervention program developed for children with hearing impairments and their families have already been summarized within the discussion of the 1994 position statement of the Joint Committee on Infant Hearing. For additional information about Part H, refer to Power-deFur and Harvey (1994).

CLINICAL AUDIOLOGIC ASSESSMENT OF INFANTS AND YOUNG CHILDREN

In order for effective intervention to begin, it is imperative that an infant's hearing be carefully assessed (Gravel, 1994). Gravel (1994) suggested that a comprehensive audiologic assessment serves several purposes. First, it provides a baseline against which the results of subsequent evaluations can be compared. This allows the clinician to monitor the stability of any permanent or intermittent hearing loss. Second, any medical or surgical management of the young child is facilitated by the evaluation. Third, an accurate and complete assessment of the hearing loss provides a basis for the selection of hearing aids and other amplification devices. This has become particularly crucial given the use of prescriptive amplification selection procedures that rely on the accuracy of hearing thresholds across the speech frequency range. Finally, a timely, comprehensive assessment provides parents with unequivocal information, which should facilitate the process of accepting the hearing loss.

Guidelines for the Audiologic Assessment of Children from Birth Through 36 Months of Age*

In accordance with the recommendations contained in the "Guidelines for Audiologic Screening of Newborn Infants Who Are at Risk for Hearing Impairment" (ASHA, 1989), the ASHA Committee on Infant Hearing developed "Guidelines for the Audiologic Assessment of Children from Birth Through 36 Months of Age" (ASHA, 1991). Pursuant to the screening guidelines (ASHA, 1989), this document sets forth procedures for the audiologic evaluation of infants and young children identified through screening programs or referred directly to audiologists for hearing assessment. The mandate for developing these guidelines was derived from several sources, including Public Law 102-119, which includes a discretionary program designed to address the special needs of handicapped children from birth through 3 years of age. Previously described in this chapter, this program emphasizes the need for appropriate assessments and for personnel qualified to provide these services.

Background

The ASHA committee (1991) emphasized several points in its background summary. First, responses should be replicable and there should be agreement among measures, or assessment should be continued until consensus is reached. The use of any test alone is discouraged. Corroboration of test results through case history, parent report, and observations of behavior is crucial to assessing the

---

*ASHA Committee on Infant Hearing (1991).

functional use of hearing. Second, effective diagnosis and management should include involvement of the parent–caregiver at all stages, enabling families to be active participants rather than passive recipients. Finally, the goal of assessment is to define precisely the type, degree, and configuration of the hearing impairment for each ear. However, the need for such precision should not preclude the initiation of intervention, including the selection and fitting of amplification (eg, hearing aids and FM systems) and other assistive devices. Accordingly, ongoing assessment is considered part of the management process. In addition, it should be recognized that single-point assessment does not adequately address the issue of progressive hearing loss. When progressive hearing loss is suspected, routine re-evaluation in conjunction with otologic management is essential.

Procedures

Principles that guided the development of the ASHA committee's recommendations (1991) for assessment procedures are described in the following sections.

Individualized Timely Assessment Protocol

It is essential that assessment tools be chosen that are appropriate for the neurodevelopmental state of the young child. Although serial evaluations yield the best information on which to base management decisions, the diagnosis and habilitation of a hearing loss should not be delayed because of an inability to reliably complete any particular test.

Use of Frequency-Specific Stimuli

Responses to pure tones, frequency-modulated tones, or narrow bands of noise should be obtained in behavioral testing, regardless of the response levels obtained to broadband signals (eg, speech, music, or environmental sounds). Because high-frequency spectral energy (above 1000 Hz) is critical to speech perception, audiologic assessment of children should always include stimuli that allow the evaluation of sensitivity in this frequency range. The committee suggested that, at a minimum, thresholds be obtained at 500 Hz and 2000 Hz to allow for the selection of appropriate amplification. Frequency-specific stimuli also are recommended for ABR assessment. The use of click stimuli alone is not sufficient for the estimation of audiometric configuration. ABR thresholds for clicks generally correlate well with behavioral thresholds in the high-frequency range (above 1000 Hz). ABR thresholds for low-frequency stimuli (eg, tone pips) should be used to estimate hearing sensitivity in other frequency regions.

Ear-Specific Assessment

Ear-specific assessment is the goal for both behavioral and electrophysiologic procedures because a unilateral hearing loss, even in the presence of a normally hearing ear, may place a child at considerable developmental risk. The ear not being tested should be masked as necessary.

*Determination of Middle Ear Status by Bone Conduction
and Acoustic Immittance Measurements*

When air-conduction thresholds obtained by either behavioral or electro-physiologic methods are found to be elevated, estimates of bone-conduction sensitivity should be completed. In contrast, acoustic immittance measurements should be accomplished during each test session to assist in the determination of middle ear status.

Assessment Protocol for Children from Birth Through 4 Months of Age

Reliable procedures for the behavioral assessment of infants who are developmentally or chronologically 4 months of age and younger (age adjusted for prematurity) do not exist at the present time. The suggested methods for evaluating the hearing of infants in this age group are the ABR (using both click and low-frequency stimuli) and acoustic immittance tests, in combination with case history, parent–caregiver report, and behavioral observation of the infant's responses to a variety of sounds. Behavioral observation is intended for corroboration of the parent–caregiver's impressions of the infant's hearing ability rather than for threshold determination.

An ABR threshold should be obtained and a latency–intensity function should be plotted for each ear. Responses to both clicks and low-frequency stimuli must be obtained in order to provide an estimate of audiometric configuration. When the air-conducted ABR is elevated, an ABR to bone-conducted stimuli should be considered.

Tympanograms and acoustic reflexes should be obtained for both ears. For the purpose of obtaining acoustic reflex thresholds, probe frequency higher than 226 Hz should be considered. Additional acoustic reflex measurements using broadband noise stimuli may provide useful information about auditory status.

Assessment Protocol for Children 5 to 24 Months of Age

Behavioral techniques, in combination with acoustic immittance measures, are often sufficient for the comprehensive assessment of children who are chronologically or developmentally 5 to 24 months of age (adjusted for prematurity). VRA should be used to assess hearing sensitivity for speech and frequency-specific stimuli. Word recognition measures should be applied at suprathreshold levels as early as possible in accordance with the child's language limitations. ABR audiometry is recommended when the validity or adequacy of behavioral test results is limited or the neurologic integrity of the brainstem auditory pathways is in question. Tympanograms and acoustic reflex measurements should be obtained for both ears.

Assessment Protocol for Children 25 to 36 Months of Age

Behavioral techniques, in combination with acoustic immittance measures, are often sufficient for the comprehensive assessment of children who are chronologically or developmentally 25 to 36 months of age. Conditioned play audiometry, TROCA or VROCA, or VRA should be used depending on the child's ability to perform the necessary task. Frequency-specific thresholds should be determined at the octave frequencies of 500 to 4000 Hz (at a minimum). Thresholds should be determined for each ear by air conduction. Bone-conduction thresholds should be determined when air-conduction thresholds are elevated. A threshold for speech, using a closed-set (picture-point, object-point, or repetition) response task, also should be obtained.

A formal assessment of word recognition ability using standardized tests such as the Word Intelligibility by Picture Identification (WIPI) test, the Northwestern University Children's Perception of Speech (NU-CHIPS) test, or the Pediatric Speech Intelligibility (PSI) test is recommended whenever possible. When a standardized test cannot be used, an attempt should be made to informally assess word recognition ability by using objects or body parts within the child's demonstrated receptive vocabulary. In the latter case, results should be reported descriptively and not quantitatively, because such tests are nonstandardized measures of word recognition ability. ABR audiometry is recommended when the validity or adequacy of behavioral test results is limited or the neurologic integrity of the brainstem auditory pathways is in question. Tympanograms and acoustic reflex thresholds should be obtained for both ears.

Personnel and Scope of the Assessment

Audiologic assessment is performed by an ASHA-certified audiologist who is responsible for the administration and interpretation of behavioral, electrophysiologic, and acoustic immittance measures. Audiologic assessment includes making recommendations regarding audiologic follow-up and management, including candidacy for use, fitting, and dispensing of amplification and alternative communication devices. Audiologic assessment also includes professional interpretation of case history and test results, parent–caregiver counseling, screening for delays in communication or other areas of development, and, when appropriate, referral to allied professionals such as the primary care physician, medical specialist, speech-language pathologist, or psychologist. In areas where programs that address the special needs of children with hearing impairment are in place (in accordance with Public Law 102-119), the audiologist and parent–caregiver are members of the multidisciplinary team and participate in decisions regarding child and family needs. Where no such programs exist, guidance should be provided regarding available education and intervention options so that the parent–caregiver can make informed decisions.

GUIDELINES FOR MAKING AUDIOLOGIC REFERRALS

The assessment of hearing in neonates, infants, and toddlers should be performed only by audiologists, preferably those with experience in pediatric testing. As Roush and McWilliam (1990) stated, the complexities involved in evaluating the hearing of young children, although well known to audiologists, sometimes are underestimated by professionals from other disciplines. For example, children with mild or moderate degrees of impairment or those with high-frequency hearing loss may, on the basis of informal assessment, appear to have normal hearing. This, however, does not imply that speech-language pathologists and health care professionals do not have a role in the early identification of hearing loss. On the contrary, speech-language pathologists and health care professionals fulfill a critical role by referring infants and young children who may have hearing impairments for audiologic evaluation.

The unique background and training of speech-language pathologists allows them to bring extensive knowledge regarding early communication, language, and speech development to the task. That is, speech-language pathologists can rely on their knowledge of developmental milestones in preverbal communication, language, speech, and audition as a basis for making referrals. They also can make use of case history information as it pertains to an increased risk for hearing loss. For example, the risk indicators published in the 1994 position statement of the Joint Committee on Infant Hearing, included in Table 4.3, should alert clinicians to the possible presence of hearing loss. In addition, it is important for speech-language pathologists to be cognizant of the fact that, in general, children who are assessed for developmental problems of any nature are at increased risk for hearing loss. Speech-language pathologists and health care professionals should question parents–caregivers about their child's behavior as it relates to sound. Several general screening questions are included in the Appendix as examples. Table 4.4 lists signs that may signal communication delay or hearing impairment in neonates, infants, and toddlers.

Finally, it must be emphasized that parental concern regarding a child's hearing is *always* a reason for referral. In this regard, speech-language pathologists can be supportive of parents who may not have received adequate or accurate information from their child's physician. On occasion, physicians may trivialize parental concern regarding a child's hearing or may be uninformed about the audiologic techniques available for evaluating the hearing of infants and young children.

UNDERSTANDING THE PEDIATRIC AUDIOLOGIC ASSESSMENT REPORT

Although speech-language pathologists may understand the basic audiologic procedures routinely used to assess the hearing of adults and older children, they may not be as comfortable with the less conventional measures used in the assessment of infants and toddlers. It is critical that speech-language pathologists understand the pediatric hearing assessment report because they may be called on by parents and other professionals to answer questions about its contents and because the information it contains must be incorporated into treatment plans developed for children and their families. It is hoped that the following comments will assist speech-language pathologists and health care professionals in under-

Table 4.4 "Red flags" that may signal communication delay or hearing impairment

Indicators of Communication Delay in Neonates and Infants:
1. Failure to respond to and/or localize auditory and visual stimuli
2. Failure to cuddle
3. Lack of eye contact
4. Poor sucking/swallowing
5. Tactile defensiveness (especially oral)
6. Hypotonia (low tone)—floppy baby, droopy facial features
7. Hypertonia (high tone)—stiff baby
8. Lack of nonverbal interaction between child and caregiver
9. Exceptionally quiet (passive)
10. Exceptionally irritable (cannot be consoled)

Indicators of Communication Delay in Toddlers:
1. Lack of intentional communication in a 12-month-old child (communication does not have to be verbal or symbolic at this time). For example, a child initially makes eye contact with an adult and then, by means of gestures or vocalization, indicates that an object or event is desired.
2. No spoken or signed words by an 18-month-old child.

Indicators of Hearing Impairment:
1. An infant (birth to approximately 4 months) fails to startle to loud, sudden noises
2. By 4 months of age, an infant fails to "listen" to a familiar voice
3. By 8 months of age, an infant fails to turn his or her head toward soft sounds
4. By 12 months of age, an infant has not developed the ability to localize a sound source or has started to babble and then stops without further development
5. At any age, an infant whose auditory behavior appears inconsistent or whose auditory development is significantly different from other infants.
6. *Most important red flag*—parental concern about their infant's hearing and/or communication development

(ASHF [1989], used with permission.)

standing some of the variations on conventional procedures that often are used in pediatric testing.

Auditory Brainstem Response

For infants in the neonatal period through the chronologic or developmental age of 4 months, audiologic reports are likely to include patient history, ABR results, acoustic immittance findings, and impressions of behavioral responses to sound. At a minimum, ABR results should be obtained for air-conducted click stimuli. The need for protocols that include frequency-specific stimuli, such as tone pips, has already been stated. If the audiologic report reveals that *only* clicks were used as stimuli, the audiometric configuration is unknown and low- or mid-frequency hearing loss can neither be ruled out nor assumed.

An ABR threshold for each ear may be reported, or a pass–fail criterion level may be used (eg, 30 dB nHL or 40 dB nHL). The use of a pass–fail criterion level is associated more closely with screening protocols but sometimes may be reported within the context of clinical assessment. ABR thresholds have been estimated to exceed behavioral thresholds in the 1000- to 4000-Hz range by approximately 10 to 15 dB. That is, hearing in the 1000- to 4000-Hz range is estimated to be better than the ABR threshold by 10 to 15 dB. Thus, using a pass–fail criterion of 30 or 40 dB nHL could allow a mild hearing loss to go undetected.

If the threshold for air-conducted stimuli is elevated, testing may be performed using bone-conducted stimuli to determine the type of hearing loss (ie, conductive, sensorineural, or mixed). Information regarding the type of hearing loss also may be obtained by plotting a latency–intensity function, in which peak latency (the time that elapses between presentation of the stimulus and the appearance of each waveform component, measured in milliseconds) at each different stimulus intensity level is plotted and compared with normative values obtained for infants of the same age. Latency varies inversely with stimulus intensity. In other words, as the stimulus presentation level is attenuated and hearing threshold is approached, the latency of the response is increasingly prolonged. The pattern of the latency–intensity function can provide information regarding the type of hearing loss. If neither bone-conduction testing nor a latency–intensity function is performed, information about the type of hearing loss and middle ear status will be provided by immittance results.

The latency of the ABR decreases with maturation through the age of 12 to 18 months post-term (term being 38 to 40 weeks gestational age). Because the ABR changes so rapidly during early life, it is essential that age-appropriate norms be used when interpreting ABR findings. Moreover, it is essential to correct for gestational age; that is, the infant's chronologic age must be adjusted for prematurity. Although waveforms are first discernible at 28 to 30 weeks postconceptual age (28 to 30 weeks gestation, not after birth), the latencies of premature infants are prolonged when compared with those of a term newborn.

Auditory brainstem response testing is most efficiently performed with the infant or young child in deep sleep. Because very young infants sleep a great deal of the time, testing often can be accomplished during periods of natural sleep. However, as infants approach the age of 6 months, they spend less time sleeping and it is frequently necessary to use sedation to induce sleep.

Tympanometry

Tympanometric findings generally are described and interpreted qualitatively, for example, "the tympanogram was normal, suggesting normal middle ear function"; "the tympanogram was flat, suggesting the presence of middle ear effusion"; or "the tympanogram revealed negative pressure, suggesting eustachian tube dysfunction." However, tympanograms sometimes are described by type. A commonly used classification system is that proposed by Jerger (1970), in which:

- A *Type A* tympanogram is associated with normal middle ear function
- A *Type B* tympanogram is flat and associated with the presence of effusion
- A *Type C* tympanogram is characterized by a peak in the negative pressure range and associated with eustachian tube dysfunction (and often developing or resolving middle ear effusion)
- A *Type A$_d$* tympanogram is characterized by abnormally high compliance and associated with ossicular discontinuity
- A *Type A$_s$* tympanogram is characterized by abnormally reduced compliance and associated with stiffness and possible ossicular fixation

Acoustic Reflex Thresholds

Acoustic reflex thresholds are absent or obscured in the presence of middle ear pathology in the ear where the response is measured (ie, the probe ear). The conductive abnormality either prevents the stapedius muscle from contracting or precludes detection of the reflex at the tympanic membrane because of increased stiffness or compliance. The acoustic reflex also is absent when the stimulus used to elicit the reflex is presented to an ear with a conductive hearing loss greater than approximately 30 dB HL (ie, when there is a conductive hearing loss in the ear receiving the stimulus used to elicit the acoustic reflex). The stimulated ear may be the probe ear (ipsilateral stimulation, or uncrossed acoustic reflex) or the opposite ear (contralateral stimulation, or crossed acoustic reflex). The presence of a conductive hearing loss of greater than 30 dB HL in the stimulated ear prevents the stimulus from reaching the cochlea at a level loud enough to elicit the reflex. Conversely, the reflex is likely to be present when an ear with a sensorineural hearing loss of up to 85 dB HL is stimulated. This is because loudness recruitment, a phenomenon peculiar to a cochlear pathology, increases the sensation of loudness in an ear with cochlear hearing loss. Given this information, acoustic reflex data can assist in determining whether a hearing loss is conductive or sensorineural. That is, if the acoustic reflex is present when the stimulated ear has a hearing loss that exceeds 30 dB HL, the loss is likely to be sensorineural rather than conductive.

Behavioral Testing

A report is likely to include patient history information relevant to the development of auditory behavior, reported reactions to environmental sounds, the caregiver's impressions of the child's hearing, and any factors that increase the child's risk for hearing loss. The audiologist may include his or her impressions of the history, his or her observations of the child's behavior, and comments regarding whether the test findings are consistent with the other information available. It should be noted that the audiologic evaluation of infants and young children rarely is complete after one session. It is likely that the report summarizes a series of sessions or is one of several in an ongoing series.

Assessment of children who are chronologically or developmentally 5 to 24 months of age is likely to include VRA, immittance testing, and ABR results if behavioral results are incomplete, inconclusive, or unreliable. In obtaining thresholds with VRA procedures, ear-specific information (ie, obtained under earphones) is desirable; however, often it is possible only to obtain soundfield information (ie, stimuli are presented through loudspeakers) because young children are reluctant to wear earphones. When responses are obtained in the soundfield (check the key to symbols on the audiogram), they represent the hearing sensitivity of only the better ear.

It has been reported that responses obtained from infants and young children using VRA procedures are approximately 10 to 15 dB poorer than those obtained from adult listeners (Nozza & Wilson, 1984; Wilson & Thompson, 1984). For this reason, some audiologists refer to responses obtained from infants and young children as *minimum response levels* rather than thresholds. In any case, the responses shown on the audiogram are likely to be at slightly suprathreshold levels.

When air-conduction responses are elevated, unmasked bone-conduction responses, at a minimum, should be obtained. Additional information regarding middle ear status is provided by immittance measures.

The report is likely to include some information regarding sensitivity to speech stimuli, perhaps in the form of a speech awareness threshold (SAT) or a speech detection threshold (SDT). In either case, responses to the presence of speech stimuli probably were obtained with VRA procedures. There may be occasions in which *only* responses to speech are reported, because some children will respond to speech but not to pure tones. Because speech is a broadband signal, such responses do not provide sufficient information regarding audiometric configuration and should not be considered complete. Responses to frequency-specific stimuli must be obtained as soon as possible.

For children approaching 24 months, it may be possible to obtain an informal speech recognition threshold (SRT) using body parts and articles of clothing as stimuli, combined with a pointing response. The presentation level of the stimuli can be varied until an estimate of threshold is determined. When using this informal procedure, one should determine that the words used as stimuli are within the child's receptive vocabulary. It is also important that the audiologist attempt to use only one-syllable words so that suprasegmental cues are not given. At this age it also may be possible to obtain an informal SRT using pictured spondees (two-syllable words with equal stress on both syllables) or objects that represent spondees, combined with a pointing response. Again, it is necessary first to determine that the words to be used as stimuli are within the child's receptive vocabulary.

Assessment of children who are chronologically or developmentally 25 to 36 months of age generally involves behavioral techniques and immittance measures. Children may be capable of participating in TROCA or VROCA or conditioned play audiometry. Again, testing should not be considered complete unless frequency-specific thresholds for at least the octave frequencies of 500 to 4000 Hz are obtained for each ear. Bone conduction thresholds should be obtained, if possible, when air-conduction thresholds are elevated.

In addition to SRTs, perhaps obtained with the modifications previously described, a formal assessment of word recognition ability (formerly known as speech discrimination ability) is recommended by means of standardized tests such as the WIPI, NU-CHIPS, or PSI. These tests use a closed-set, picture-pointing response format in which words, carefully selected to be within the vocabularies of young children, are used as stimuli. Although none relies on a verbal response, each is subject to the limitations imposed by the child's developing language skills, and this should be taken into account when reporting and interpreting the results as reflective of word recognition ability (rather than receptive language ability). When interpreting the results of these tests, one should remember that scores obtained using a closed-response set format will be slightly better than those obtained using an open-response set format, as is typically used with adults.

Finally, word recognition scores often are obtained at optimal presentation levels to determine the child's potential for word recognition under ideal listening conditions. However, at other times, scores may be obtained at conversational levels, even in the presence of competing noise. Under these conditions, it is likely that scores will be lower, particularly if the child has a hearing loss. It is critically important that speech-language pathologists consider presentation levels and the conditions under which scores were obtained in order to interpret them correctly.

The model for pediatric audiologic assessment proposed in the ASHA (1991) guidelines reviewed earlier in this chapter incorporates a variety of procedures that provide the audiologist with a means for examining the reliability and validity of test outcomes. That is, the audiologist must look for concordance among outcomes of the procedures included in the test battery (Gravel, 1994). According to Gravel (1994), disparity in the results signals the need to reassess conclusions, reanalyze test findings, or seek additional information. The model includes the parent or caregiver in the evaluation process. It is important to incorporate direct, informal, and parental observations of the infant's auditory function throughout the audiologic assessment process (Gravel, 1994).

SUMMARY AND CONCLUSIONS

In 1993, C. Everett Koop, former surgeon general of the United States, wrote:

> Hearing impairment in infants interferes with the normal development of language, the skill that sets humans apart from all other animals. Because language develops so rapidly during the first few months of life, the longer a child's hearing loss goes undetected, the worse the outcome is likely to be.

Koop (1993) emphasized that the tragic results of hearing impairment in infancy can be prevented or substantially lessened if intervention is initiated early enough. Early identification, diagnosis, and habilitation of hearing loss in young children is critical, whether the hearing loss is unilateral or bilateral; sensorineural, mixed or conductive; mild, moderate, severe, or profound (Mauk & Behrens, 1993). Despite the recognized value of early identification of hearing loss, only 3 to 5 percent of all newborns in the United States are screened (Bess & Hall, 1992). Although the commitment to neonatal and infant hearing screening has come a long way and is evolving rapidly, the average age at which young children with hearing loss are identified is still unacceptable (Mauk & Behrens, 1993).

Koop (1993) reported that in 1989 he challenged parents, physicians, state agency staff, and researchers to work together to find better ways to identify young children with hearing losses. He set a public goal that by the year 2000, all children with hearing impairments would be identified before they were 12 months of age. This goal has been echoed in the U.S. Department of Health and Human Services report, *Healthy People 2000*. With a public policy focus at the national level, in conjunction with the implementation of Public Law 102-119, there is good reason to believe that early identification and intervention efforts will become more comprehensive and better coordinated. The responsibility for developing and providing comprehensive early identification and intervention services to all infants with hearing impairments falls, in great part, to speech-language-hearing professionals. We must redouble our efforts on behalf of all children in need of our services.

REFERENCES

American Speech-Language-Hearing Association (1989). Guidelines for audiologic screening of newborn infants who are at risk for hearing impairment. *Asha, 31,* 89-92.

American Speech-Language-Hearing Association (1991). Guidelines for the audiologic assessment of children from birth through 36 months of age. *Asha, 33* (Suppl. 5), 37-43.

American Speech-Language-Hearing Foundation (1988). *How does your child hear and talk?* Rockville: American Speech-Language-Hearing Association.

American Speech-Language-Hearing Foundation (1989). *Speaking of prevention: A resource guide for speech-language pathologists and audiologists.* Rockville: American Speech-Language-Hearing Foundation.

Bess, F. H., & Hall, J. W., III. (1992). *Screening children for auditory function.* Nashville: Bill Wilkerson Center Press.

Bess, F. H., & Tharpe, A. M. (1984). Unilateral hearing impairment in children. *Pediatrics, 74,* 206-216.

Brackett, D., Maxon, A. B., & Blackwell, P. M. (1993). Intervention issues created by successful universal newborn hearing screening. *Seminars in Hearing, 14,* 88-104.

Chomsky, N. (1966). *Aspects of the theory of syntax.* Cambridge: MIT Press.

Commission on Education of the Deaf (1988). *Toward equality: Education of the deaf.* Washington, DC: U.S. Government Printing Office.

Dennis, J. M. (1987). Using the auditory brainstem response in the operating room as a means of detection and prevention of hearing loss in infants and children. *Seminars in Hearing, 8,* 115-123.

Downs, M. P. (1986). The rationale for neonatal hearing screening. In E. T. Swigart (Ed.), *Neonatal hearing screening* (pp. 3-16). San Diego: College Hill Press.

Downs M. P. (1994). The case of detection and intervention at birth. *Seminars in Hearing, 15,* 76-83.

Downs, M. P., & Hemenway, W. G. (1969). Report on the hearing screening of 17,000 neonates. *International Audiology, 8,* 72-76.

Downs, M. P., & Sterritt, G. M. (1964). Identification audiometry for neonates: A preliminary report. *Journal of Auditory Research, 4,* 69-80.

Doyle, W. J. & Webster, D. B. (1991). Neonatal conductive hearing loss does not compromise brainstem auditory function and structure in Rhesus monkeys. *Hearing Research, 54,* 145-151.

Durieux-Smith, A., Picton, T., Edwards, C., Goodman, J. T., & MacMurray, B. (1985). The Crib-O-Gram in the NICU: An evaluation based on brain stem electric response audiometry. *Ear and Hearing, 6,* 20-24.

Eichwald, J., & Mahoney, T. (1993). Apgar scores in the identification of sensorineural hearing loss. *Journal of the American Academy of Audiology, 4,* 133-138.

Elssman, S., Matkin, N., & Sabo, M. (1987). Early identification of congenital sensorineural hearing impairment. *Hearing Journal, 40,* 13-17.

English, K. (1992). States' use of a high-risk register for the early identification of hearing impairment. *Asha, 34,* 75-77.

Gerkin, K. P., & Downs, M. P. (1984). The high risk register for newborn hearing programs. *Seminars in Hearing, 5,* 9-16.

Goldberg, B. (1993). Universal screening of newborns: An idea whose time has come. *Asha, 35,* 63-64.

Gravel, J. S. (1994). Auditory assessment of infants. *Seminars in Hearing, 15,* 100-113.

Hosford-Dunn, H., Johnson, S. Simmons, B., Malachowski, N., & Low, K. (1987). Infant hearing screening: Program implementation and validation. *Ear and Hearing, 8,* 12-20.

Houle, G. R., & Hamilton, J. L. (1991). Public Law 99-457: A challenge to speech-language pathologists and audiologists. *Asha, 33,* 51-60.

Jacobson, J. T. (1990). Issues in newborn ABR screening. *Journal of the American Academy of Audiology, 1,* 121-124.

Jacobson, J., & Morehouse, R. (1984). A comparison of auditory brainstem response and behavioral screening in high risk and normal newborn infants. *Ear and Hearing, 5,* 253, 254.

Jerger, J. (1970). Clinical experience with impedance audiometry. *Archives of Otolaryngology, 92,* 311-324.

Jerger, J. (1993). Toward universal screening. *Journal of the American Academy of Audiology, 4,* Editorial.

Johnson, J. L., Mauk, G. W., Takekawa, K. M., Simon, P. R., Sia, C. C. J., & Blackwell, P. M. (1993). Implementing a statewide system of services for infants and toddlers with hearing disabilities. *Seminars in Hearing, 14,* 105-119.

Johnson, M. J., Maxon, A. B., White, K. R., & Vohr, B. R. (1993). Operating a hospital-based universal newborn hearing screening program using transient evoked otoacoustic emissions. *Seminars in Hearing, 14,* 46-56.

Joint Committee on Infant Hearing (1982). 1982 position statement. *Asha, 24,* 1017-1018.

Joint Committee on Infant Hearing (1991). 1990 position statement. *Asha, 33* (Suppl. 5), 3-4.

Joint Committee on Infant Hearing (1994). 1994 position statement. *Audiology Today, 6,* 6-9.

Kemp, D. T., & Ryan, S. (1993). The use of transient evoked otoacoustic emissions in neonatal hearing screening programs. *Seminars in Hearing, 14,* 30-45.

Koop, C. E. (1993). We can identify children with hearing impairment before their first birthday. *Seminars in Hearing, 14,* Foreword.

Kuhl, P. K., Williams, K. A., Lacerda, F., Stephens, L. N., & Lindbloom, B. (1992). Linguistic experience alters phonetics perception in infants by six months of age. *Science, 255,* 606-608.

Lenneberg, E. H. (1967). *Biological foundations of language.* New York: Wiley.

Levitt, H., McGarr, N. S., & Geffner, D. (1987). *Development of language and communication skills in hearing impaired children* (Monograph No. 26). Rockville, MD: American Speech-Language-Hearing Association.

Mahoney, T. M., & Eichwald, J. G. (1987). The ups and "downs" of high risk hearing screening: The Utah statewide program. *Seminars in Hearing, 8,* 155-163.

Martin, F. N. (1994). *Introduction to audiology* (5th ed.). Englewood Cliffs, NJ: Prentice Hall.

Mauk, G. W., & Behrens, T. R. (1993). Historical, political, and technological context associated with early identification of hearing loss. *Seminars in Hearing, 14,* 1-17.

Mauk, G. W., White, K. R., Mortenson, L. B., & Behrens, T. R. (1991). The effectiveness of screening programs based on high-risk characteristics in early identification of hearing impairment. *Ear and Hearing, 12,* 312-319.

Moore, J. M., Thompson, G., & Folsom, R. C. (1992). Auditory responsiveness of premature infants utilizing visual reinforcement audiometry (VRA). *Ear and Hearing, 13,* 187-194.

National Institutes of Health (1993). Early Identification of Hearing Impairment in Infants and Young Children. *NIH Consensus Statement, 11,* 1-24.

Northern, J. L., & Downs, M. P. (1991). *Hearing in children* (4th ed.). Baltimore: Williams & Wilkins.

Norton, S. J. (1993). Application of transient evoked otoacoustic emissions to pediatric populations. *Ear and Hearing, 14,* 64-73.

Nozza, R. J., & Wilson, W. R. (1984). Masked and unmasked pure-tone thresholds of infants and adults: Development of auditory frequency selectivity and sensitivity. *Journal of Speech and Hearing Research, 27,* 613-622.

Pappas, D. G. (1983). A study of high-risk registry for sensorineural hearing impairment. *Archives of Otolaryngology—Head and Neck Surgery, 91,* 41-44.

Power-deFur, L., & Harvey, J. (1994). Legal basis for early intervention services. *Seminars in Hearing, 15,* 65-75.

Public Law 94-142 (1975). Education of the Handicapped Act.

Public Law 99-457 (1986). Education of the Handicapped Act Amendments.

Public Law 102-119 (1991). Individuals with Disabilities Act Amendments.

Roush, J., & McWilliam, R. A. (1990). A new challenge for pediatric audiologists: Public Law 99-457. *Journal of the American Academy of Audiology, 1,* 196-208.

Ruben, R. J., & Rapin, I. (1980). Plasticity of the developing auditory system. *Annals of Otology, Rhinology, and Laryngology, 89,* 303-311.

Thompson, G., & Weber, B.A. (1974). Responses of infants and young children to behavioral observation audiometry (BOA). *Journal of Speech and Hearing Disorders, 39,* 140-147.

Turner, R. G. (1990). Recommended guidelines for infant hearing screening: Analysis. *Asha, 32,* 57-61.

U.S. Department of Health and Human Services (DHHS) (1990). *Healthy people 2000: National health promotion and disease prevention objectives.* Washington, DC: Public Health Service.

Vohr, B. R., White K. R., Maxon, A. B., & Johnson, M. J. (1993). Factors affecting the interpretation of transient evoked otoacoustic emission results in neonatal hearing screening. *Seminars in Hearing, 14,* 57-72.

Weber, H. (1987). Ten years of searching for the hearing impaired infant in rural Colorado. *Seminars in Hearing, 8,* 149-154.

Webster, D. B., & Webster, M. (1977). Neonatal sound deprivation affects brain stem auditory nuclei. *Archives of Otolaryngology, 103,* 392-406.

Webster, D. B., & Webster, M. (1979). Effects of neonatal conductive hearing loss on brainstem auditory nuclei. *Annals of Otology, Rhinology, and Laryngology, 88,* 684-688.

Webster, D. B., & Webster, M. (1980). Mouse brainstem auditory nuclei development. *Annals of Otology, Rhinology, and Laryngology, 68* (Suppl. 89), 254-256.

Welsh, R., & Slater, S. (1993). The state of infant hearing impairment identification programs. *Asha, 35,* 49-52.

White, K. R., & Behrens, T. R. (1993). Preface. *Seminars in Hearing, 14.*

White, K. R., Vohr, B. R., & Behrens, T. R. (1993). Universal newborn hearing screening using transient evoked otoacoustic emissions: Results of the Rhode Island hearing assessment project. *Seminars in Hearing, 14,* 18-29.

Widen, J. E. (1993). Adding objectivity to infant behavioral audiometry. *Ear and Hearing, 14,* 49-57.

Wilson, W. R., & Thompson, G. (1984). Behavioral audiometry. In J. Jerger (Ed.), *Pediatric audiology* (pp. 1-44) San Diego: College Hill Press.

Wright, L. B., & Rybak, L. P. (1983). Crib-o-Gram (COG) and ABR: Effect of variables on test results. *Journal of the Acoustical Society of America, 74* (Suppl. 1), 540-544.

Yellin, M. W. (1993). Auditory brain stem response (ABR) audiometry in the neonatal nursery. *Seminars in Hearing, 14,* 155-162.

APPENDIX

The following are examples of questions clinicians should ask caregivers about their child's responses to sound and his or her early communication development. If caregivers answer "no" to more than one question in their child's age category, the child should be referred for audiologic evaluation.

At Birth

Hearing and Understanding
Does your child listen to speech?
Does your child startle or cry at noises?
Does your child awaken at loud sounds?

Talking
Does your child make pleasure sounds?
When you play with your child, does he or she look at you, look away, and then look again?

0 to 3 Months

Hearing and Understanding
Does your child turn to you when you speak?
Does your child smile when spoken to?
Does your child seem to recognize your voice and quiet down if crying?

Talking
Does your child repeat the same sounds a lot (cooing, gooing)?
Does your child cry differently for different needs?
Does your child smile when she or he sees you?

4 to 6 Months

Hearing and Understanding
Does your child respond to "no"? Changes in your tone of voice?
Does your child look around for the source of new sounds (eg, the doorbell, vacuum, dog barking)?
Does your child notice toys that make sounds?

Talking
Does your child's babbling sound more speech-like with lots of different sounds, including *p, b,* and *m*?
Does your child tell you (by sound or gesture) when he or she wants you to do something again?
Does your child make gurgling sounds when left alone? When playing with you?

7 Months to 1 Year

Hearing and Understanding
Does your child enjoy games like peek-a-boo and pat-a-cake?
Does your child turn or look up when you call his or her name?
Does your child listen when spoken to?
Does your child recognize words for common items like "cup," "shoe," "juice"?
Has your child begun to respond to requests ("Come here," "Want more?")?

APPENDIX *(continued)*

7 Months to 1 Year *(continued)*

Talking

Does your child's babbling have both long and short groups of sounds such at "tata upup bibibibi?"

Does your child imitate different speech sounds?

Does your child use speech or noncrying sounds to get and keep your attention?

Does your child have one or two words (bye-bye, dada, mama, no) although they may not be clear?

1 to 2 Years

Hearing and Understanding

Can your child point to pictures in a book when they are named?

Does your child point to a few body parts when asked?

Can your child follow simple commands and understand simple questions ("Roll the ball," "Kiss the baby," "Where's your shoe?")?

Does your child listen to simple stories, songs, and rhymes?

Talking

Is your child saying more and more words every month?

Does your child use some one- or two- word questions ("where kitty?" "go bye-bye?" "what's that?")

Does your child put two words together ("more cookie," " no juice," "mommy block")?

Does your child use many different consonant sounds at the beginning of words?

2 to 3 Years

Hearing and Understanding

Does your child understand differences in meaning ("go–stop"; "in–on"; "big–little"; up–down")?

Does your child continue to notice sounds (telephone ringing, television sounds, knocking at the door?)

Can your child follow two requests ("get the ball and put it on the table")?

Talking

Does your child have a word for almost everything?

Does your child use two- to three-word "sentences" to talk about and ask for things?

Do you understand your child's speech most of the time?

Does your child often ask for or direct your attention to objects by naming them?

From the American Speech and Hearing Foundation 1988 brochure, "How Does Your Child Hear and Talk?" Used with permission.

5 ⌐⌐

Hearing Screening for School-Aged Children, Adults, and the Elderly

Lida G. Wall

Audiologists are the professionals responsible for establishing hearing screening programs, training volunteers, and supervising the hearing screening, but frequently the professional who administers the hearing screening test is the speech-language pathologist or school health nurse. Screening guidelines, scope of practice, and personal preferences usually restrict these professionals to pure-tone air-conduction audiometry for screening hearing. However, in consultation with and usually under the supervision of an audiologist, other aspects of an identification program may be undertaken. Suggested protocols for how to screen for hearing impairment and middle ear disorders; when to rescreen and refer; and what screening tests and equipment are most efficient for school-aged children, for adults, and for the elderly are covered in this chapter. For school-aged children and adults, screening procedures are very similar, but the primary type of hearing loss identified changes from conductive in young children to sensorineural in adults. For elderly people (those 65 years of age and older), the same screening protocol is used but is supplemented with self-report test instruments.

Hearing Screening

Most states have mandatory laws pertaining to hearing screening programs for school-aged children and have been operating screening programs for several decades. However, state mandates for neonatal and elderly hearing screenings are not in place in most states. State laws that pertain to hearing screening for school-aged children may (1) state when the screening should be initiated and who should be screened, (2) indicate what equipment or procedures are approved by the governing state department (education or health), (3) state the age or grade levels to be screened, (4) indicate the criteria for referral, and (5) provide approved forms for keeping records of the tests and follow-up measures recommended for the identified problems (ODH, 1987).

The enactment in 1986 of Public Law 99-457 (Education of the Handicapped Act Amendments) has provided the impetus for development of state neonatal screening programs for early intervention for infants and toddlers. The enactment reauthorized the Education of the Handicapped Act (Public Law 94-142) passed in 1975. The Early Intervention Program for Infants and Toddlers with Handicaps law (Public Law 99-457) encouraged early intervention for the 0- to 5-year-old population and expanded the provision of Public Law 94-142. As a result, departments of education and health in many states are developing guidelines for assisting with early intervention programs. The identification guidelines and recommendations for hearing in 0- to 3-year-old children are contained in Chapter 4. The pure-tone screening procedures described in the first half in this chapter are intended for school-aged children (those 5 years and older). The need for identification is important and has a potential impact on approximately 8 million school-aged children (Berg, 1986) who have some type of hearing loss. Of course, prevention of the hearing loss is preferable to remediation of the problem. A tutorial on prevention of communication disorders is available (ASHA, 1991) and is recommended for further reading. Speech-language pathologists who work in the school system have an opportunity to collaborate with classroom teachers as well as with special education teachers regarding the communication needs of all children and particularly the needs of children with hearing impairments.

Screening versus Identification

The term *identification audiometry* was popularized after an American Speech-Language-Hearing Association (ASHA) conference and resultant monograph entitled *Identification Audiometry* (Darley, 1961). The term is used to mean finding (identifying) a person who has a clinically significant hearing problem. The more commonly preferred term in medical and health organizations is *screening*. It is used to refer to a test applied to large populations to find individuals with specific disorders (Chaiklin et al, 1982). Both of these terms, *hearing screening* and *identification audiometry*, are used interchangeably throughout this chapter.

PREREQUISITES OF A SCREENING PROGRAM

Before an identification program is initiated, decisions must be made regarding the disorder to be screened, the procedures to be used, and the resources available. Screening programs are tremendous undertakings that involve a large, specifically defined population to be screened; a sufficient number of individuals in the population who are expected to be affected by the disorder; the availability of an accurate, reliable screening test; well-trained personnel to administer the screening test; an adequate number of professionals available for follow-up evaluations and treatment of the identified disorder; and a mechanism to ensure that people identified as having a disorder will comply with the screening recommendations (Bluestone et al, 1986; Cadman et al, 1984; Cross, 1985). As is apparent, administering the screening test is only one component of a comprehensive hearing identification program. Although the speech-language pathologist or school nurse may not be involved in all aspects of a hearing identification program, awareness of the program components is beneficial for proper referral and follow-up.

Incidence and Prevalence

The terms *incidence* and *prevalence* are important in identification programs. A brief explanation of each term is included here, but for an excellent in-depth discussion of the concepts, the reader is referred to Marge (1991). According to Marge, *incidence* refers to the number of new occurrences of a disorder or disease in a population within a designated time period. Once the number of new cases of the disorder or disease is known, the number of individuals exposed to the risk for development of the disorder or disease during the same limited time period needs to be determined. To calculate the incidence of the disorder or disease, the number of new cases is divided by the number of individuals in the population exposed to the risk for development of the disease or disorder, and the result is multiplied by 1000. The answer provides the estimated number of cases per 1000 people. In the determination of incidence, individuals found to have the disease at the beginning of the designated time period are excluded. Only people in whom the disease develops during the test period are included in the incidence.

Prevalence, on the other hand (Marge, 1991), provides an estimate of the number of individuals within a population who have a disorder or disease during a specified time. The number of cases of a disorder or disease determined to be present in a specified population at a defined time is divided by the number of people in the population at the same time. The result is multiplied by 1000 to determine the prevalence. According to Marge (1991) prevalence is affected by two factors; the duration of the disease under study and the number of individuals in the population who have had the disease in the past.

Hearing Disorders in the School-Aged Population

In a target population of school-aged children, the question to be answered before a screening program is initiated is whether sufficient numbers of school-aged children have an educationally handicapping hearing impairment or suffer from middle ear disease. In other words, are there ample numbers of cases of middle ear disease present in this population (prevalence) or adequate numbers of new cases of middle ear disease (incidence) occurring on a regular basis in the school-aged population to justify mass screening? Furthermore, it should be determined if there are adverse consequences associated with the hearing problem that, when identified and treated, would show clear and measurable benefits to early intervention. Benefits of screening, such as a reduction of the physical and psychological effects of a hearing loss, may be difficult to calculate. These benefits, however, must be balanced against the cost of not screening and leaving the middle ear disease untreated or the hearing impairment undetected along with the potential medical and educational consequences.

Middle Ear Disease and Conductive Hearing Loss

The most common cause of conductive hearing loss in children is otitis media with effusion (OME) (Brooks, 1981). The National Center for Health Statistics (1978) indicated that middle ear effusion is the most common diagnosis among young children who visit pediatricians. The prevalence of OME among children varies widely and is influenced by a variety of factors, including age, race, heredity, sex, climate, and socioeconomic status. A Boston study indicated that 71 percent of the 2565 children in the study had experienced at least one episode of OME by the age of 3 years, and 33 percent had experienced three or more episodes (Bluestone et al, 1986). These statistics suggest that OME is a common problem among children (see Chapter 2) that should be addressed in any comprehensive screening program (Jerger, 1986). However, not all professionals involved in screening for OME believe that early screening is beneficial or that it has any preventive effect on hearing loss or ear disease (Augustsson et al, 1990).

Brooks (1981), on the other hand, argued that early identification of conductive hearing losses associated with OME is necessary because some cases of OME do not resolve spontaneously, and the possible complications of OME, although rare, can become serious. Another reason for identifying OME is its potential impact on educational and communication skills. Unfortunately, no definitive statements on middle ear disease and language learning can be made, but Hall and Hill (1986) speculated on the basis of several case studies that otitis media can have deleterious educational effects on children. They suggested that at least five variables (age of onset, severity of hearing loss, child's intelligence, child's personality, and child's environment) contribute to the seriousness of the effect.

Sensorineural Hearing Loss

Although less common, sensorineural hearing losses are also important to identify in screenings. Several investigators (Frasier, 1971; Punch, 1983; Roeser & Northern, 1981; Schein & Delk, 1974; Shea, 1981; Simmons, 1978; Stewart & Bergstrom, 1974) indicated that 1 in 1000 newborns have a congenital profound hearing loss and about 1 in 380 have a clinically significant hearing impairment. Children born with sensorineural losses, especially the subtle types such as unilateral sensorineural hearing impairment, may not be identified by the age of 3 years (Simmons, 1978). Bess (1985) reported that children and adults with mild hearing losses (less than 25 decibels hearing level [dB HL]) experience greater difficulty with educational progress and with communication than was previously believed. When identified, children with minimal hearing impairment, whether unilateral or bilateral, should receive assistance to aid communication and learning (Bess, 1985). From these few reports, it is apparent that hearing impairment and middle ear disease occur frequently in the school-aged population and that the benefit of identification for treatment is substantial enough to justify hearing screening.

Screening Tests

It is not an easy task to efficiently screen large numbers of children and to ensure that a high number of positive identifications are made without increasing the number of false identifications. Choosing a test that is rapid, efficient, and appropriate for the target population is important. If the primary goal of the hearing identification program is to identify school-aged children who have a hearing impairment that might interfere with communication and education, the most efficient and effective test would be manual pure-tone audiometry. Manual pure-tone audiometry is a valid and reliable tool for finding hearing impairment, but it is not an efficient screening tool for identifying middle ear disease (Eagles et al, 1967; Melnick et al, 1964). Pure-tone audiometry may miss ears with middle ear disease, and a noisy test environment may make pure-tone audiometry less than effective for identifying middle ear disease.

If school-aged children are the target population and middle ear disease is to be screened, an appropriate screening protocol includes immittance testing. Acoustic immittance is an excellent screening tool for identifying middle ear disease (Stach & Jerger, 1987), but it may produce a high overreferral rate by identifying children whose middle ear condition would resolve naturally. Moreover, it is not an adequate screening tool for identifying sensorineural hearing impairment.

Although each of these two screening instruments has certain limitations, they are still the instruments of choice for screening. Under ideal circumstances, a comprehensive hearing screening program incorporates both pure-tone audiometry and acoustic immittance measurements to identify children in need of services. Unfortunately, few hearing identification programs use both pure-tone testing and acoustic immittance measurements.

Pass–Fail Criteria

Good screening tests must have well-defined pass–fail criteria. Appropriately defined pass–fail criteria help ensure that the test is sensitive enough to identify a child with a hearing problem but does not fail a child without a hearing problem. To pass a screening test implies that the person screened does not have the disorder or is free of the disease. In reality, however, passing a pure-tone screening test does not mean a child is free of middle ear disease nor does it mean the child does not have a mild hearing impairment. Rather, passing simply means that the middle ear disease or hearing impairment for which the child was screened was not severe enough to be picked up by the pass–fail criteria decided on for the screening test. For example, if the pass–fail criteria defined a response of 30 dB HL or better at 8000 Hz as passing, a child with a mild hearing loss of 25 dB HL at 8000 Hz would pass the test in spite of the hearing loss. When defining the criteria for the test, it may have been decided that a threshold of 25 dB HL at 8000 Hz would not require further medical evaluation and treatment and would not require any special educational provision for daily activities. Therefore, it would not be efficient to fail a child with this amount of hearing loss. Conversely, a child who is free of ear disease and hearing impairment may instead fail a hearing screening because of factors unrelated to hearing sensitivity. For example, a child may not understand the instructions or may be distracted and fearful, or environmental noise may exceed permissible levels and render the tones inaudible.

Reliability and Validity

A screening test must be reliable so that repeat screenings produce the same results. For example, a test is considered reliable if it can be given to one child by the same screener at different times and yield the same information each time. A test is also considered reliable if it can be given to one child by more than one screener and continue to yield the same information.

Validity is an equally important consideration for a screening test. A valid screening test should measure the quality it was intended to measure and should be used for the purpose for which it was designed. For example, if a screening test is designed to measure middle ear disorders (tympanogram) and it is used for the purpose of detecting inner ear disorders (sensorineural hearing loss), the test is not measuring what it was intended to measure and the results would not be considered valid. Tympanograms, however, when administered appropriately and for the intended purpose of identifying middle ear dysfunction, are valid.

Sensitivity and Specificity

Under ideal circumstances, a screening test is sensitive to a designated disorder all of the time and only infrequently falsely identifies the disorder when it is not present. Sensitivity of a screening test can be increased to identify all individuals within a population who have the disorder; at the same time, however, care must be taken not to increase test sensitivity at the expense of incorrectly identifying individuals who do not have the disorder. Increasing the sensitivity (positive identification of the hearing problem) of a test increases not only the number of identified individuals but also the number of incorrectly identified individuals (false–positive finding) because these two measurements are interrelated. Changes in one measurement alter the outcome of the other. *Sensitivity* then is defined as the ability of a test to find the disease in a person who in fact has the

Table 5.1 Sensitivity and Specificity of Hearing Screening Results and the Medical Diagnosis of Ear Disease

Hearing Screening	Diseased Ears	Nondiseased Ears
Pass (negative)	11	65
Fail (positive)	36	8

disease (Thorner & Remein, 1982). A screening test that is extremely sensitive to middle ear disorders should identify a person as having a middle ear disorder (a positive result). *Specificity is* defined as the ability of a test to correctly identify a person who is free of middle ear disease (a negative result). If the person has the disease but is identified as disease free, then the test result is false–negative. The results of any screening test should be subjected to a sensitivity and specificity evaluation. The simplified example (Table 5.1) illustrates the complementary relationship between sensitivity and specificity and false–positive and false–negative rates.

To calculate the sensitivity of screening procedures, the number of diseased ears that failed the hearing screening (36) is added to the number of diseased ears that passed the hearing screening (11). This total (47) is divided into the number of diseased ears that failed the screening (36) and the result is multiplied by 100. The sensitivity for this example, then, is 77 percent. To determine the specificity of the screening, the number of nondiseased ears that passed the screening (65) is added to the number of nondiseased ears that failed the screening (8). This total (73) is divided into the number of nondiseased ears that passed the screening (65) and the result is multiplied by 100. The specificity is 89 percent for this example. Two excellent detailed reviews of the relationship between sensitivity and specificity can be found in Jacobson and Jacobson (1987) and Thorner and Remein (1982).

Program Evaluation

Screening programs need to be reviewed periodically to ascertain the effectiveness of the program and to determine if the efficiency can be improved. It is possible that the number of new patients identified, referred, and treated is so small that preventive screening costs cannot be justified and the available resources must be used to benefit greater numbers. Costs of screening programs include tangible expenses such as those associated with administering the screening and referring for follow-up treatment or therapy, but these costs must be weighed with other intangible costs, such as anxiety caused by a falsely identified child. Both children and parents experience anxiety and frustration when faced with a falsely identified hearing loss. However, the cost of the program must be evaluated in terms of the potential consequences of an untreated medical or educational problem.

SCREENING PROCEDURES

The ASHA Committee on Audiometric Evaluation (1985) has published guidelines for rapid and efficient identification of hearing impairment by means of pure tones and, in conjunction with a Working Group on Acoustic Immittance Measurements, published Guidelines for Screening for Hearing Impairment and Middle Ear Disorders (ASHA, 1990). These guidelines can be obtained from ASHA and can provide an information base for screening strategies. Unfortunately, the recommended hearing screening guidelines and components of an identification program do not always reach screeners such as speech-language pathologists and school or public health nurses. A national survey (Wall et al, 1985) of practices and procedures in the school systems indicated that guidelines for comprehensive screening programs were needed. These guidelines are now available but must be made accessible to the proper personnel.

Personnel and Training

As indicated in the Guidelines for Identification Audiometry (ASHA, 1985), a screening program for the identification of hearing loss or middle ear disease is the responsibility of an audiologist. However, even though the mandatory responsibility and supervision of an identification program remains with an audiologist, it does not always mean that the audiologist performs the actual screening test. It is more likely that the audiologist is responsible for (1) training other personnel to administer the screenings and rescreenings, (2) ensuring the proper equipment is used and calibrated, (3) monitoring the screening procedures, (4) interpreting the results, and (5) making the proper referrals to professionals. The speech-language pathologist and health nurse most frequently are identified as the practitioners responsible for completing the actual screening in the school system and may also be responsible for assuring recommendations are followed and treatment received.

Training of the Screener

Two different surveys (Garstecki, 1978; Wall et al, 1985) of audiometric practices and procedures in schools have indicated that the personnel most frequently responsible for hearing screenings in the schools are nurses (65 percent) and speech-language pathologists (34 percent) and only a few other people such as technicians, parents, and volunteers participate in actual screenings. Unfortunately some (23 percent) of the respondents indicated no training was provided for the screeners, but of those who did receive the training, nearly half (47 percent) reported the training was voluntary. The speech-language pathologist, as a primary hearing screener in the schools, is one of the few professionals with ready access to the ASHA Guidelines for Identification Audiometry and the Guidelines for Screening for Hearing Impairment and Middle Ear Disorders; the public health or school nurse or paraprofessional may not have access to the guidelines. Furthermore, because guidelines and procedures, as well as test equipment, are modified periodically, ongoing education for hearing screening should be available for personnel involved in the screenings.

The training program should cover a number of topics ranging from anatomy and physiology of the hearing mechanism, hearing disorders and hearing loss, equipment and calibration requirements, practicum in otoscopy, pure-tone and acoustic immittance screening techniques, referral sources, and follow-up for screenings to forms, record keeping, and counseling. The training sessions, under the direction of an audiologist, should include an opportunity for screeners to perform the procedures. For practical and effective programs, training should include both lecture information and a practicum on a wide variety of topics to ensure that screeners receive needed information and develop appropriate skills. The information could be presented by an audiologist in a two-day training session. The first day would include lectures and videotapes on various topics, and the second day would be devoted to actual screening procedures, equipment, and practicum experiences. Specifics of a sample identification and training program (Wall & Bührer, 1987) are presented in Appendix 5.1.

Equipment

Most identification programs (98 percent) use pure-tone audiometry for screening hearing, but many (30 percent) use acoustic immittance or other screening instruments (5 percent) in combination with the pure-tone testing (Wall et al, 1985). However, new screening instruments continually become available and need to be evaluated. Although these new instruments may prove to be beneficial, problems arise for newly developed screening instruments when manufacturing standards are not available. Therefore, if new screening instruments are to be used, the operating characteristics of the instrument must be established. The supervising audiologist who is aware of instrument differences and has calculated the operating characteristics of each instrument may need to be consulted regarding instrument performance before the actual screenings are conducted.

Programs that use pure-tone audiometry in combination with immittance are the most effective for screening for hearing loss and middle ear disease, but supplementing pure-tone audiometry with other instrumentation may have some value. A screening instrument called an acoustic reflectometer (Teele & Teele, 1984), which was designed to evaluate the presence of middle ear fluid, does not require a hermetic seal in the ear canal and can be used when a child is crying. The acoustic reflectometer is shaped like an otoscope and is handheld. The examiner simply reads numbers on a vertical display. The larger the number, the greater the possibility that middle ear effusion is present. Teele and Teele (1984) reported the

Table 5.2 ASHA 1985 Guidelines for Pure-Tone Hearing Screening

Test Frequency	Intensity Level	Pass–Fail Criteria
1000, 2000, 4000 Hz (with acoustic immittance)	20 db HL	Failure to respond to any test presentation in either ear
500, 1000, 2000, 4000 Hz (without acoustic immittance)		

(Reprinted from ASHA (1990) Guidelines for Hearing Impairment and Middle Ear Disorders, as modified, with permission from Northern and Downs, Williams & Wilkins, 1991.)

reflectometer to be a valuable tool for finding middle ear effusion and to complement traditional methods for identifying middle ear effusion (Bührer et al, 1985; Schwartz & Schwartz, 1987). However, the reflectometer has been found to be a less effective screening tool than immittance audiometry (Bührer et al, 1985; Holmes et al, 1989; Wall et al, 1986). It has been suggested that the instrument should not be used to diagnose other pathologic conditions of the ear (Schwartz & Schwartz, 1987).

Many other devices are available for screening hearing sensitivity and middle ear function; all devices, however, should be evaluated carefully before purchase or use. Research has not been conducted on many of these new instruments; therefore, screeners are responsible for keeping themselves updated regarding the technologic developments and performance of screening instruments.

Pure-Tone Audiometry

Frequency

The ASHA guidelines (1985) suggest the frequencies of 500 Hz (if ambient noise allows), 1000 Hz, 2000 Hz, and 4000 Hz for screening hearing at an intensity level of 20 dB HL (Table 5.2). However, these guidelines are not used consistently by many programs. According to respondents in a survey (Wall et al, 1985), the frequencies used for screening were 250 Hz (24 percent), 500 Hz (80 percent), 1000 Hz (95 percent), 2000 Hz (95 percent), 4000 Hz (95 percent), 6000 Hz (32 percent), and 8000 Hz (31 percent). The inclusion of 250 Hz and 500 Hz as test frequencies for an identification program conducted in high ambient noise environments is inappropriate because of masking effects on the stimulus frequency. The inclusion of 6000 Hz is inappropriate because of interactions between the earphone and ear canal (Villchur, 1970).

Intensity

Signal levels for screening also vary according to respondents. Even though better agreement with the ASHA guidelines was found, no uniform signal level was reported. The survey respondents (85 percent) indicated that the most frequently used screening level was 20 or 25 dB HL, but the level of choice ranged from 15 to 30 dB HL and varied with frequency (Wall et al, 1985).

Fail–Rescreen

Lack of response to any frequency at the screening level in either ear is considered failure according to the current guidelines (ASHA, 1985). However, the screener should be aware that it is not uncommon to have a high fail rate after only one screening. A second screening is thus extremely important and can reduce the over-referral rate by 30 to 50 percent (Melnick et al, 1964; Wilson & Walton, 1974). A rescreening should be performed no longer than 2 weeks after the first screening (ASHA, 1985).

Acoustic Immittance

Standards (American National Standards Institute [ANSI], 1987) have been written for aural acoustic immittance instruments that assist in standardizing the instruments and the measurement units. Screening guidelines (ASHA, 1990) help standardize terminology and are modified to respond to changes in technology. The Guidelines for Screening for Hearing Impairment and Middle Ear Disorders (ASHA, 1990) incorporate suggestions from the Guidelines for Identification Audiometry (ASHA, 1985) with previous Guidelines for Acoustic Immittance Screening of Middle Ear Function (ASHA, 1979) in an attempt to reduce overreferral problems associated with acoustic immittance measurement, particularly the acoustic reflex measurement. The 1990 guidelines recommend that information regarding hearing status and middle ear function be obtained from four major sources—hearing history (ear pain or infection), visual inspection of the ear, identification audiometry (screen at 1000, 2000, 4000 Hz at 20 dB HL) and tympanometry. Referral criteria (Table 5.3) and a referral flow chart (Figure 5.1) are contained in the 1990 ASHA guidelines. They are particularly helpful for screening with pure-tone audiometry and acoustic immittance. These referral criteria suggest that if ear pain or discharge is present or if visual inspection suggests abnormalities, an immediate referral should be made for medical or audiologic attention. If the person being tested does not pass the audiometric screening, a repeat screening is scheduled. If the person does not pass the second screening, a referral is made. If the person passes the second screening, the tympanometric results are evaluated for peak and gradient. If the tympanometric peak and gradient measurements are abnormal, then a referral is made or tympanometric measures are repeated within 4 to 6 weeks. The interested reader can find a discussion of the advantages and disadvantages of these guidelines in Roush et al (1992).

Table 5.3 ASHA Referral Criteria

History
• Otalgia
• Otorrhea

Visual Inspection of the Ear
• Structural defect of the ear, head, or neck
• Ear canal abnormalities
  – Blood or effusion
  – Occlusion
  – Inflammation
  – Excessive cerumen, tumor, foreign material
• Eardrum abnormalities
  – Abnormal color
  – Bulging eardrum
  – Fluid line or bubbles
  – Perforation
  – Retraction

Identification Audiometry
• Failure of air-conduction screening at 20 dB HL at 1, 2, or 4 kHz in either ear
  (ASHA, 1985; these criteria may require alteration for various clinical settings and
  populations).

Tympanometry
• Flat tympanogram and equivalent ear canal volume (VEC) outside normal range
• Low static admittance (Peak Y) on two successive occurrences in a 4- to 6-week
  interval
• Abnormally wide tympanometric width (TW) on two successive occurrences in a
  4- to 6-week interval.

(Reprinted from ASHA Referral Criteria, 1990, with permission of the American Speech-Language-
Hearing Association.)

Problems Encountered with Pure-Tone and Acoustic Immittance Screening

Problems that screeners encounter routinely (Roeser & Northern, 1988) whether screening with pure-tone audiometry or acoustic immittance are found in Table 5.4. First-time screeners would do well to become familiar with these potential problems.

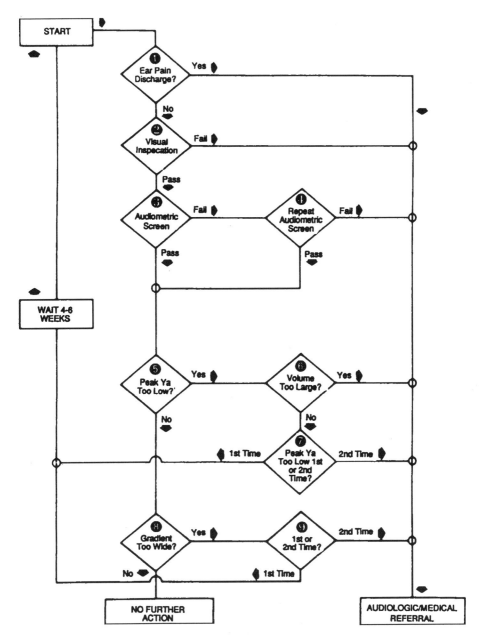

FIGURE 5.1 Flow-chart for steps to follow when screening with pure-tone audiometry and immittance measures. The time frame for referral and suggestions for rescreening are included.

Table 5.4 Pitfalls to Avoid in Hearing and Immittance Screening

Hearing Screening Pitfalls

- Child observing dials. This should be avoided at all times because children respond to the visual cues. The most appropriate position to seat the child is at an oblique angle, so the tester and audiometer are out of the child's peripheral vision.
- Examiner giving visual cues (facial expression, eye or head movements).
- Incorrect adjustment of the headband and incorrect earphone placement. Care must be taken to place the earphones carefully over the ears so that the protective screen mesh of the earphone is directly over the entrance of the external auditory canal. Misplacement of the earphone by only 1 inch can cause a threshold shift as great as 30 to 35 dB.
- Vague instructions
- Noise in the test area
- Overlong test sessions. The screening should require only 3 to 5 minutes. If a child requires more time than this, the routine screening should be discontinued, and a short rest taken. If the child continues to be difficult to test, play conditioning should be used.
- Too long or too short a presentation of the test tone. The test stimulus should be presented for 1 to 2 seconds. If the stimulus is for a shorter or longer time than this, inaccurate responses may be obtained.

Immittance Screening Pitfalls

- Clogged probe and probe tip. The probe and probe tips must be kept free of cerumen.
- Probe tip too large or too small. Each ear canal is different and may require a different-sized probe tip. Use of the correct size for each child avoids possible errors.
- Head movement, swallowing, or eye blinks. The child should be kept still during testing; sudden abnormal movement during testing may be interpreted as a reflex.
- Probe tip against ear canal wall. The probe tip must be inserted directly into the ear canal, and when the canal is not straight, the tip must be kept away from the canal wall.
- Debris in ear canal. The ear canal should be inspected before testing to ensure that it is clear.

(Reprinted from Roeser & Northern, 1988, with permission of Thieme Medical Publishers, Inc.)

Otoscopic Inspection

If the speech-language pathologist or school nurse is involved in a screening program for hearing loss and middle ear disorders, and if acoustic immittance screening is included, otoscopic inspection should be included as part of the training. The otoscopic inspection is not intended to provide diagnostic clues, but is intended to assist the individual in landmark recognition of the canal and tympanic membrane to inspect for structural anomalies, to determine if foreign bodies, tumors, or excessive cerumen are present, and to visually ascertain if there are indications of middle ear disease that need immediate medical attention. Otoscopic inspection requires experience and training to avoid overlooking many conditions of the external and middle ear. Visual inspection is required for immittance screening and it should be performed before the probe tip is inserted.

Audiologic and Otologic Referral

If a child fails two pure-tone screenings, a referral should be made. Of course, depending on whether acoustic immittance measurements are used, other referral criteria should be considered (see Table 5.3). The referral process may vary according to the procedures of the school districts or health departments involved. However, general referral procedures may include distribution of information to an audiologist, an otologist, an educator, and a parent. Referrals to an otologist mean that the child receives a complete otologic examination and possibly additional hearing testing. If surgical or medical treatment is needed to manage the hearing problem, remedial steps are taken. Referrals to an audiologist means the child receives a complete hearing evaluation to determine the type and degree of hearing impairment as well as the recommended remedial steps required.

Several outcomes of the audiologic evaluation are possible. First, it is possible that the hearing results indicate normal hearing in spite of failure of two hearing screenings. Second, the results could indicate the need for a medical referral that was not apparent during the screening. Third, the results could indicate the need for amplification or special classroom provisions.

Under ideal circumstances, referral after the screening would be made to a facility where both audiologic and otologic services are available. Frequently, however, this is not the case. If the administrator of the screening program is able to determine that an immediate medical referral is needed, the choice regarding the appropriate physician must be made. In many programs, the traditional referral is to the family physician or pediatrician. This referral may not be the most appropriate when otologic services are needed. An alternative could be to refer the patient to an otolaryngologist with appropriate notification to the family physician or pediatrician. In most cases, however, the medical referral may not be appropriate as the initial referral (Roeser & Northern, 1988). If the audiologist responsible for the screening program determines that an immediate medical referral is not needed, a complete audiologic evaluation is the appropriate referral. In larger school systems or programs administered by health departments, audiologic services may be available within the system. Regardless of the type of services available, identified children should have a complete evaluation and receive treatment. If complete evaluations and diagnoses are not available and medical treatment or amplification cannot be provided, conducting a screening program may not be an appropriate endeavor.

Parental and Educational Follow-up

Parents and educators should be made aware of the process of referral and of the potential outcomes of the process. Informed parents are more likely than uninformed parents to follow referral recommendations and are less likely to be anxious regarding their child's welfare. Informing parents can be accomplished by written reports of the results or by phone calls. Feedback from the involved professionals and the parents should be requested. This type of information would help determine whether the recommendations are followed and whether the screening program is effective in identifying the hearing problem.

Educators should be informed of the hearing problem. If hearing impairment or middle ear disease is found, the educator should be informed regarding the appropriate classroom modifications. If the hearing impairment is determined to be fluctuating, seating in the classroom may be an appropriate environmental modification. If the hearing impairment is more severe, amplification, assistive listening devices, or room noise modification may be more appropriate than preferential seating alone (see Chapters 7 and 8).

IDENTIFICATION PROGRAMS FOR OLDER ADULTS

One of the prerequisites for justifying the establishment of a screening program is to determine if a large population exists with a sufficient number of individuals potentially affected by the disorder. The elderly population, 65 years and older, has a sufficient proportion of individuals with potential hearing losses—certainly enough to justify a screening program. According to Cox (1988), the U.S. Bureau of the Census reports the elderly population has been growing fairly rapidly over the past 90 years. It is projected that the elderly population will continue to grow and increase in proportion to the total population. Cox reported that in 1900, 3 million people were older than 65 years and comprised approximately 4 percent of the total population. In 1980, 20 million people were older than 65 years and comprised 10 percent of the total population. It is projected that by the year 2000 there will be 36 million people 65 years of age and older, who may comprised as much as 13 percent of the total population. These figures suggest that the first prerequisite of a screening program—a large population—is met.

The next question to consider is whether a sufficient proportion of people in the elderly population have a hearing loss. Fein (1983) estimates that the elderly population constitutes 43 percent (8 million Americans) of the present hearing-impaired population with the expectation that this proportion will increase to 59 percent by the year 2050. Estimates of the prevalence of hearing impairment vary considerably depending on the criteria used to determine the presence of a hearing loss. For example, if the "low fence" (minimum intensity level) for determining a hearing impairment is greater than 26 dB HL for the average of the thresholds at 500 Hz, 1000 Hz, and 2000 Hz, according to Nerbonne (1988) the prevalence of hearing impairment would range from 30 to 48 percent in the population 65 to 74 years of age. As this low fence of 26 dB HL is raised (to 40 dB HL, for example) or lowered (to 20 dB HL, for example), the proportion of older people defined as having a hearing impairment increases or decreases accordingly. Regardless of whether the low or high end of the estimate is assumed, it is apparent that one of the most common health problems among older adults is hearing impairment (Nerbonne, 1988). Therefore, with a large and increasing number of older adults affected by a hearing loss, two prerequisites of a screening program have been met. The remaining concerns involve finding a good screening test and qualified people to administer the test and make recommendations for follow-up.

As of 1993, agreement had not been reached regarding hearing screening guidelines or protocol to be used for older adults. This controversy exists even though hearing impairment is known to have a high prevalence among older adults and even though hearing loss is known to be closely associated with increased isolation, confusion, and depression (Shadden, 1988). An attempt to develop guidelines (ASHA, 1985) for screening for hearing impairments in older adults was not successful. Agreement could not be reached regarding the signal level to be used, the signal frequencies to be screened, and the pass–fail criteria to be used. Until the results of data-based research are available regarding signal level and pass–fail criteria, speech-language pathologists and health care professionals involved in screening activities with this older population may need to consult with an audiologist to determine the appropriate signal frequency and level to be used. Issues surrounding the screening of adults and older persons is discussed in a report by an Ad Hoc Committee on Hearing Screening in Adults (ASHA, 1992).

Objectives of a Hearing Screening Program for Adults

Objectives of a screening program designed for adults older than 65 years are different from objectives selected for screening a school-aged population or an adult population younger than 65 years (Marge, 1991). For adults who are not retired and who are between 18 and 65 years of age, hearing status should be assessed if a hearing problem is suspected or on entry into the workforce and thereafter during employment. Moreover, information regarding the hazards of noise exposure should be provided as part of the identification program. For adults older than 65 years, information should be provided about the auditory system and how to recognize the symptoms associated with a hearing loss that is either already present or is gradually developing. Furthermore, hearing screenings should be conducted and information made available to retirement communities and centers regarding services and treatments which are available and accessible (Marge, 1991). However, for all adults aged 18 and older, the hearing screening protocol has two major objectives: identification of hearing problems that need medical attention, and identification of hearing problems that are handicapping (Schow, 1991).

Hearing Screening Instruments

Alternatives to pure-tone audiometry screening include two types of self-report questionnaires. One type of self-report instrument attempts to predict hearing loss and the other type attempts to predict the degree of handicap associated with the hearing loss. Before 1970, attempts to screen hearing with self-report instruments centered on predicting hearing loss, but they later shifted to predicting handicap.

Hearing Screening Inventory

A self-report screening instrument, the Hearing Screening Inventory (HSI), was developed by Coren and Hakstian in 1992. The instrument was designed to be used for group testing and to predict hearing loss. The authors reported that the results of the test correlate quite highly with pure-tone thresholds of the better ear and indicate good test–retest stability. The advantages of this instrument are many. It is brief; it is reliable; the results correlate with pure-tone sensitivity; test administration is easy; scoring is straightforward; and the test can be administered to large groups. The test (Appendix 5.2) provides an excellent alternative for speech-language pathologists and health care professionals to use to in lieu of pure-tone audiometry to screen the hearing of older people.

Hearing Handicap Inventories

After the 1970s and until the recent HSI screening instrument was developed, self-report instruments focused on self-reported hearing handicaps (Ventry & Weinstein, 1982). In other words, people reported how handicapping the hearing loss was relative to their everyday activities. These self-report instruments can be used alone or in conjunction with pure-tone audiometry and tympanometry. The first of these questionnaires (Appendix 5.3) is the Self-Assessment for Communication (SAC) (Schow & Nerbonne, 1982), and the second is the Hearing Handicap Inventory for the Elderly—Screening Version (HHIE-S) (Ventry & Weinstein, 1983; Weinstein, 1986). The HHIE-S included in this chapter (Appendix 5.4) is a screening instrument, but a more complete inventory form is available (Ventry & Weinstein, 1982). For those who desire a short screening instrument to measure self-perceived handicap, however, the HHIE-S is a good choice and has been shown to have good test–retest reliability (Newman et al, 1991).

Combinations of Screening Instruments for Older Adults

Older adults may benefit from a combination of screening instruments (pure-tone audiometry, acoustic immittance, self-report questionnaires for sensitivity or handicap), even though many of the instruments are designed to be used alone. Because a healthy older adult does not have a high incidence of middle ear disease and is generally regarded as at low risk for middle ear disease, a self-report handicap–disability index coupled with pure-tone audiometry or the HSI screening instrument may be appropriate choices. For this combination of instruments a self-perceived assessment and a threshold estimate are obtained. Schow (1991) suggested that when pure-tone audiometry is used, the frequencies of 1000 Hz, 2000 Hz, and 4000 Hz should be screened at 25 dB HL. Thus, even though the pure-tone thresholds may suggest a hearing loss, if the self-perceived handicap is minimal, no further action may be necessary. Knowing the person's perception of the problem helps in the recommendation of successful rehabilitation strategies. If the person perceives the hearing loss to have a considerable impact on daily activities, recommendations for rehabilitation are more likely to be followed. If, on the other hand, no disability is perceived even in the presence of a hearing loss, it is highly unlikely the client would follow the rehabilitation recommendations.

Although acoustic immittance measures such as tympanometry may not be routinely used with a group of healthy older adults, selective older-adult populations should be screened with immittance measurements according to the Guidelines for Screening for Hearing Impairment and Middle Ear Disorders (ASHA, 1990). Schow (1991) recommended that immittance measures be added to the screening protocol if the elderly population to be screened resides in a nursing home. He also suggested using the frequencies described earlier but increasing the screening level for pure-tone audiometry to 40 dB HL. He also recommended administration of the SAC for anyone older than 18 years and the HHIE-S for all people older than 65 years. Thus, for selected adult populations, three instruments in addition to the case history may be needed to screen for hearing sensitivity, hearing handicap, and middle ear function.

Recommendations and Referrals

If a person passes the screening tests discussed previously, no further action is necessary, according to Schow (1991), because the probability of a hearing impairment and associated medical problem is low. If, however, one portion of the screening battery is failed, at least three alternatives are possible. One alternative is to retest the person in one year because this person is considered to be at risk for a hearing problem. A second alternative is to make a referral to an audiologist or medical practitioner (Schow, 1991). If, however, the speech-language pathologist or health care professional is using the HSI for screening, the appropriate referral is to an audiologist, who can obtain a complete hearing evaluation.

Until such time as guidelines for hearing screening for adults and elderly are available, the speech-language pathologist or health care professional, in consultation with the supervising audiologist, needs to make decisions on the basis of the disorder to be screened, the screening instrument available, the intent of the screening, and the availability of follow-up resources to assess the effectiveness of a screening protocol (Cadman et al, 1984).

Screening Program Evaluation

An Ad Hoc Committee on Hearing Screening in Adults (ASHA, 1992) summarized hearing screening considerations for older adults in a recent report. Within the report, the committee summarized seven major points advocated by Cadman et al (1984), which can be used for evaluating a hearing screening program. The points rephrased into questions can be used effectively for most screening programs. The questions are as follows: (1) Has it been demonstrated that the program is effective? (2) Are services for treatment available and affordable? (3) Is the impact of the hearing loss sufficient to warrant screening? (4) Is a good screening instrument available? (5) Will the program reach the population it is designed to benefit? (6) Is there an available health care system that can absorb the patients? (7) Is there reasonable expectation that the referral recommendations will be followed? The committee report provides an excellent review for speech-language pathologists and health care professionals involved in hearing screening programs for older adults.

Once the screening has been completed and a person is identified as having a hearing impairment, information regarding hearing aids and assistive listening devices should be explained (see Chapters 7 and 8). Of course, depending on the circumstances and the degree of the hearing loss, speechreading and other alternative modes of communication should be described (see Chapter 9). It is also possible that for some older people speech therapy may be appropriate.

In all remediation plans undertaken or explained, a significant other should be involved. The significant other, such as a spouse, can learn along with the person with the hearing impairment about the hearing aid or assistive listening device. Both people are thus provided with information about which environmental situations prove to be difficult for communication. The interested reader is referred to Schow (1991) and the ASHA (1992) report for greater detail regarding prevention guidelines for school-aged children, adults, and the elderly.

REFERENCES

American National Standards Institute (1987). Specifications for instruments to measure aural acoustic impedance and admittance (aural acoustic immittance). ANSI S3.39-1987. New York: American National Standards Institute.

American Speech-Language-Hearing Association (1979). Guidelines for Acoustic Immittance Screening of Middle-Ear Function. *Asha, 21,* 283-288.

American Speech-Language-Hearing Association (1985). Guidelines for Identification Audiometry. *Asha, 27,* 49-53.

American Speech-Language-Hearing Association (1990). Guidelines for Screening for Hearing Impairment and Middle Ear Disorders. *Asha, 32* (Suppl. 2), 17-24.

American Speech-Language-Hearing Association (1991). The prevention of communication disorders tutorial. *Asha, 33* (Suppl. 6), 15-41.

American Speech-Language-Hearing Association Ad Hoc Committee on Hearing Screening in Adults (1992). Considerations in screening adults/older persons for handicapping hearing impairments. *Asha 34,* 81-87.

Augustsson, I., Nilson C., & Engstrand, I. (1990). The preventive value of audiometric screening of preschool and young school children. *International Journal of Pediatric Otorhinolaryngology, 20,* 51-62.

Berg, F. S. (1986). Characteristics of the target population. In F. S. Berg, J. C. Blair, J. H. Vlehweg, & A. Wilson-Vlotman (Eds.), *Educational audiology for the hard of hearing child* (pp. 1-24). New York: Grune & Stratton.

Bess, F. H. (1985). The minimally hearing-impaired child. *Ear and Hearing, 6,* 43-47.

Bluestone, C. D., Fria, T., Arjona, S., et al. (1986). Controversies in screening for middle ear disease and hearing loss in children. *Pediatrics, 77,* 57-70.

Brooks, D. N. (1981). Otitis media in infancy. In G. T. Mencher & S. E. Gerber (Eds.). *Early management of hearing loss.* New York: Grune & Stratton.

Buhrer, K., Wall, L. G. & Shuster, L. (1985). The acoustic reflectometer as a screening device: A comparison. *Ear and Hearing, 6,* 307-314.

Cadman, D., Chambers, L., Feldman, W., & Sackett, D. (1984). Assessing the effectiveness of community screening programs. *Journal of the American Medical Association, 251,* 1580-1585.

Chaiklin, J. B., Ventry, I. M., & Dixon, R. F. (1982). *Hearing measurement.* Reading, MA: Addison-Wesley.

Coren, S., & Hakstian, A. R. (1992). The development and cross-validation of a self-report inventory to assess pure-tone threshold hearing sensitivity. *Journal of Speech and Hearing Research, 35,* 921-928.

Cox, H. (1988). Social realities of aging. In B. Shadden (Ed.), *Communication behavior and aging: A source book for clinicians* (pp. 43-57). Baltimore: Williams & Wilkins.

Cross, A. W. (1985). Health screening in schools. *Journal of Pediatrics, 107,* 487-493.

Darley, F. (1961). Identification audiometry. *Journal of Speech and Hearing Disorders,* (Suppl. 9).

Eagles, E., Wishik, S., & Doerfler, F. (1967). Hearing sensitivity and ear diseases in children: A prospective study. *Laryngoscope* (Monograph), 1-274.

Fein, D. (1983). Projections of speech and hearing impairments to 2050. *Asha, 11,* 31.

Frasier, G. R. (1971). The genetics of congenital deafness. *Otolaryngology Clinics of North America, 4,* 227-247.

Garstecki, D. (1978). A survey of school audiologists. *Asha, 20,* 291-296.

Hall, D. M. B., & Hill, P. (1986). When does secretory otitis media affect language development? *Archives of Disease in Childhood, 61,* 42-47.

Holmes, A., Muir, K., & Kemker, F. J. (1989). Acoustic reflectometry versus tympanometry in pediatric middle ear screenings. *Language-Speech-Hearing Services in Schools, 20,* 41-49.

Jacobson, J. T., & Jacobson, C. A. (1987). Application of test performance characteristics in newborn auditory screening. *Seminars in Hearing, 8,* 133-141.

Jerger, J. F. (1986). Controversies in screening for middle ear disease and hearing loss in children. *Pediatrics, 77,* 21-23.

Lichtenstein, M. J., Bess, F. H., & Logan S. A. (1988). Performance of the Hearing Handicap Inventory for the Elderly (Screening Version) against differing definitions of hearing impairment. *Ear and Hearing, 9,* 208-211.

Marge, M. (1991). Guidelines for the prevention of communication disorders: Concepts, principles and models. *Seminars in Hearing, 12,* 93-115.

Melnick, W., Eagles, E. L., & Levine, H. S. (1964). Evaluation of a recommended program of identification audiometry with school-age children. *Journal of Speech Hearing Disorders, 29,* 3-13.

National Center for Health Statistics (1978). *Office visits to pediatricians.* Hyattsville: National Ambulatory Care Services.

Nerbonne, M. (1988). The effects of aging on auditory structures and functions. In B. Shadden (Ed.), *Communication behavior and aging: A source book for clinicians* (pp. 137-161). Baltimore: Williams & Wilkins.

Newman, C., Weinstein, B., Jacobson, G. P., & Hug, F. A. (1991). Test-retest reliability of the hearing handicap inventory for adults. *Ear and Hearing, 12,* 355-357.

Northern, J. L., & Downs, M. P. (1991). Screening for hearing disorders. *Hearing in children* (pp. 231-283). Baltimore: Williams & Wilkins.

Ohio Department of Health (ODH) (1987). *Policies for hearing conservation programs for children: Requirements and recommendations.* Report No. 0269.13, 1-20.

Punch, J. (1983). The prevalence of hearing impairment. *Asha, 25,* 27.

Roeser, R. J., & Northern, J. L. (1988). Screening for hearing loss and middle ear disorders. In R. J. Roeser & J. Downs (Eds.), *Auditory disorders in school children: The law, identification, remediation* (pp. 120-150). New York: Thieme-Stratton.

Roush, J., Drake, A., & Sexton, J. E., (1992). Identification of middle ear dysfunction in young children: A comparison of tympanometry screening procedures. *Ear and Hearing, 13,* 63-69.

Schein, J. D., & Delk, M. L. (1974). *The deaf population of the United States.* Silver Spring: National Association of the Deaf.

Schow, R. (1991). Considerations in selecting and validating an adult/elderly hearing screening protocol. *Ear and Hearing, 12,* 337-348.

Schow, R. L., & Nerbonne, M. A. (1982). Communication screening profile: Use with elderly clients. *Ear and Hearing, 3,* 135-147.

Schwartz, D., & Schwartz, R. (1987). Validity of acoustic reflectometry in detecting middle ear effusion. *Pediatrics, 29,* 739-742.

Shadden, B. (1988). Perceptions of daily communicative interactions with older persons. In B. Shadden, (Ed.), *Communication behavior and aging: A sourcebook for clinicians* (pp. 12-38). Baltimore: Williams & Wilkins.

Shea, D. R. (1981). The hearing impaired infant: Primary care. In G. T. Mencher & S. E. Gerber (Eds.), *Early management of hearing loss.* New York: Grune & Stratton.

Simmons, F. B. (1978). Identification of hearing loss in infants and young children. *Otolaryngology Clinics of North America, 11,* 19-26.

Stach, B. A., & Jerger, J. F. (1987). Techniques for acoustic-reflex measurement and analysis. *Seminars in Hearing, 8,* 356-367.

Stewart, J. M., & Bergstrom, L. (1974). Familial hand abnormality and sensorineural deafness, a new syndrome. *Journal of Pediatrics, 78,* 102-110.

Teele, D. W., & Teele, J. (1984). Detection of middle ear effusion by acoustic reflectometry. In D. J. Lim, C. D. Bluestone, J. O. Klein, et al (Eds.), *Recent advances in otitis media with effusion (* pp. 237-238). Burlington: Decker.

Thorner, R. M., & Remein, Q. R. (1982). Principles and procedures in the evaluation of screening for disease. In J. B. Chaiklin, I. M. Ventry, & R. F. Dixon (Eds. *), Hearing measurement* (pp. 408-421). Reading:, MA: Addison-Wesley.

Ventry, I., & Weinstein, B. (1982). The Hearing Handicap Inventory for the Elderly: A new tool. *Ear and Hearing, 3,* 128-134.

Ventry, I., & Weinstein, B. (1983). Identification of elderly people with hearing problems. *Asha, 25,* 37-47.

Villchur, E. (1970). Audiometer-earphone mounting to improve inter-subject and cushion-fit reliability. *Journal of the Acoustical Society of America, 48,* 1387-1396.

Wall, L. G., & Bührer, K. (1987). Hearing identification of the preschool child: A proposed training program. *Folia Phoniatrica, 39,* 145-152.

Wall, L. G., Naples, G., Bührer, K., & Capodanno, C. (1985). A survey of audiological services with the school system. *Asha, 27,* 31-34.

Wall, L. G., Shuster, L. I., Bührer, K., & Lutes, R. A. (1986). Reliability and performance of the acoustic reflectometer. *Journal of Family Practice, 23,* 443-447.

Weinstein, B. (1986). Validity of a screening protocol for identifying elderly people with hearing problems. *Asha, 5,* 41-45.

Weinstein, B., & Ventry, I. (1983). Audiometric correlates of the Hearing Handicap Inventory for the Elderly. *Journal of Speech and Hearing Disorders, 48,* 379-384.

Wilson, W. R., & Walton, W. K. (1974). Identification audiometry accuracy: Evaluation of a recommended program for school-age children. *Language, Speech, and Hearing Services in the Schools, 5,* 132-142.

SUGGESTED READING

Allonen-Allie, N, & Florentine, M. (1990). Hearing Conservation Program in Massachusetts' vocational/technical schools. *Ear and Hearing, 11,* 237-40.

Lankford J. E., & West D. M. (1993). A study of noise exposure and hearing sensitivity in a high school woodworking class. *Language, Speech, and Hearing Services in the Schools, 24,* 167-173.

Mauk, G. W., & Behrens, T. (1993). Historical, political, and technological context associated with early identification of hearing loss. *Seminars in Hearing, 14,* 1-17.

Maurok, D. M., Mangold, L. S. (1990). Hearing conservation for upper primary grade school students. Presented at the NIH Consensus Development Conference on Noise and Hearing Loss.

APPENDIX 5.1

Sample Training Program

A. Introduction: Role of the speech-language pathologist in early identification and screening programs

1. To understand the unique position of speech-language pathologists in early identification of children at risk for communicative handicaps.

2. To understand the importance of early identification of communicative impairments and the potential effects on educational, social, and emotional development.

3. To understand the role of the speech-language pathologist and audiologist in providing services for children with communicative disorders.

4. To describe professional ethics and their application to the speech-language pathologists who provide hearing screenings.

B. Anatomy and physiology of the speech and hearing mechanisms

1. To review major anatomic divisions within the auditory system.

2. To understand how acoustic energy is transmitted and transformed into neural impulses through the mechanisms of the outer, middle, and inner ear.

C. Hearing disorders and associated hearing losses

1. To review the difference between conductive and sensorineural hearing losses.

2. To become familiar with disorders of the outer, middle, and inner ear and associated hearing impairments in preschool children.

3. To understand the role of the audiologist and otolaryngologist in the treatment of hearing disorders.

D. Hearing screening procedures and equipment

1. Otoscopy

a. To review the appropriate position for placement and viewing of the external auditory meatus and tympanic membrane.

b. To know special procedures for performing an otoscopic examination of 2- to 3-year-old children.

c. To know how to recognize obstructions, such as cerumen, before performing audiometric and immittance tests.

2. Pure-tone audiometry

a. To know the importance and be able to perform daily calibration checks to troubleshoot for equipment malfunction.

b. To understand the importance of a regular electroacoustic calibration.

c. To understand the problems associated with ambient noise levels and the effect on test results.

d. To understand the importance of earphone placement and how to gain a child's acceptance of the headset.

   e. To understand the importance of instructions and the level of language to be used with 2- to 3-year-old children.
   f. To learn effective behavioral response conditioning procedures.
   g. To understand the ASHA guidelines for hearing screening frequencies and intensities and recommended screening and rescreening procedures.
   h. To understand pass–fail criteria for screening and rescreening.
3. Acoustic immittance testing
   a. To be able to set up and calibrate the acoustic immittance bridge.
   b. To know how to obtain a tympanogram and acoustic reflex thresholds.
   c. To understand the importance of earphone and probe placement and how to gain a child's acceptance.
   d. To know the ASHA recommended guidelines for acoustic immittance test procedures.
   e. To understand pass–fail criteria and associate them with pure-tone results.

E. Practicum
   1. Otoscopy
      a. To demonstrate preparation of a child for an otoscopic screening.
      b. To demonstrate otoscopic screening procedures for young children.
   2. Pure-tone air-conduction audiometry
      a. To set up equipment and demonstrate how to prepare a child for a pure-tone screening test.
      b. To demonstrate performance of a pure-tone screening test with young children using appropriate conditioning and reinforcement procedures.
   3. Acoustic immittance screening
      a. To set up equipment for an acoustic immittance test and demonstrate preparation of a child for tympanometry testing.
      b. To demonstrate performance of an acoustic immittance test with young children.

F. Referral and follow-up for hearing screenings
   1. To know and be able to apply criteria for determining whether a child passes, does not pass, or should receive a rescreening.
   2. To understand the importance of audiologic and medical for children who do not pass hearing screenings.
   3. To identify local referral sources appropriate to the type of hearing disorder.
   4. To be able to explain the results of the screening and recommendations for referral and follow-up to the child's parents.
   5. To identify local referral sources appropriate for the age of the child.

(Reprinted and modified from Wall and Bührer, 1987, with permission of S. Karger AG, Basel.) The original training program was designed for skills to be developed by nurses.

APPENDIX 5.2

Hearing Screening Inventory

Instructions: This questionnaire deals with a number of common situations. For each question you should select the response that describes you and your behaviors best. You can select from among the following response alternatives: N = never (or almost never), S = seldom, O = occasionally, F = frequently, A = always (or almost always)

Simply circle the letter that corresponds to your choice. (If you normally use a hearing aid, answer as if you were not wearing it.)

1. Are you ever bothered by feelings that your hearing is poor?
   N S O F A
2. Is your reading or studying easily interrupted by noises in nearby rooms?
   N S O F A
3. Can you hear the telephone ring when you are in the same room in which it is located?
   N S O F A
4. Can you hear the telephone ring when you are in the next room?
   N S O F A
5. Do you find it difficult to make out the words in recordings of popular songs?
   N S O F A
6. When several people are talking in a room, do you have difficulty hearing an individual conversation?
   N S O F A
7. Can you hear the water boiling in a pot when you are in the kitchen?
   N S O F A
8. Can you follow the conversation when you are at a large dinner table?
   N S O F A

Please answer the following questions using G = good, A = average, S = slightly below average, P = poor, and V = very poor. Circle the letter that corresponds to your choice.

9. Overall I would judge the hearing in my RIGHT ear to be
   G A S P V
10. Overall I would judge the hearing in my LEFT ear to be
    G A S P V
11. Overall I would judge my ability to make out speech or conversation to be
    G A S P V
12. Overall I would judge my ability to judge the location of things only by the sound they are making to be
    G A S P V

Scoring Instructions: Responses are scored 1 = never, 2 = seldom, 3 = occasionally, 4 = frequently, and 5 = always (1 = good to 5 = very poor). The total score is simply the sum of the 12 responses (items 2, 3, 4, 7, and 8 are reverse-scored.)

(From Coren and Hakstian, 1992. Copyright SC Psychological Enterprises, Ltd, Vancouver, BC, Canada. Reprinted by permission of the American Speech-Language-Hearing Association.)

APPENDIX 5.3

Self-Assessment of Communication

Please select the appropriate number ranging from 1 to 5 for the following questions. Circle only one number for each question. If you have a hearing aid, please fill out the form according to how you communicate when the hearing aid is not in use.

Various Communication Situations

1. Do you experience communication difficulties in situations when speaking with one other person? (For example, at home, at work in a social situation, with a waitress, a store clerk, a spouse, a boss.)
   1) Almost never (or never)
   2) Occasionally (about one-fourth of the time)
   3) About half of the time
   4) Frequently (about three-fourths of the time)
   5) Practically always (or always)

2. Do you experience communication difficulties in situations when conversing with a small group of several people? (For example, with friends or family, co-workers, in meetings or casual conversations, over dinner or while playing cards)
   1) Almost never (or never)
   2) Occasionally (about one-fourth of the time)
   3) About half of the time
   4) Frequently (about three-fourths of the time)
   5) Practically always (or always)

3. Do you experience communication difficulties while listening to someone speak to a large group? (For example, at church or in a civic meeting, in a fraternal or women's club, at an educational lecture).
   1) Almost never (or never)
   2) Occasionally (about one-fourth of the time)
   3) About half of the time
   4) Frequently (about three-fourths of the time)
   5) Practically always (or always)

4. Do you experience communication difficulties while participating in various types of entertainment? (For example, television, radio, plays, night clubs, musical entertainment)
   1) Almost never (or never)
   2) Occasionally (about one-fourth of the time)
   3) About half of the time
   4) Frequently (about three-fourths of the time)
   5) Practically always (or always)

APPENDIX 5.3 *(continued)*

5. Do you experience communication difficulties when you are in an unfavorable listening environment? (For example, at a noisy party, where there is background music, when riding in an automobile or a bus, when someone whispers or talks from across the room)

    1) Almost never (or never)

    2) Occasionally (about one-fourth of the time)

    3) About half of the time

    4) Frequently (about three-fourths of the time)

    5) Practically always (or always)

6. Do you experience communication difficulties when using or listening to various communication devices? (For example, telephone, telephone ring, doorbell, public address system, warning signals, alarms)

    1) Almost never (or never)

    2) Occasionally (about one-fourth of the time)

    3) About half of the time

    4) Frequently (about three-fourths of the time)

    5) Practically always (or always)

Feelings about Communication

7. Do you feel that any difficulty with your hearing limits or hampers your personal or social life?

    1) Almost never (or never)

    2) Occasionally (about one-fourth of the time)

    3) About half of the time

    4) Frequently (about three-fourths of the time)

    5) Practically always (or always)

8. Does any problem or difficulty with your hearing upset you?

    1) Almost never (or never)

    2) Occasionally (about one-fourth of the time)

    3) About half of the time

    4) Frequently (about three-fourths of the time)

    5) Practically always (or always)

Other People

9. Do others suggest you have a hearing problem?

    1) Almost never (or never)

    2) Occasionally (about one-fourth of the time

    3) About half of the time

    4) Frequently (about three-fourths of the time)

    5) Practically always (or always)

10. Do others leave you out of conversations or become annoyed because of your hearing?

    1) Almost never (or never)
    2) Occasionally (about one-fourth of the time)
    3) About half of the time
    4) Frequently (about three-fourths of the time)
    5) Practically always (or always)

Raw Score _____ × 2 = _____ − 20 _____ × 1.25 = _____

(From Schow and Nerbonne, 1982. Reprinted with permission of the American Speech-Language-Hearing Association, 1992.)

Interpretation of Scores

SAC Raw Score Interpretation	Handicap Range	Referral
10-18	Normal (no handicap)	No referral
19-26	Slight handicap	Possible referral
27-38	Mild to moderate handicap	Referral, intervention
39-50	Severe handicap	Strong referral, intervention

(Reprinted from *Asha*, 34, 1992, with permission of the American Speech-Language-Hearing Association and Schow and Nerbonne, 1990.)

APPENDIX 5.4

Hearing Handicap Inventory for the Elderly Screening Version (HHIE-S)

Please answer *Yes, No,* or *Sometimes* to each of the following items. Do not skip a question if you avoid a situation because of a hearing problem. If you use a hearing aid, please answer the way you hear *without* the aid.

E- 1. Does a hearing problem cause you to feel embarrassed when meeting new people?

E- 2. Does a hearing problem cause you to feel frustrated when talking to members of your family?

S- 3. Do you have difficulty hearing when someone speaks in a whisper?

E- 4. Do you feel handicapped by a hearing problem?

S- 5. Does a hearing problem cause you difficulty when visiting friends, relatives, or neighbors?

S- 6. Does a hearing problem cause you to attend religious services less often than you would like?

E- 7. Does a hearing problem cause you to have arguments with family members?

S- 8. Does a hearing problem cause you difficulty when listening to television or radio?

E- 9. Do you feel that any difficulty with your hearing limits or hampers your personal or social life?

S- 10. Does a hearing problem cause you difficulty when in a restaurant with relatives or friends?

Interpretation of Scores

HHIE-S Raw Score Interpretation	Handicap Range	Post Hoc Probability of Hearing Impairment *
0-8	No handicap/no referral	13%
10-24	Mild to moderate	50%
26-40	Severe	84%

*Data from Lichtenstein et al, 1988, as reprinted in *Asha, 34,* 1992, with permission of the American Speech-Language-Hearing Association.

(Questionnaire from Ventry and Weinstein, 1983, with permission of the American Speech-Language-Hearing Association)

6

Interpretation of Clinical Test Results

Kevin M. Fire

Although detailed assessment of auditory function is not the responsibility of speech-language pathologists, health care professionals, and educators, it is important that they understand the results of an auditory evaluation to effectively plan patient care. This chapter describes the tests that compose a routine audiometric test battery, explains some of the tests that are used to establish the site of an auditory pathologic condition, and combines the results of the clinical tests into a clinical test battery that provides the typical findings associated with various auditory impairments.

ROUTINE CLINICAL TEST BATTERY

Pure-Tone Testing

Pure-tone audiometry is the basic evaluation used to establish auditory threshold sensitivity. For clinical purposes, auditory threshold can be described as the lowest intensity level at which a person can detect the presence of a stimulus a certain percentage of the time. This percentage is typically taken to be 50 percent (three of six correct detections of the stimulus) (ANSI, 1986). In pure-tone testing, thresholds are established by both air-conduction and bone-conduction testing. Air-conduction testing provides a measurement of the integrity of the entire auditory pathway (Yantis, 1985). Bone-conduction testing bypasses the outer and middle ear and indicates the status of the cochlea and the acoustic nerve (the sensorineural portion of the auditory system) with some influences by the middle ear (Tonndorf, 1972).

The air- and bone-conduction threshold responses are recorded on a chart called an audiogram (Figure 6.1), which is a graph of auditory threshold for each frequency tested (American Speech-Language-Hearing Association [ASHA], 1990a). The chart is in two dimensions; frequency in Hertz (Hz) is on the abscissa,

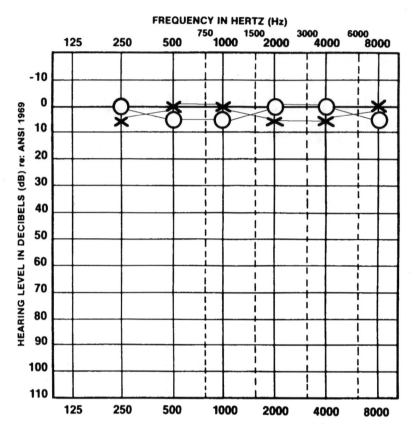

FIGURE 6.1 Example of a pure-tone audiogram used in clinical testing. The threshold responses are consistent with normal auditory sensitivity. Air- and bone-conduction thresholds overlap and are within normal limits (less than 20 dB).

and intensity in decibels hearing level (dB HL) is on the ordinate. The frequency is generally listed across the top of the chart, from lowest frequency on the left (typically 125 Hz) to highest frequency on the right (typically 8000 Hz). Intensity of the stimulus is on the left side of the chart, with the lowest intensity at the top (typically –10 dB HL) and the highest intensity (typically 110 dB HL) at the bottom of the graph. The thresholds via air conduction and bone conduction for each ear are represented on the graph. The audiogram in Figure 6.1 shows normal air-conduction thresholds for right (o) and left (x) ears respectively. If a symbol for threshold is located farther down on the chart, a higher-intensity stimulus was needed to find auditory threshold. This finding is consistent with abnormal auditory sensitivity at the tested frequency.

A hearing loss demonstrated during air-conduction testing could be due to a dysfunction at any point along the peripheral auditory pathway. There could be a problem in the outer ear, middle ear, inner ear, eighth cranial nerve, or, less

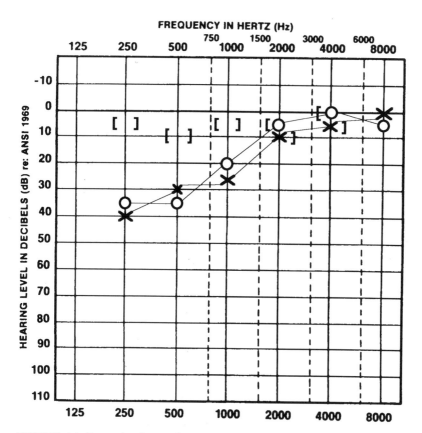

FIGURE 6.2 Example of a conductive hearing loss. Bone-conduction thresholds are within the normal range, and air-conduction thresholds indicate a low-frequency hearing loss.

commonly, a disorder in the auditory pathway in the lower brainstem. A hearing loss found during air-conduction testing could also be due to a dysfunction in more than one of these auditory structures at the same time. Air-conduction testing in isolation can tell the examiner if a hearing loss is present, the ear with the loss of hearing, the frequencies involved, and the relative magnitude of the auditory dysfunction.

An important piece of information not established by air-conduction testing is the location of the auditory dysfunction. Bone-conduction testing, used in combination with air-conduction testing, can help differentiate between abnormalities of the conductive mechanism and the sensory or neural mechanism (Dirks, 1964a).

A person with normal auditory sensitivity when tested by bone conduction and with a loss of hearing when tested by air conduction demonstrates a dysfunction in the outer or middle ear. Because this loss is in the conductive apparatus of the auditory system, it is termed a *conductive hearing loss* (Figure 6.2).

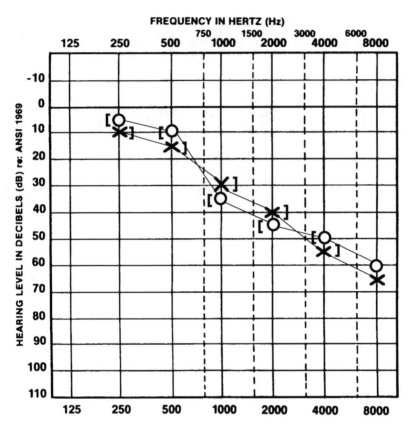

FIGURE 6.3 Example of a sensorineural hearing loss. Air- and bone-conduction thresholds overlap but are not within a normal range for frequencies from 1000 Hz to 8000 Hz.

If there is a considerable difference (10 dB or greater) in thresholds when testing by air conduction and by bone conduction (with air-conduction thresholds showing a greater hearing loss) there is said to be an air-bone gap. The air-bone gap is simply the difference between air-conduction and bone-conduction thresholds. Thus, if a person has an air-conduction threshold of 45 dB HL and a bone-conduction threshold of 20 dB HL at a given frequency, there is a 25 dB air-bone gap. The air-bone gap gives a measurement of the contribution of the conductive component of the hearing loss. If reliable and accurate thresholds are established, air-conduction thresho'ds can be at a higher level (ie, poorer hearing sensitivity) than bone-conduction thresholds, but bone-conduction thresholds cannot be considerably higher (poorer hearing sensitivity) than air-conduction thresholds. A difference of 5 dB is not considered clinically significant. If, however, bone-conduction thresholds are elevated relative to air-conduction thresholds, the accuracy of the test results should be questioned.

If there is a loss of hearing while testing by bone conduction and similar auditory thresholds are revealed by air conduction, the dysfunction is typically located in the inner ear and acoustic nerve. These parts of the peripheral auditory system are called the sensory and neural structures, respectively, and a hearing loss that is due to dysfunction of these structures is called a sensorineural hearing loss (Figure 6.3). A sensorineural loss can be defined as thresholds of 25 dB HL or greater at any test frequency and air- and bone-conduction thresholds that do not differ from each other by more than 5 dB. Pure-tone threshold testing does not typically isolate whether a hearing loss is due to sensory or neural dysfunction, or both, but special tests described later in this chapter have been developed for this purpose.

If there is a loss of auditory sensitivity while testing by bone conduction, a sensorineural component to the hearing loss is indicated. If auditory thresholds are poorer when testing by means of air conduction than by bone conduction, there is a conductive component. It logically follows that if there is a hearing loss when testing by bone conduction, and the hearing is worse during testing by air conduction, there is evidence of both conductive and sensorineural hearing loss. Such a hearing loss is said to be a mixed hearing loss (Figure 6.4).

Degree of Hearing Loss

Several terms are used to describe the severity of an auditory impairment. Often, in describing the severity of a hearing loss an arithmetical mean of the thresholds at 500 Hz, 1000 Hz, and 2000 Hz (ANSI, 1989) is used. There are differing opinions as to the range of auditory sensitivity considered normal. Some authors believe that normal hearing sensitivity includes thresholds of 25 dB HL and lower (Goodman, 1965). Clark (1981), in a modification of the Goodman system, described a pure-tone average (mean thresholds of 500 Hz, 1000 Hz, and 2000 Hz) of −10 to 15 dB as encompassing the normal range of hearing sensitivity and 16 to 25 dB constituting a slight hearing loss. Both classification systems are in agreement for degree of hearing losses that would be classified as falling in the mild range and of greater severity.

These systems attempt to classify the communicative deficit that may result from a hearing loss, but it should be remembered that the impact of a hearing loss on a person is subject to considerable individual variation. Thus, the reader is cautioned against interpreting this terminology too literally. Figure 6.5 illustrates an example of ranges of hearing impairment.

If the thresholds fall in the ranges from 26 dB HL to 40 dB HL, the person is said to have a *mild* loss of auditory sensitivity. A person with this degree of hearing impairment likely has difficulty hearing faint speech and the quietest phonemes and hearing in noisy listening conditions.

If the thresholds fall between 41 and 55 dB HL, the loss is called a *moderate* hearing loss. If this loss involves the primary speech frequencies, the person

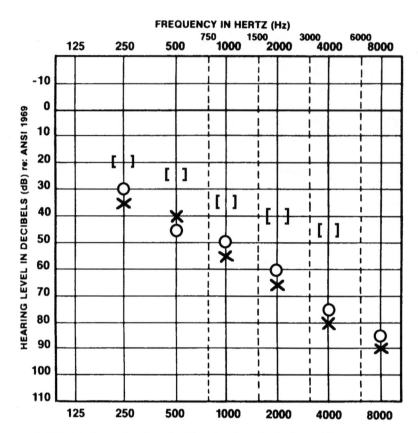

FIGURE 6.4 Example of a mixed hearing loss. Both air- and bone-conduction thresholds are abnormal, and there is a difference in thresholds between the air- and bone-conduction responses (air-bone gap).

frequently has difficulty understanding most parts of speech, even in favorable listening conditions.

If most thresholds range from 56 to 70 dB HL, the hearing loss is *moderately severe*. A person with this loss has great difficulty understanding spoken communication, even if the speech is loud and the listening conditions are favorable.

Auditory thresholds that range between 71 and 90 dB HL are consistent with a *severe* hearing loss. A person with a severe hearing loss likely understands speech only with the assistance of amplification.

If the auditory thresholds are 91 dB HL or greater, the hearing loss is termed a *profound* loss. If this degree of impairment includes the primary speech frequencies, the person likely has an extreme communication handicap, even with appropriate amplification (see Figure 6.5).

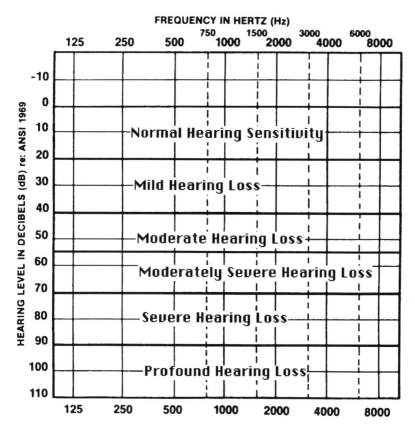

FIGURE 6.5 Example of the different severities of hearing loss based on pure-tone thresholds.

Configuration of Hearing Loss

The severity of a hearing loss is not the only aspect of an audiogram. The overall shape of the audiogram is also described. This is termed the *slope* or *configuration* of the audiogram and gives a general impression of the amount of hearing loss at various frequencies. If the auditory thresholds are similar at each frequency tested, that is, the loss of hearing is nearly the same across the frequency range evaluated, the slope is said to be *flat* (Figure 6.6). If the thresholds are progressively worse in the high frequencies, the configuration is said to be *sloping* (Figure 6.7). If the thresholds are higher (greater impairment) in the low frequencies, the configuration is termed *rising* (Figure 6.8). Poorer auditory sensitivity in the mid-frequencies is termed *trough-shaped* (Figure 6.9). This may also be referred to as a *cookie-bite* configuration. Many clinics use other descriptive terms to describe the configuration of a hearing loss. These may include *ski-slope*, *falling*,

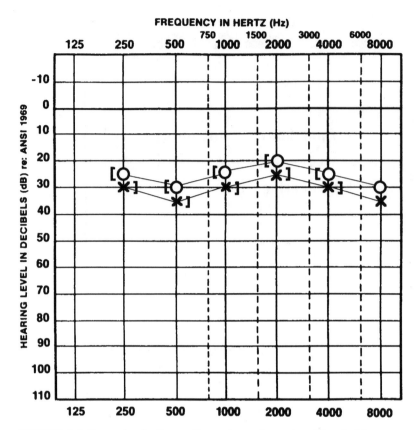

FIGURE 6.6 Example of a flat audiometric configuration. Threshold responses change only minimally across frequencies tested.

sharply dropping, and precipitous, among others (Figure 6.10). It is important to remember that these terms describe the overall shape of the audiogram, and can suggest the relative loss of hearing at given frequencies. An example of another classification system for the configuration of audiograms may be found in Kaplan et al (1993). This system is detailed in Table 6.1 on page 183.

Tests of Speech Understanding

Auditory impairments interfere with the understanding of speech. For this reason, speech materials are typically included as part of a hearing evaluation. These tests are designed to evaluate the impact of the auditory dysfunction on the understanding of speech. These clinical speech evaluations can be classified as either threshold or suprathreshold tests.

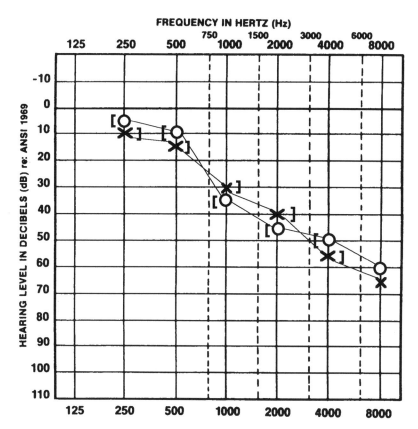

FIGURE 6.7 Example of a sloping or falling audiometric configuration. Threshold responses are better in the low frequencies than in the high frequencies.

Threshold Tests

The concept of pure-tone auditory threshold sensitivity testing has correlates in speech testing. The purpose of speech threshold testing is to establish the lowest intensity level at which a person can perceive speech a specified percentage of time (ASHA, 1988). Speech threshold testing typically consists of two kinds of evaluations, speech detection threshold (SDT) and speech recognition threshold (SRT).

SDT may be defined as the lowest intensity level at which a person can detect the presence of speech a specified percentage of time. SDT may also be termed speech awareness threshold. The listener cannot understand the meaning of the speech message, but can only perceive the signal is present (Martin & Dowdy, 1986).

Speech detection threshold testing is typically established with sentence stimuli. The intensity of the speech signal is raised and lowered by the examiner,

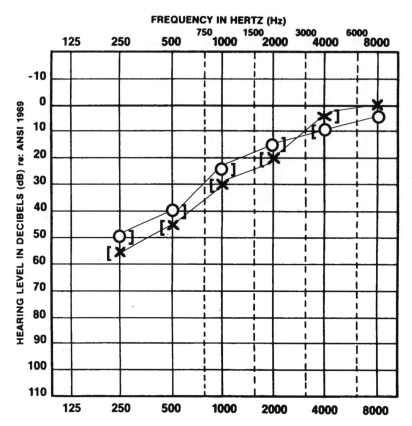

FIGURE 6.8 Example of a rising audiometric configuration. Threshold responses are poorer in the low frequencies than in the high frequencies.

and the listener indicates awareness of the presence of the signal. The point at which the listener detects the presence of the speech 50 percent of the time is typically considered the SDT.

Speech recognition threshold is the lowest level at which a listener can understand or identify speech stimuli 50 percent of the time. This testing is used for clinical purposes much more frequently than SDT. The speech recognition threshold is typically found at a level about 8 to 9 dB above the SDT (Chaiklin, 1959).

The most common stimuli used to elicit SRT are spondees. Spondees are two-syllable words with equal emphasis on both syllables. Typical English words that can be produced with equal emphasis on both syllables include *toothbrush*, *whitewash*, *hotdog*, *cowboy*, and *nightlight*. The Central Institute for the Deaf (CID) Auditory Test W-1 (Hirsh, 1952) is a list of 36 spondees. These words are of relatively common usage and of approximately the same auditory difficulty.

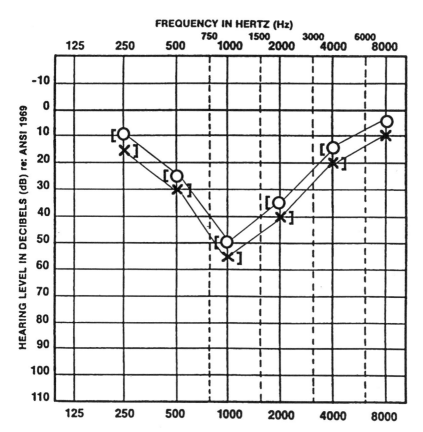

FIGURE 6.9 Example of a trough-shaped or cookie-bite configuration. Threshold responses are normal for both the low and high frequencies but are below the normal range for the center frequencies.

As spondaic stimuli are used routinely to establish SRT, these results may also be termed the *spondee threshold*, which means SRT is established when spondaic words are used as stimuli. These stimuli may be presented by a monitored live voice using a microphone or recorded tapes or compact disks. The use of prerecorded stimuli in speech testing is preferable because it eliminates speaker variability, which may influence results. SRT typically correlates with the average of the pure-tone thresholds at 500, 1000, and 2000 Hz (Carhart, 1971). The arithmetical mean of these three frequencies has been termed the pure-tone average (PTA). SRT may not correlate well with PTA if the configuration of the hearing loss is such that thresholds change dramatically through the frequencies used to calculate the PTA. In that case, a two-frequency PTA (PTA2) may more closely approximate (5 dB) SRT. The PTA2 is found by taking the arithmetical average of the better two thresholds at 500, 1000, and 2000 Hz.

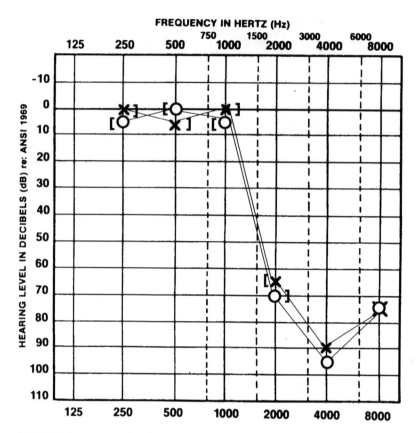

FIGURE 6.10 Example of a ski-slope audiometric configuration. Threshold responses are normal in the low frequencies but drop sharply to below the normal range for the center and high frequencies.

Suprathreshold Speech Testing

Typical clinical procedures investigate not only the lowest level at which a person can reliably identify speech but also the accuracy of speech identification at some level above threshold. These tests may be called *speech discrimination, speech identification,* or *speech recognition* testing. This testing provides useful information about the impact of the hearing loss on speech understanding, assists in the proper selection of amplification systems, gives information concerning the site of a lesion in the auditory system, and provides an indication of the speech sounds that may be the most difficult for a person to perceive.

A variety of speech tests are used to assess speech understanding. The type of test and the presentation level should be indicated on the test results. The speech-language pathologist, educator, or health care professional should understand the purpose of the tests and the meaning of the results, particularly if speech therapy is part of the recommended follow-up care.

Table 6.1 Classification System to Describe Audiometric Configuration

Term	Description
Flat	Less than 5 dB rise or fall per octave
Gradually falling	5–12 dB decrease per octave
Sharply falling	13 dB or more decrease per octave
Abruptly falling	Flat or gradually falling, then sharply falling
Rising	5 dB or more increase per octave
Trough	20 dB or greater loss at 1000 Hz and 2000 Hz than at 500 and 4000 Hz
Miscellaneous	Does not fit any of the above

(Reprinted with permission from Kaplan et al, 1993. Copyright © 1993 by Allyn and Bacon.)

Monosyllabic Stimuli for Speech Recognition Testing

A number of stimulus–word lists contain a series of monosyllabic words. These lists are typically phonetically balanced (PB); that is, the phonetic elements in the stimulus words occur in the list in the same proportion as they occur in connected English discourse. These monosyllabic word lists typically contain 50 stimulus words each.

The first PB stimulus–word list to achieve widespread clinical use was the PAL PB-50 word lists created at the Psychoacoustic Laboratories at Harvard University (Egan, 1948). There are many similarities between these original stimulus–word lists and other lists commonly used in clinics today. Typically the stimulus list is phonetically balanced (PB) and contains words that are monosyllabic, in common usage, and used in a speech recognition (open response set) paradigm.

Another common set of speech recognition stimuli is the CID W-22 word lists. These lists were developed from Egan's PB list, but many of the stimulus words from the original lists were eliminated for relative difficulty or because listeners were not familiar with them (Hirsh et al, 1952).

The Northwestern University NU-6 word lists are similar to the PB-50 and W-22 lists, with an important exception. These word lists are *phonemically* balanced; that is, the proportion of sounds in the 50-word list is based on the occurrence of sounds in connected speech, not written English. The creators of this set of stimuli asserted that a speech identification test should logically be representative of the occurrence of the elements of connected speech (Tillman & Carhart, 1966).

Other monosyllabic word lists are in common clinical use. The California Consonant Test is a speech discrimination test that primarily is reflective of high-frequency hearing ability (Owens & Schubert, 1977). This test and the Modified Rhyme Test (Griffiths, 1967) are more accurately called speech discrimination tests, in that the stimulus word is chosen from a set of response alternatives, the response foils varying only by a single phoneme.

The Phonetically Balanced Kindergarten (PBK-50) (Haskins, 1949) lists are PB stimuli using monosyllabic words that should be familiar to children older than about $3\frac{1}{2}$ years. The Word Intelligibility by Picture Identification (WIPI) Test (Ross & Lerman, 1970) is a word discrimination test that requires the listener to point to a picture that represents the stimulus word.

Typical word identification testing is done at a suprathreshold level. Although clinical procedures may vary, word identification testing may be conducted at several levels of presentation intensity. One typical level to conduct word identification testing is the intensity level of average speech. Thus, the speech stimuli are presented at 45 to 50 dB HL. This gives an indication of the person's speech understanding ability in typical communication settings. If a person has a severe loss of auditory sensitivity, it may not be logical to test word identification at this level, because the presentation level may be well below the person's auditory thresholds.

As the presentation level of speech discrimination stimuli increases above a person's absolute SRT, there is typically an improvement in speech discrimination. If a graph were made of the speech discrimination score (a percentage) and the presentation level (in dB) relative to SRT, an improvement in speech discrimination with increasing presentation level would be seen. At some point this function would level off; that is, increasing the presentation level would not lead to an increased speech understanding score. Such a plot is called a performance-intensity (PI) function (Eldert & Davis, 1951). When this plot is established with PB stimuli, it is termed a *PI-PB function*. The stimulus presentation level associated with maximum word identification performance is termed *PBmax* (Eldert & Davis, 1951).

PI-PB functions have diagnostic value. A person with normal hearing shows a function that reveals improved speech understanding with increasing intensity up to PBmax. Further increases in the intensity of presentation are associated with word identification equal to PBmax. A person with a conductive hearing loss shows a similar pattern. For both types of listeners, PBmax is at or near 100 percent.

A person with a sensorineural hearing loss shows a slightly different pattern. The function shows an increase in word understanding with increasing presentation level up to PBmax. PBmax with this auditory dysfunction is likely to be lower than that with normal hearing or a conductive loss. This is because the speech signal is distorted by the damage in the auditory system. The reduction in PBmax depends on the severity and configuration of the loss. Speech discrimination scores are equal to PBmax or slightly reduced if the presentation level continues to be increased (Jerger & Jerger, 1971).

A person with a lesion on the acoustic nerve or in the central auditory pathway contralateral to the ear tested shows a pattern considerably different from those described earlier. Word identification performance improves with increased presentation level above the SRT. PBmax itself may be rather low. An increase in presentation level above PBmax leads to a reduction in word identification scores. This reduction in performance with an increase in presentation level is termed *rollover*. It is a finding often associated with a retrocochlear lesion on the same side as the ear showing the rollover (Rintelmann, 1991).

Establishment of PBmax can be time-consuming. Many studies have shown that PBmax is achieved with typical speech identification materials at approximately 30 to 40 dB above the listener's SRT (30 to 40 dB sensation level [SL]) (Martin, 1991). Therefore, to save time, speech recognition materials are presented at only one intensity, 40 dB SL, to obtain an estimate of PBmax. Thus, a clinician can quickly determine the speech understanding ability of a listener at the probable optimal presentation level.

Sentence Tests Used to Test Speech Understanding

Several sentence tests are used for evaluating speech understanding. The rationale behind using sentences for stimuli is that listeners do not typically listen to speech as isolated words but in connected discourse. Sentence testing, therefore, seems more indicative of typical communication interactions.

The first sentence test to be extensively used in clinical settings was the CID Everyday Sentence Test (Davis & Silverman, 1978). Because of problems with reliability (scores may vary significantly from one administration of this test to another), this test is not extensively used at this time. The Speech Perception in Noise (SPIN) (Kalikow et al, 1977) test is a series of sentences presented in the presence of background noise. The final word in the sentence is the stimulus word that requires identification by the listener. Half of these sentences contain contextual information so that the final word is highly predictable. The other half does not contain contextual information that aids in the identification of the final word. Thus, word identification can be evaluated, as can the relative contribution of contextual linguistic information.

The Synthetic Sentence Identification (SSI) (Speaks & Jerger, 1965) test consists of ten synthetic sentences of seven words each. These synthetic sentences are third-order sentential approximations (each word is linguistically dependent on the two words preceding it). These sentences are presented to the listener with a competing message either in the same ear as the stimuli or in the contralateral ear. The listener is required to identify from a list of alternatives the sentence presented. This test is typically used in the assessment of central auditory function.

Another purpose of speech testing is to determine the most comfortable loudness level (MCL) (Kopra & Blosser, 1968) and the uncomfortable loudness level (UCL) (Martin, 1991). MCL is simply the level at which a listener prefers to listen to speech. UCL is the intensity at which speech is too loud to be tolerable for more than a short time. These tests are typically used as part of a hearing aid evaluation to determine the optimum setting for the amplification device.

Masking

At certain presentation levels, it is possible that the ear not being tested is actually being stimulated (cross-hearing). Whenever the presentation level exceeds the bone-conduction threshold of the ear not being tested by more than the interaural attenuation value, cross-hearing must be suspected (Chaiklin, 1967). Interaural attenuation is the decrease in the amplitude of the signal as it crosses the head to the contralateral ear (Martin, 1991). Essentially, the stimulus causes vibrations in the skull that can stimulate the cochlea of the ear not being tested. Thus, all cross-hearing occurs by means of bone conduction.

When a stimulus is presented by means of air conduction, the reduction in the signal as it crosses the skull varies from about 40 to 65 dB. To be conservative (and clinically cautious), most clinicians take the interaural attenuation value for air-conduction testing to be 40 dB. Thus, when the presentation level by air conduction is at a level 40 dB or greater than the bone-conduction threshold of the ear not being tested, masking is indicated.

When a stimulus is presented by means of bone conduction, the entire skull is set into vibration. If the entire skull is set into vibration, both cochleae are being stimulated. There is no reduction in the amplitude of the signal as it crosses over to the cochlea of the ear not being tested. Thus, the interaural attenuation value when the signal is presented by means of bone conduction is considered to be 0 dB.

The most efficient masking noise used during pure-tone testing is a narrow band of noise centered on the test frequency (Goldstein & Newman, 1985). Although white noise can be used as a masker, the frequencies in white noise that are far removed from the stimulus frequency do not contribute to masking. They only serve to make the masker louder and more annoying.

During speech testing the masker used is called *speech noise*. This is a spectrally shaped noise that is similar to the frequency content of speech. That is, much of the energy in speech noise is in the frequencies below 1000 Hz and there is progressively less energy in the higher frequencies.

It is important to remember that skill in masking techniques is often necessary to establish reliable thresholds. This is particularly true when there is an air-bone gap or a considerable difference in sensitivity between the two cochleae. The speech-language pathologist should become familiar enough with masking techniques and requirements so that the results of a hearing test can be examined to determine if masking was performed when necessary. Unmasked thresholds should be evaluated with a high index of suspicion as to the accuracy of the findings if cross-hearing is possible.

TESTS FOR AUDITORY SITE OF PATHOLOGIC CONDITION

A number of tests may be described to a professional working with the hearing impaired population. It is not the intention of this section to describe these clinical procedures in the same detail as was used for the routine clinical tests. However, the practicing professional should have some idea as to the purposes of the test procedures, and this section provides a reference.

Objective Tests for Abnormalities of the Outer and Middle Ear

A routine part of clinical evaluations includes an objective assessment of the transmission of the sound energy through the conductive mechanism. Resistance to the flow of acoustic energy through the auditory system is termed *acoustic impedance*. The inverse of this, that is, the ease of energy transmission through the ear, is termed *acoustic admittance*. The term *immittance* is used to describe all measurements of energy transmission through the conductive mechanism of the ear (ASHA, 1978).

Dysfunction of the conductive portion of the ear causes a hearing loss by altering the transmission of sound through the conductive apparatus. An objective measurement of the transmission of sound through the ear can be useful clinically to test for a conductive abnormality.

The three clinical immittance measurements in common use include tympanometry, static admittance, and acoustic reflex. Tympanometry measures the transmission of energy through the ear at various air pressures. Static admittance gives an indication of the overall mobility of the tympanic membrane and ossicular chain. Acoustic reflex testing measures small changes in the immittance of the conductive mechanism associated with reflexive contraction of a muscle in the middle ear when the listener is exposed to sound of moderate or high intensity.

Immittance measurements are obtained by use of an electroacoustic immittance meter. This instrument is connected to a tube that fits securely in the ear. The tube is covered with a small plastic probe and provides an airtight seal when placed in the ear canal, isolating the ear canal from the outer environment. The probe has three openings. One is a receiver opening that delivers either a 220-Hz or 660-Hz tone to the ear. The second connects to an air pump used to vary the air pressure in the ear canal. The third opening is for a microphone that measures the sound pressure in the ear canal.

If the conductive mechanism has low impedance, much of the sound energy delivered by the receiver passes through the system, and the microphone records low sound pressure in the ear canal. If the system has high impedance, much of the sound delivered by the receiver does not transmit through the conductive mechanism and the microphone records a high amount of sound pressure in the external ear.

A tympanogram is obtained by measurement of the transmission of sound energy through the ear at various air pressures (ASHA, 1990b). A tympanogram is a graph with the admittance of the ear represented on the Y axis in cubic centimeters (cc) or milliliters (mL) and the air pressure on the X axis in deca-Pascals (daPa) or millimeters of water (mm H$_2$0) (Figure 6.11). If the air pressure in the ear canal is high or low relative to the air pressure in the middle ear, the conductive mechanism tends to stiffen. This is evident on the tympanogram by a reduction in admittance. When the air pressure in the ear canal is equal to the air pressure in the middle ear, the conductive mechanism transmits sound efficiently that is, admittance is higher.

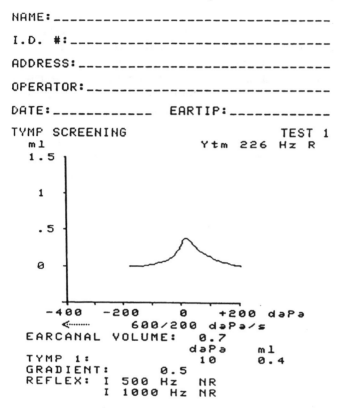

GSI 33
Middle-Ear Analyzer

NAME: _____

I.D. #: _____

ADDRESS: _____

OPERATOR: _____

DATE: _____   EARTIP: _____

TYMP SCREENING   TEST 1
                         Ytm 226 Hz R

EARCANAL VOLUME: 0.7
                         daPa   ml
TYMP 1:   10   0.4
GRADIENT: 0.5
REFLEX: I 500 Hz   NR
          I 1000 Hz   NR

FIGURE 6.11 Example of a Type A tympanogram. The static admittance is 0.4 cc, the peak is at +10 daPa, and the ear canal volume is 0.7 cc. All of these values are within the normal range.

When there is a pressure difference between the outer ear and the middle ear, sounds are somewhat muffled because of the increase in impedance in the conductive mechanism caused by stiffening of the middle ear system. Therefore, sounds of low frequency do not transmit through the system efficiently. When the eustachian tube opens, the impedance of the system drops, and sound travels through more efficiently. The subjective effect is that one can hear better when the pressure is equalized.

The transmission of sound through the conductive apparatus at various sound pressures demonstrates how a tympanogram can give an indirect measurement of the pressure in the middle ear. As illustrated in the foregoing example, when the air pressure in the external ear and that in the middle ear are equalized, admittance is highest, and sound travels through the system most efficiently. Thus, on a graph of air pressure versus admittance, the air pressure where maximum admittance is found corresponds to the air pressure of the middle ear space.

A normal tympanogram shows maximum admittance at atmospheric pressure (see Figure 6.11). This is represented on the graph as 0 daPa. This value is relative to ambient air pressure; that is, 0 daPa is the same pressure as ambient air pressure; +200 daPa is 200 daPa above ambient air pressure. If there is negative pressure in the middle ear space, the point of maximum admittance is a value below 0 daPa (Margolis & Shanks, 1985). The opposite is true for increased pressure in the middle ear. The range of normal values of peak pressure extends from –150 daPa to +100 daPa. If there is a clinically significant restriction in the mobility of the conductive mechanism, a point of maximum admittance may not be found. That is, the admittance of the conductive mechanism may be quite low regardless of changes in the air pressure of the external ear.

Static admittance measurements involve comparing the admittance of the ear at a high air pressure (typically +200 daPa) and comparing this value to the maximum admittance of the system (Margolis & Shanks, 1985). The air pressure in the ear canal is first increased to +200 daPa. This increased air pressure has the effect of stiffening the conductive mechanism, which results in a large amount of the sound energy to be reflected off the tympanic membrane. The immittance meter therefore shows low admittance. The air pressure is adjusted to find the point where sound energy transmits through the system the best, that is, the point of maximum admittance. The difference in admittance between these two points is termed the *static admittance*. This measurement gives an indication of the mobility of the tympanic membrane–ossicular chain system. The normal values for static admittance range from about 0.3 to 2.5 milliliters of water. Static admittance also can be described as the height of the peak on the tympanogram (ASHA, 1990b).

A conductive loss may be associated with either high or low static admittance, depending on the cause of the loss. A conductive loss caused by a restriction in the mobility of the conductive mechanism shows low static admittance. In some cases, a point of maximum admittance may not be found at all. Possible causes for this finding include a fixation of the ossicles or fluid in the middle ear space. A conductive loss may be associated with extremely high static admittance. If there is an air-bone gap and very high static admittance, a disarticulation of the ossicular chain is suspected.

Several characteristic types of tympanograms associated with middle ear function have been described (Feldman, 1976). A person with normal hearing and normal conductive function typically has a normal tympanogram. This is defined as a peak admittance in the normal pressure range with the height of the peak (the static admittance) also falling within the normal range. This is often termed a Type A tympanogram (see Figure 6.11). A person with a sensorineural hearing loss has dysfunction in the inner ear, not the conductive apparatus, and he or she would have a Type A tympanogram.

A conductive or a mixed loss shows abnormalities on the tympanogram for the affected ear. A tympanogram that shows the point of maximum admittance at a normal pressure but a low static admittance is called a *Type As (shallow)*

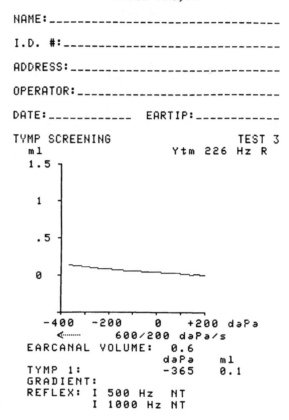

FIGURE 6.12

Example of a Type B (flat) tympanogram. There is no peak, so there is no indication of middle ear mobility. The ear canal volume is within normal limits. A common pathology associated with this type of tympanogram is otitis media.

tympanogram. Type As is consistent with restricted middle ear mobility. A tympanogram that shows the point of maximum admittance at a normal pressure but an abnormally high static admittance is called a *Type Ad (deep) tympanogram.* Excessive admittance may be caused by a disarticulation of the ossicles or a flaccid tympanic membrane. A tympanogram on which a point of maximum admittance cannot be found, that is, a flat tympanogram, is called a *Type B tympanogram* (Figure 6.12). Type B tympanogram is often found with otitis media or adhesions in the middle ear. A tympanogram on which the static admittance is normal but the point of maximum admittance is at an abnormally low pressure (for example, –290 daPa) is called a *Type C tympanogram* (Figure 6.13). A Type C tympanogram is consistent with abnormally low middle ear pressure and may be indicative of early stages of otitis media or eustachian tube dysfunction.

An immittance meter also typically reports the volume of air in front of the probe. This is referred to as the ear canal volume. Patterns in the tympanogram

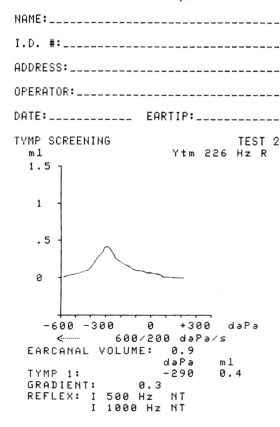

GSI 33
Middle-Ear Analyzer

NAME: _____

I.D. #: _____

ADDRESS: _____

OPERATOR: _____

DATE: _____ EARTIP: _____

TYMP SCREENING   TEST 2
   ml   Ytm 226 Hz R
  1.5

   1

   .5

   0

       -600 -300   0   +300   daPa
        <········   600/200 daPa/s
    EARCANAL VOLUME: 0.9
                      daPa   ml
    TYMP 1:   -290   0.4
    GRADIENT: 0.3
    REFLEX: I 500 Hz   NT
              I 1000 Hz   NT

FIGURE 6.13
Example of a Type C tympan-
nogram. All of the values are
within the normal range except
for peak pressure, which is at
an abnormally low level (–290
daPa). A common disorder
associated with this type of
tympanogram is eustachian
tube dysfunction.

should be interpreted in light of the ear canal volume of the ear tested. The normal range for ear canal volume is about 0.4 to 1.0 cc for children and 0.6 to 1.5 cc for adults.

If there is a flat tympanogram with a normal ear canal volume (see Figure 6.12), the abnormality is likely in the middle ear space (such as otitis media with effusion). If a flat tympanogram is found with a reduced ear canal volume (Figure 6.14), one should suspect blockage in the ear canal (such as cerumen occlusion). A flat tympanogram with an abnormally large ear canal volume (Figure 6.15) is consistent with an opening in the tympanic membrane (which may be caused by a traumatic perforation or an open ventilating tube).

Several parameters of the tympanogram other than static admittance, peak pressure, and ear canal volume may be reported. These include tympanogram width (TW) and tympanogram gradient. TW is defined as the width of the tympanogram (in daPa) at one-half the peak height. One measure of tympanogram gradient that can be used is the slope of the tympanogram. Research indicates that

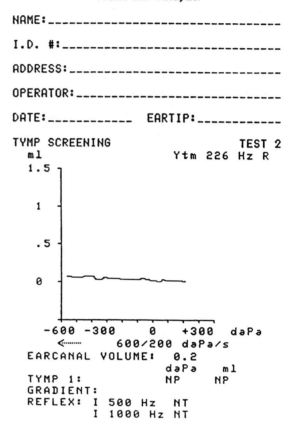

FIGURE 6.14

Example of a Type B (flat) tympanogram. The ear canal volume is abnormally small.

these measurements may provide information that assists in the early detection of otitis media (ASHA, 1990b). A tympanogram that is very wide or has a low gradient is often associated with the early stages of otitis media.

Acoustic Reflex Test

When moderately intense sound is presented to humans, a bilateral reflexive contraction of the stapedius muscle can be measured (Metz, 1946). When the stapedius muscle contracts, it stiffens the ossicular chain. This stiffening causes a measurable increase in the stiffness of the conductive mechanism. This contraction of the stapedius muscle has been termed the *acoustic reflex*.

Most people with normal auditory systems demonstrate an acoustic reflex to pure-tone stimuli at levels ranging from 70 to 105 dB HL (Metz, 1946). The reflex occurs bilaterally; that is, when the stimulus is presented to one ear, contraction of the stapedius muscle can be measured in both ears. This bilateral reflex arc

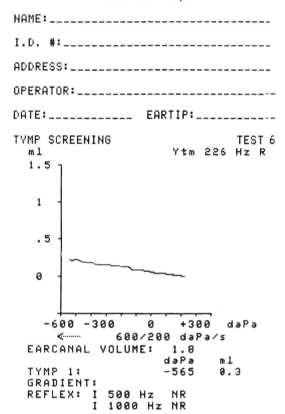

FIGURE 6.15
Example of a Type B (flat) tympanogram. The ear canal volume is abnormally large.

involves the acoustic nerve on the side of stimulation (the sensory component of the reflex), the brainstem (from the level of the cochlear nucleus to the superior olivary complex), and the facial nerve bilaterally (the motor segment of the reflex) (Borg, 1973). Measurement of the elicited reflex provides a noninvasive, objective means of evaluating several important neurophysical structures.

The following characteristic patterns of results of acoustic reflex testing are consistent with several types of auditory abnormalities.

1. The acoustic reflex generally is absent in the ear with a conductive abnormality (Jerger & Hayes, 1980). This is because the change in stiffness associated with the acoustic reflex may not be detectable in an ear with already low admittance. This is often the case in an ear in which the ossicular chain or tympanic membrane has severely restricted mobility.

2. The reflex is not elicited if the stimulus is too low in intensity. Therefore, in the ear contralateral to a conductive hearing loss, the reflex may be found at an abnormally high intensity level when the ear with the conductive loss is stimulated. This

is because the conductive loss attenuates the signal that reaches the cochlea (Jerger & Hayes, 1980).

3. A reflex may be absent or abnormal in an ear with abnormalities associated with the stapedius or tensor tympani muscles.

4. When an ear with a cochlear hearing loss is stimulated, acoustic reflexes may be elicited at a fairly low SL (40-55 dB SL). Eliciting an acoustic reflex at low SLs is thought to be an objective correlate of recruitment (an abnormally large growth in the loudness of a signal with a corresponding increase in intensity) (Metz, 1952). The exact cause of recruitment is unknown, but this finding is associated with cochlear dysfunction.

5. A dysfunction in the acoustic nerve of the stimulated ear may lead to absent reflexes or to reflexes of low amplitude. A higher-intensity stimulus may be needed to elicit the reflex (Jerger et al, 1974). Another common finding is that the reflex rapidly decays once it is elicited.

6. The facial nerve supplies the motor innervation to the stapedius muscle. If there is dysfunction in the facial nerve, a reflex will not be measured on the side of the dysfunction (Jerger et al, 1983). Reflexes on the contralateral side are not affected.

7. Lower brainstem abnormalities are associated with normal ipsilateral reflexes, but abnormal or absent contralateral reflexes (Jerger, 1980). This occurs when either ear is stimulated.

8. Central auditory disorders associated with dysfunction in the auditory cortex or corpus callosum do not adversely affect the acoustic reflex (Jerger, 1980).

Behavioral Tests of Abnormalities of the Outer and Middle Ear

Two of the behavioral tests used to establish the presence of conductive abnormalities are the Bing and Weber tests. These tuning-fork tests were originally developed by physicians to help establish the presence of a conductive hearing loss. Today these tests are often performed using a tuning fork or bone vibrator (Martin, 1991). Several other tuning-fork tests were also used for this purpose, but today they are seldom used and are not discussed herein.

The Bing and Weber tests are based on the occlusion effect. The occlusion effect is an increase in loudness of bone-conducted sounds associated with a conductive hearing loss. The Weber test also depends on the Stenger effect. This effect describes the phenomenon that occurs when stimuli of the same frequency and phase but different amplitude are presented to both cochleae at the same time. The stimulus is heard only on the side of the cochlea that receives the stimulus of higher amplitude.

The Weber test is performed by placing a bone oscillator or a tuning fork on the forehead of the listener. The subject is told to report in which ear the sound is louder. If the subject hears the sound louder in the ear with reported poor hearing sensitivity, the hearing loss is likely conductive in that ear. The occlusion effect causes an increase in loudness of the bone-conducted stimulus on the side with the conductive hearing loss, and the Stenger effect causes the lateralization of the signal to that ear. The occlusion effect is much more noticeable for low-frequency sounds; thus, the Weber test is typically performed at 500 Hz and below.

If the stimulus lateralizes to the ear with better hearing sensitivity, the hearing loss is likely sensorineural in nature. This lateralization is due to the Stenger effect because of the better sensitivity of the unimpaired cochlea.

The Bing test is performed by placing the bone oscillator or the tuning fork behind the subject's pinna on the mastoid process or on the forehead. The external ear canal is then occluded, and the listener is asked if the stimulus sound changes in any way. If the sound changes, then the examiner has produced an occlusion effect, and the hearing in that ear is likely either normal or there is a sensorineural loss. If no change is noted, an occlusion effect already exists, and there is probably a conductive or mixed hearing loss. Like the Weber test, the Bing test is performed with low-frequency stimuli. The Bing and Weber tests are not typically performed in isolation but are used in conjunction with other tests. These results can provide evidence that supports pure-tone and immittance findings.

Objective Measurements of Cochlear Abnormality

Many times, behavioral test results cannot be reliably obtained from a listener. The listener may be too young to cooperate, may not be able to understand or perform the response task, or may not truthfully respond to the stimuli. In these situations, it is desirable to use measurements of auditory function that do not depend on volitional or conditioned responses from the subject. Immittance measurements (tympanometry and static admittance) are objective evaluations that allow the examiner to make judgments about the physiologic characteristics of the conductive mechanism. Several measurements also exist to help describe the function of the sensory mechanism in the cochlea.

Acoustic Reflexes

As described earlier, a reflexive contraction of the stapedius muscle occurs upon the presentation of acoustic stimuli of moderate to high intensity. The presence of the reflex provides objective evidence that the cochlea and reflex arc are responding to auditory stimuli. The acoustic reflex is generally elicited between 70 and 100 dB HL, which is also 70 dB to 100 dB above the normal auditory threshold (SL of 0 dB). In this case, both HL and SL are the same—70 dB. If a cochlear lesion is present and there is a sensorineural hearing loss, the acoustic reflex may occur at lower than expected (70 to 100 dB HL) intensity levels. For example, if a sensorineural hearing loss is 40 dB HL and an acoustic reflex is elicited at 90 dB HL, the reflex is only 50 dB SL (50 dB over the pure-tone audiogram thresholds of 40 dB HL) instead of the anticipated 70 to 100 dB SL. The occurrence of an acoustic reflex at expected intensity levels but reduced SL is consistent with a cochlear lesion (Metz, 1952).

Electroacoustic Measurements

Electrocochleography

Another method of objectively evaluating cochlear function involves the use of auditory evoked potentials. One procedure for evaluating the neuroelectrical activity in the cochlea is called electrocochleography (ECoG) (Jacobson & Hyde, 1985). This test consists of measuring electrical activity in the cochlea by means of a small electrode placed either in the ear canal or through the tympanic membrane (and in contact with the promontory). Characteristic patterns of the evoked ECoG waveforms are associated with cochlear lesions, particularly Ménière's disease.

Auditory Brainstem Response

A second procedure for evaluating neuroelectrical activity is the auditory brainstem response (ABR) (Jewett & Williston, 1971). The ABR is an averaged electrical wave generated from auditory structures within the acoustic nerve, the brainstem, and the midbrain. This is an extremely sensitive test for brainstem abnormalities and acoustic nerve dysfunction. It has also been found to be useful as an objective audiometric assessment of transmission of neuroelectrical impulses through the auditory system from the cochlea through the brainstem. An ABR evaluation yields a series of positive and negative waves on a graph. The amplitude of the wave (measured as voltage) is on the Y axis, and time is the X axis (Figure 6.16). The wave amplitude and latency (time they appear on the chart) are evaluated for normal or abnormal function. Absolute latency and the amount of time between wave peaks (the interpeak latency) are evaluated. There are six or seven identifiable wave peaks in a typical ABR. These are numbered I through VII but usually only I through V are evaluated. Because wave V is particularly identifiable, its latency is commonly reported.

An understanding of where the wave peaks are generated is helpful in understanding characteristic ABR patterns associated with different abnormalities in the auditory system (Moller et al, 1981). The generator sites of the commonly observed wavepeaks are as follows. Wave I is generated at the cochlear end of cranial nerve VIII. Wave II is generated at the medial (near the cerebellopontine angle) end of cranial nerve VIII. Waves III and IV seem to originate in the pons. Wave V arises from the midbrain. The generator sites of waves VI and VII are unknown at this time.

A typical ABR evaluation to assess audiologic or neurologic function is conducted in the following manner. The subject is told to relax (and may even

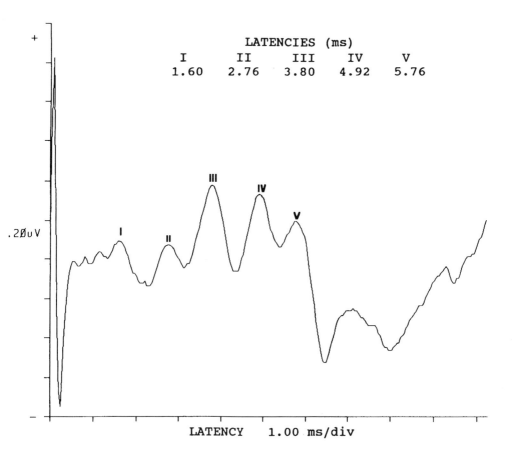

FIGURE 6.16 Example of averaged neuroelectrical brainstem responses. The major peaks are numbered I through V.

sleep) during the evaluation. Electrodes are attached to the skin of the scalp and perhaps the earlobes. Clicks or other brief acoustic stimuli are presented to the test ear at a rate of 11 to 60 stimuli per second for approximately 2000 presentations. The ABR test equipment averages the electrical activity of the neural structures for a very brief time period (approximately 10 msec) after each of the clicks. In this way, all neuroelectrical activity not associated with the click stimuli is averaged out. The final averaged waveform provides information about the auditory system in the frequency range from 1000 to 4000 Hz.

The ABR pattern of results depends on the status of the auditory system (Jerger & Jerger, 1983). If hearing is normal, the absolute latencies of the waves are likely to be normal, even at low presentation levels. If a conductive loss is present, a higher-intensity stimulus is needed to establish replicable ABR waves. If there is a sensory loss, wave V is absent at a low stimulus presentation level but is present with near normal latency at higher presentation levels. Wave I may remain delayed with a cochlear loss. A neural loss is often associated with longer than normal absolute latencies for waves II through VII. Interpeak latencies for waves I through III are typically longer than normal. This is consistent with increased transmission time through the acoustic nerve and loss of the synchronous firing of the neurons of the acoustic nerve. A lesion in the brainstem may show different ABR patterns depending on the location of the lesion. These patterns include normal wave I through III interpeak latency with prolonged wave III through V interpeak latency, or total obliteration of the waves after wave I.

Otoacoustic Emissions

A test of cochlear function called *cochlear otoacoustic emissions* is being evaluated for possible clinical use (Johnson et al, 1983). It has been known since the late 1970s that the cochlea produces sounds (Kemp, 1978). These spontaneous sounds are measured as part of this test procedure. It has since been learned that these emissions can be evoked by presenting auditory stimuli to the ear (see Chapter 1). Furthermore, a cochlear hearing loss changes these evoked otoacoustic emissions. Research is currently underway to investigate the use of otoacoustic emissions as an objective test of cochlear function. Early results are promising, but the technique is not without its shortcomings.

Behavioral Tests of Cochlear Function

Before the development of electrophysiologic methods of objectively assessing cochlear function, several behavioral tests were used to differentiate between sensory and neural abnormalities. These tests are based on several common behavioral findings associated with dysfunction of the sensory or neural units of the auditory system but are rarely used in clinics. Therefore, no expected clinical findings are discussed, and the tests are only described briefly.

Recruitment

Recruitment is defined as an increase in the perception of loudness with a corresponding increase in the intensity of sound. Several clinical tests were developed to evaluate this phenomenon, which is usually associated with cochlear abnormality. The Alternate Binaural Loudness Balance (ABLB) (Fowler, 1937) test of recruitment for unilateral sensorineural loss and the Alternate Monaural Loudness Balance (AMLB) (Reger, 1936) test of recruitment were designed to compare the growth of loudness at a frequency with normal sensitivity with the growth of loudness at a frequency with impairment. The ABLB compares the growth of loudness for the same frequency for two ears (impaired in one ear but not the other) while the AMLB compares loudness growth for a frequency with normal sensitivity to an impaired frequency in the same ear. For both tests, a rapid growth of loudness at the frequency of impairment was determined to be consistent with a cochlear hearing loss.

Difference Limen for Intensity

The smallest intensity change that can be detected between two signals is called the *difference limen for intensity* (DLI). Clinical evaluations have shown that if a signal is presented at about 20 dB SL to a person with a sensorineural hearing loss, the listener is typically able to make DLI discriminations on the order of about 1 dB. This finding led to the development of the Short Increment Sensitivity Index (SISI) (Jerger, 1962). In this test, a 1-dB intensity increment was superimposed on a 20-dB SL pure-tone carrier signal. If a listener detected the presence of the 1-dB increase in intensity more than 70 percent of the time, a cochlear abnormality was thought to be likely.

Behavioral Tests of Neural Function

If a person with an intact auditory system listens to an unvarying, continuous acoustic signal, the signal eventually is no longer heard. This gradual fading away of the perception of a signal is termed *adaptation*. An auditory dysfunction associated with a lesion of the eighth cranial nerve often leads to abnormal adaptation. This loss of perception to an unvarying signal is often quite rapid.

Abnormal adaptation has led to the development of a number of tone-decay tests (Green, 1985). These tests are discussed in general because they are administered in a similar manner. A typical tone-decay test consists of presenting a continuous signal to an impaired ear. The listener is instructed to respond as long as the signal is heard. The starting presentation level varies among different tests, but may range from 5 to 20 dB SL. A stopwatch is used to time the length of response by the listener. When the subject no longer hears the signal, the intensity is increased, and the timing is started again. A person with normal hearing maintains perception of the signal for at least 1 minute. An eighth-nerve abnormality generally is associated with tone decay of 25 dB or more in 1 minute.

Objective Tests of Neural Abnormalities

Auditory Brainstem Response

The ABR is a very sensitive objective test for pathologic conditions from the acoustic nerve through the brainstem. Pathologic conditions that involve cranial nerve VIII produce several changes in normal ABR results. If function of the acoustic nerve is only slightly impaired, there may be a decrease in the absolute latencies of waves II through VII. There would be a large increase in interpeak latency between waves I through V and I through III, but there would not likely be abnormal interpeak latency between peaks III through V. This finding is consistent with an increased transmission time of information through cranial nerve VIII. Severe dysfunction of the acoustic nerve may cause the absence of all wave peaks beyond wave I.

Acoustic Reflex Decay

An objectively measured correlate to the abnormal adaptation associated with an eighth-nerve lesion is rapid decay of the acoustic reflex when the stimulus is presented on the side of the disorder. With a neural impairment, the reflex amplitude often decays to less than 50 percent of its amplitude within 10 seconds of elicitation of the reflex. Administering the reflex-decay test is straightforward. The threshold for the acoustic reflex is determined. The stimulus intensity is then increased 10 dB over this level. The stimulus is then presented for 10 seconds. Decrease of the reflex amplitude to less than 50 percent of its maximum value is consistent with dysfunction of the acoustic nerve. With clinically significant neural abnormality, the decay likely occurs in the first 5 seconds of stimulus presentation.

Central Auditory Dysfunction

A number of behavioral tests can be administered to investigate function of the central auditory nervous system. Whereas dysfunction in the peripheral auditory system often produces effects that have a dramatic impact on verbal communication, the symptoms of central auditory dysfunction may be quite subtle. People with dysfunction limited to the central auditory structures may show completely normal peripheral hearing. The effects of a central auditory disorder may appear to be inconsistent, manifesting most noticeably under less than ideal listening conditions.

Because of the nature of central auditory disorders, routine clinical evaluations may not be sensitive to the typical symptoms. Special tests have been developed to measure performance of the central auditory mechanism. Many of these tests use a speech message that is acoustically degraded in some way. Methods used to increase the sensitivity of speech material to central auditory nervous system status include low-pass filtering, competing messages (both ipsilaterally and contralaterally), interrupting the message, temporally altering the message, and mixing the signal with noise. By providing an acoustically impoverished speech message, these tests can demonstrate decreases in performance of the central auditory system (see Chapter 13).

Low-Pass Filtered Speech

Recognition of low-pass filtered speech has been shown to be markedly reduced in the ear contralateral to a lesion in the temporal lobe (Bocca et al, 1954). There may be no differences between the ears in recognition of nonfiltered speech, but the more challenging filtered speech materials reveal the dysfunction.

Binaural Fusion

Binaural fusion consists of separating the spectral components of a speech signal into a high- and a low-frequency band. One band is delivered to one ear, the other band to the opposite ear. Speech identification would be very poor if only one of the frequency bands were used. If the brainstem is functioning appropriately, the two spectral bands can be combined into a meaningful message. A low rate of recognition of these materials is indicative of a brainstem lesion (Matzger, 1959).

Competing Sentence

Several central auditory tests make use of a competing message to increase the difficulty of the task. The Competing Sentences Test (Ivey, 1969) delivers a target sentence to one ear at 35 dB above SRT and a competing sentence to the other ear at 50 dB SL. People with normal central auditory function can easily respond to the target sentence. The performance in the ear contralateral to a temporal lobe lesion is often very low. Children with learning disabilities often show difficulty with this task.

Synthetic Sentences with Ipsilateral or Contralateral Message

Synthetic sentences (Speaks & Jerger, 1965) are often paired with a competing message. These may be ipsilateral competing messages (SSI-ICM) or contralateral competing messages (SSI-CCM). The level of the competing message is often varied to give several message-to-competition ratios (MCR). People with lesions of the brainstem typically show large differences in ear performance under the ICM paradigm. Furthermore, in the presence of a brainstem lesion, the ICM condition shows a greater performance deficit than the CCM condition. Under the CCM condition, people with cortical lesions show reduced performance when the target message is contralateral to the lesion.

Staggered Spondaic Word Test

Another common central auditory test is the Staggered Spondaic Word Test (SSW) (Katz, 1962). This test consists of pairs of spondees with staggered onsets to each ear but overlapped in time for part of the spondee. The spondees are temporally overlapped in presentation so that the final syllable of the first word is presented to one ear at the same time as the initial syllable of the second word is presented to the other ear. Poor scores on this test suggest a cortical lesion on the side opposite the reduced score.

Other Central Tests

Other central auditory measurements include presenting digits to both ears simultaneously (the Dichotic Digits Test) (Dirks, 1964b), alternating speech between the ears, and temporally compressing PB words (Bocca, 1958). The typical finding of these evaluations is reduced performance contralateral to the side of the lesion.

None of the behavioral tests for central auditory abnormality alone is sensitive and specific enough to allow an accurate diagnosis of all central auditory nervous system disorders. It is therefore a clinically accepted procedure to give these evaluations as part of a test battery.

Objective Measurements of Central Auditory Dysfunction

Important clinical information can be obtained from objective measurements of the status of the central auditory structures. Evoked potential testing provides an objective, noninvasive technique to measure the transmission of neural information through the auditory system. The ABR provides a sensitive measurement of the transmission of information through the level of the midbrain.

Auditory Evoked Potentials

ABR findings depend on the location of the lesion. An abnormality in the lower brainstem would likely lead to normal latencies for wave I and wave II, with a prolonged latency or absence of later wave peaks (wave III, wave V). The interpeak latencies of waves III through V and I through V would also likely be longer than normal. A lesion in the upper brainstem would likely cause an absence of or an increase in the absolute latency of waves after wave III. A diffuse brainstem lesion may lead to an absence of all waves beyond wave I.

It should be noted that brainstem lesions also can cause abnormalities in the early waves (I and II). If these waves are generated along the acoustic nerve, how can brainstem abnormality affect them? This may be explained in the case of a space-occupying lesion. For example, a neoplasm may displace the brainstem enough to cause a disruption in the transmission of information along cranial nerve VIII.

Middle Latency Responses

Although ABR testing is extremely sensitive to disease of the midbrain, it is not sensitive to dysfunction in the higher structures of the auditory nervous system. There are, however, evoked potential measurements that are sensitive to dysfunction in the higher centers. The Auditory Middle Latency Response (AMLR) (Fifer & Sierra-Irizarry, 1988) evaluation is performed in much the same way as ABR testing. The listener is alert but inactive, and a series of 1000 to 2000 clicks or tone bursts are presented to average a clear AMLR. In addition to information about the transmission of auditory information through upper brainstem and auditory cortical structures, this test also provides information about low-frequency hearing sensitivity (Fifer & Sierra-Irizarry, 1988). For this reason, AMLR is often used for audiologic purposes in conjunction with ABR evaluations, but the listener must be alert and cooperative. The generator sites for the AMLR in the central auditory system include the auditory cortex and perhaps upper brainstem structures.

Late Auditory Potentials

Late-occurring potentials are called *late evoked responses* (LER) or *late latency responses* (LLR). The late auditory potentials can be observed on an electroencephalogram (EEG) at a latency between 70 and 500 msec. There are multiple generator sites for these potentials throughout the central nervous system. Although there are a number of these late-occurring potentials, only a selection of them are described in this section.

In response to an auditory stimulus, a negative wave (*N1*) occurs at approximately 100 msec. This is a rather complex wave with several components, each sensitive to such things as the physical features of the stimulus and the general state of the listener (Naatanen & Picton, 1987). The *P2* (or P200) is a positive wave that occurs approximately 200 msec after presentation of the auditory stimulus.

A late potential that occurs only under special circumstances and has a peak that is large in magnitude and occurs approximately 300 msec after stimulus presentation is termed *P300*. This waveform seems to be related to the listener's recognition of an infrequently occurring stimulus (Kibbe-Michel et al, 1986). Processes of attention, auditory discrimination, memory, and semantic expectancy seem to be associated with the generation of the P300. This wave may be a neural correlate of several cognitive processes. The disadvantage of these late potentials for clinical use is the same as for the AMLR; they are state-dependent and the subject must be alert and cooperative. The subject's state limits the use of these measurements for some people for whom they are needed most.

EXPECTED CLINICAL FINDINGS

A large number of measurements may be used to evaluate the status of the auditory system. These tests are not given in isolation but are performed as part of a test battery. Each of these measurements has some disadvantages (low sensitivity, low specificity, long administration time). This section summarizes the expected clinical results of the tests previously described. The summaries are grouped according to type of hearing disorder.

Normal Auditory System

Test Results

Pure-tone air-conduction thresholds for normal hearing are found at 20 dB HL or better from 250 Hz to 8000 Hz. Pure-tone bone-conduction thresholds approximate air-conduction thresholds; they do not vary from the air-conduction findings by more than 10 dB at any frequency, and the bone-conduction thresholds are also less than 20 dB HL.

Speech-recognition thresholds are found at 20 dB HL or lower levels. The SRT is typically found within approximately 7 dB of the two- and three-frequency

PTAs. Speech recognition scores range from 90 percent to 100 percent at normal conversational levels (typically 45 to 50 dB HL). An increase in presentation level beyond PBmax is not associated with a reduction in speech identification (there is no appreciable rollover).

On otoscopic examination, the external auditory meatus is free of obstruction. A small amount of cerumen may be visible. The canal skin should be free of inflammation or discharge. The tympanic membrane should be opaque and pearl-gray. There should not be an obvious retraction, a fluid meniscus, or bubbles behind the tympanic membrane. An area of reflected light is seen in the inferior anterior quadrant. This is called the cone of light. The manubrium of the malleus and possibly the long process of the incus should be partially visible behind the tympanic membrane.

Immittance results indicate a pressure peak that occurs between +100 and −150 daPa (Type A tympanogram) and a normal static admittance. The ear canal volume ranges between 0.5 cc and 1.6 cc. The ear canal volumes of the two ears typically are within 20 percent of each other. A marked disparity in ear canal volumes between the ears may be indicative of foreign matter in the ear canal or a perforation in the tympanic membrane. Abnormally large or small volumes may provide diagnostically useful information.

Acoustic stapedial reflexes using pure-tone stimuli are elicited in both ears at approximately 70 to 105 dB HL. If broadband stimuli are used, the reflexes typically are seen at 15 to 20 dB lower stimulus levels. There is no decay in the reflex if the stimulus is continuously presented for 10 to 30 seconds. Further testing is done only if results or history indicate a need for special testing.

Central auditory tests show no reduction in performance. The listener responds within normal limits when the signal is acoustically degraded, mixed with noise, or presented with a competing stimulus either ipsilaterally or contralaterally.

Evoked potentials generated from sites in the central auditory pathways are expected to be within normal limits. Evoked potential testing shows normal wave morphology, absolute latencies, and interpeak latencies.

Intervention

There is no indication for medical intervention or aural rehabilitation for a person with a normally functioning auditory system.

Conductive Auditory Impairment

Test Results

Pure-tone air-conduction thresholds are elevated in the ear with the conductive abnormality. The slope of the audiogram varies. If the conductive loss is due to a lesion that stiffens the conductive apparatus, the air-conduction auditory sensitivity tends to be poorer in the low frequencies (a rising configuration). If the disorder tends to increase the mass of the conductive apparatus, the air-conduction thresholds tend to be worse in the high frequencies (a sloping or falling configuration). Another common pattern is a flat configuration. The rising and flat configurations are the most common patterns associated with a conductive hearing loss. The severity of the hearing loss does not exceed 60 dB HL.

Little or no loss of sensitivity is associated with a conductive hearing loss at testing by means of bone conduction. There may be a slight elevation of bone-conduction thresholds at certain frequencies depending on the cause of the conductive hearing loss. For example, otosclerosis (Chapter 3) typically is associated with increased (poorer) bone-conduction thresholds, particularly at 2000 Hz. The change in bone-conduction thresholds from normal is not due to cochlear abnormality, but rather is associated with the loss of the inertial component (the ossicles tend to lag behind the vibrations of the skull) of bone-conduction hearing.

The Weber test lateralizes to the ear with the greater air-bone gap. A unilateral conductive loss lateralizes to the ear with the loss. If there is a bilateral conductive loss, there is often (but not always) a lateralization to the ear with the poorer air-conduction sensitivity (greater air-bone gap). The Bing test is negative; the listener reports no change in the loudness of the stimulus when the ear with a conductive loss is occluded.

Tympanograms typically are abnormal. The abnormality in the tympanogram depends on the type of conductive abnormality. If the conductive loss is due to an occlusion in the outer ear, the tympanogram is flat, and there is a low ear canal volume. If the loss is due to a perforation in the tympanic membrane, the tympanogram is flat, and there is a large ear canal volume. A stiffening of the conductive mechanism is often associated with low static admittance. If the system is flaccid, perhaps because of a disarticulation of the ossicles, there will be abnormally high static admittance. Eustachian tube dysfunction or otitis media may initially be associated with a pressure peak at an abnormally low value. If fluid is present (otitis media with effusion), the tympanogram typically is flat.

Acoustic reflexes in the affected ear are usually abnormal when a conductive loss is present. The ear with the conductive loss determines which acoustic reflex is abnormal. In bilateral conductive impairment, reflexes for both ears may be absent.

The otoscopic examination may be normal or abnormal. If the conductive loss is due to a problem in the outer ear or tympanic membrane, the abnormality can typically be visualized. Fluid in the middle ear space may be visible through the tympanic membrane; a retracted tympanic membrane or a reddened, inflamed, or bulging tympanic membrane may be observed and reported. Many times a conductive hearing loss due to dysfunction in the middle ear space does not reveal abnormalities seen during an otoscopic examination.

SRTs should be in agreement with PTAs. Speech discrimination testing reveals normal performance at higher than normal presentation levels. That is, when the speech stimuli are presented at comparable SLs, a person with a conductive hearing loss shows the same performance-intensity function as a person with normal hearing. PBmax is 90 to 100 percent, and there is no appreciable rollover. An ear with a conductive hearing loss does not typically have test results for recruitment or adaptation.

Evoked potential testing, if administered for reasons other than the conductive hearing loss, shows normal wave morphology, absolute latencies, and inter-peak latencies at an SL comparable to that of a person with normal hearing. That is, the waveform latency is comparable in appearance to that of a person with normal hearing, but the presentation levels are higher than those used to test a person with normal hearing. This is due to the attenuation of the signal by the conductive hearing loss.

Behavioral central auditory assessments are not routinely administered in the evaluation of a conductive hearing loss. If behavioral tests are administered, the hearing loss shows normal, symmetric results.

Intervention

A conductive hearing loss necessitates both a medical and an audiologic referral. Treatment can involve surgical intervention, medication, monitoring of hearing status, or a combination of these.

Sensory Impairment

Test Results

Pure-tone air-conduction thresholds associated with a cochlear impairment are elevated. A loss of sensitivity also is found by bone conduction. The magnitude of the loss while testing by air conduction and bone conduction does not differ greatly. No air-bone gap is apparent.

The configuration of the auditory impairment may be of any shape, including rising, flat, trough-shaped, falling, or precipitously falling. In general, most sensory losses are associated with poorer hearing in the high frequencies. The severity of the sensory loss may also vary according to the extent of damage to the sensory structures. A relatively minor, isolated dysfunction leads to a mild loss in a restricted frequency range. Extensive cochlear damage is associated with a severe or profound loss of hearing through a wide range of frequencies.

The other clinical findings associated with a cochlear loss include an overall reduction in speech recognition or discrimination. In other words, PBmax is poorer than for a person with a conductive hearing loss or with normal auditory function. The magnitude of the reduction in speech understanding depends on the scope and severity of the impairment (because of the amount of distortion to the incoming speech signal imposed by the damage to the cochlea). A person with a mild cochlear loss may not experience a reduction in speech understanding, whereas a person with a severe or profound loss likely has very poor speech understanding. An increase in stimulus level above PBmax likely is associated with slight rollover, but not to the extent seen with a lesion that involves the acoustic nerve or the brainstem.

SRTs are elevated to levels comparable with pure-tone thresholds. A cochlear hearing loss is associated with a Type A (normal) tympanogram. For example, the peak admittance is from +100 to −150 daPa and the static admittance is normal. The peak gradient is typically normal, and the ear canal volume ranges from 0.4 to 1.7 cc. The canal volumes are similar between the ears. During an otoscopic examination the tympanic membrane and external auditory meatus appear to be normal.

Acoustic stapedial reflexes can vary according to the severity of the hearing loss. Acoustic reflexes can often be elicited with a sensory loss that is mild to moderately severe. The level at which reflexes are found may be in the range of values given for people with normal hearing even though the person with a sensory loss has increased absolute auditory thresholds. Thus, the reflexes may be elicited at a normal HL and a reduced SL. This pattern of acoustic reflexes (elicited at a reduced SL) is a strong indicator of a cochlear hearing loss. If the hearing loss is severe to profound, reflexes often cannot be elicited during stimulation of the impaired ear. A large amount of acoustic reflex decay is not associated with a cochlear hearing impairment. The Weber test lateralizes away from an ear with a sensory impairment (toward the better cochlea). When the Bing test is administered, the listener reports a change in the stimulus when the ear is occluded. This finding indicates that an occlusion effect (and therefore a conductive hearing loss) is not present in the ear.

Electroacoustic test results for cochlear hearing impairment are particularly informative. Otoacoustic emissions typically cannot be elicited at the frequencies of impairment from an ear with a cochlear loss. ECoG shows alterations in the evoked waveforms. The ABR shows an increase in the absolute latency of the wave peaks at low presentation levels. The absolute latencies approach normal values as the presentation level increases. However, the latency observed depends on the degree of loss and configuration. Adaptation of a continuous pure-tone signal (tone-decay test) occurs but does not exceed 20 dB. Thus, cochlear losses are associated with either normal adaptation (no threshold change) or a small amount of adaptation (5 to 25 dB).

Intervention

Several treatments are available for managing sensory hearing loss. Amplification (Chapter 7), assistive listening devices (Chapter 8), cochlear implants (Chapter 9), speech therapy and auditory and visual training (Chapter 10) are available for people with hearing losses.

Mixed Hearing Loss

The clinical implications for a person with a mixed hearing loss are a combination of the results for a conductive and a sensorineural loss that exist in the same ear.

Test Results

The behavioral or objective test results are the same as for a sensory impairment, but the responses are obtained at higher intensity levels because of the attenuating characteristics of the conductive component. An air-bone gap is found during pure-tone testing. Immittance findings are consistent with a conductive loss.

Intervention

Medical or surgical intervention can be effective for the conductive aspect of the mixed auditory impairment. However, it is important to understand that a sensory or neural loss continues to exist after the conductive hearing loss is treated. Therefore, rehabilitative efforts, including amplification, auditory training, visual training, and environmental modifications are appropriate for these patients even after medical and surgical intervention.

Neural Disease

A neural auditory impairment stems from dysfunction along the eighth cranial nerve. This damage may be caused by viral disease, congenital factors, anoxic episodes, space-occupying lesions, ototoxicity, or a demyelinating disease. It often is not possible to determine with routine clinical tests whether a hearing loss is due to damage in the sensory or the neural components of the auditory system. The term sensorineural hearing loss is used for an auditory dysfunction that is not due to dysfunction in the conductive or central auditory structures, and it is not known whether the primary locus of the lesion is in the inner ear or along the acoustic nerve.

Test Results

As in a cochlear hearing loss, when pure tones are presented by means of air conduction and bone conduction, there is an elevation in absolute thresholds, and the thresholds do not differ considerably; there is no air-bone gap. The configuration for neural loss (as for sensory loss) may be of any shape. In general, neural losses are associated with poorer hearing in the high frequencies, particularly early in the onset of the disease. If the disorder is due to a space-occupying lesion (such as a vestibular schwannoma), the pure-tone results generally show a unilateral or asymmetric bilateral loss with a sloping audiometric contour. If the abnormality is due to a demyelinating condition such as multiple sclerosis, the severity of the auditory dysfunction may vary according to the activity and progression (exacerbation or remission) of the disease.

The neural loss shows Weber and Bing test results similar to those described for sensory impairment. The otoscopic examination reveals a normal tympanic membrane and external auditory meatus. The other clinical findings associated with a neural loss are similar to the cochlear loss and include an overall reduction in speech recognition or discrimination, often out of proportion to the degree of sensitivity loss. PBmax is lower than for a person with normal auditory function, or a conductive or sensory loss, and may be associated with a substantial reduction in speech understanding (rollover) as the stimulus level increases. A person with a mild neural loss may not experience a considerable reduction in speech understanding.

A neural hearing loss is associated with normal tympanometric and static admittance results, as found with a cochlear hearing loss in the previous sections. The most sensitive of the immittance results for a neural loss is the acoustic reflex. Acoustic stapedial reflex findings are generally a sensitive diagnostic tool to establish the presence of neural abnormality. Reflexes may be elicited at a higher than normal level during stimulation of the affected ear, but in many cases, reflexes are absent. The reflexes (if found) are elicited at lower presentation levels when broadband noise levels are used than when pure-tone stimuli are used. Strong diagnostic evidence of a neural abnormality is obtained when there is clinically significant reflex decay to unvarying stimulation. That is, if the reflex is elicited while the affected ear is stimulated, the reflex amplitude is reduced (decays) rapidly. A decay in reflex amplitude of 50 percent over 10 seconds of stimulation is consistent with neural disease.

Electroacoustic testing results for neural abnormality, particularly ABR and acoustic reflex threshold, provide the most sensitive and specific information. Otoacoustic emissions can be elicited at the frequencies of impairment from an ear with a neural loss. ECoG does not show alterations in the evoked waveforms. The ABR shows an increase in the absolute latency of wave I. If the neural abnormality is severe enough, the entire ABR beyond wave I may be obliterated. If the waves can be elicited, there is an increase in the interpeak latency of waves I through III, and possibly an increase in the latency of waves I through III. These findings are consistent with a reduction in neural transmission along the acoustic nerve.

The primary clinical findings that separate neural impairment from sensory impairment include abnormal adaptation, poor speech recognition, decreased speech understanding with increased intensity (rollover), and abnormal evoked potentials and acoustic reflexes.

Intervention

A neural hearing loss does not present a favorable prognosis for medical or surgical intervention. If the acoustic nerve bodies have died, no medical intervention can alleviate the hearing loss. If the neural abnormality is due to a space-occupying lesion along the acoustic nerve, the lesion can be surgically removed. This may lead to a total loss of auditory function in the affected ear. If the pathologic condition is related to a medical condition, such as meningitis, that is successfully treated medically, improvement in neural function can be expected.

Because of the poor prognosis for effective medical intervention in neural dysfunction, the emphasis is on aural rehabilitation, including amplification, auditory training, visual training, and developing an environment conducive to auditory communication (see Chapters 7 and 8). However, the prognosis for successful use of amplification may be poor because of the poor speech recognition often associated with neural abnormality.

Central Auditory Dysfunction

Tests of Peripheral Auditory Function

In general, a person with a dysfunction that is isolated in the central auditory structures and pathways does not demonstrate an auditory impairment when evaluated by traditional tests of peripheral auditory function. These people often report that communication in a quiet environment is possible but that communication in a degraded acoustic environment is difficult.

Pure-tone air- and bone-conduction sensitivity thresholds and SRT are normal (less than 20 dB HL). Speech recognition scores range from 90 to 100 percent at normal conversational levels (typically 45 to 50 dB HL). An increase in presentation level beyond PBmax is not associated with a reduction in speech identification (there is no appreciable rollover).

A person with a normal peripheral auditory system demonstrates the following immittance results. The tympanogram is Type A (normal). This is defined as a pressure peak that occurs between +100 and −175 daPa and the static admittance is normal. The ear canal volume ranges between 0.4 cc and 1.7 cc. The ear canal volumes of the two ears are within 20 percent of each other. A marked disparity in ear canal volumes between the ears may indicate foreign matter in the ear canal or a perforation of the tympanic membrane.

Acoustic stapedial reflexes using pure-tone stimuli are elicited in both ears at approximately 70 to 105 dB HL. A clinically significant finding for lower brainstem abnormality is normal reflexes in the ear that is stimulated (ipsilateral) and abnormal reflexes opposite the ear being stimulated (contralateral). This finding suggests an interruption in the transmission of auditory information at the level of the cochlear nuclei to the superior olivary complex. At otoscopic examination, the external auditory meatus and the tympanic membrane are healthy.

Tests of Central Auditory Function

Behavioral tests of central auditory function are likely to be abnormal. If a decrease in performance is found, the greatest decrement in performance is contralateral to the side of the lesion. The section on behavioral tests of central auditory function detailed the sensitivity and expected findings of several common clinical tests of central auditory function.

Evoked potentials may also be abnormal. Absence of or increased interpeak and absolute latencies of waves beyond wave II are found in the ABR if the dysfunction is in the brainstem. A dysfunction in higher auditory pathways and centers manifests itself as abnormalities in later-occurring potentials.

Intervention

If the central auditory disorder is due to an acute cerebral infarction, auditory performance improves as the neurologic symptoms subside. Most central auditory disturbances are not due to such a gross physiologic dysfunction, however. For most of these patients, medical treatment holds little promise of restoration of auditory function.

Many children who demonstrate abnormal function on central auditory evaluations show improved performance with physical maturation. It has been theorized that a large number of the central auditory disturbances demonstrated by children is related to a delay in the myelinization of the corpus callosum (a large bundle of nerve tracts that connect the cerebral hemispheres).

Because medical intervention is not effective for people with central auditory dysfunction, rehabilitative efforts are focused on the other aspects of aural rehabilitation. An improvement in the signal-to-noise ratio may improve communicative function. Modification of the signal-to-noise ratio can be obtained in one of three ways. One method is to increase the intensity of the signal. The second is to reduce the level of the background noise. The last is to increase the signal and to reduce the noise. Auditory-training and assistive-listening devices may be helpful to a person with a central auditory dysfunction, not because of the increase in the intensity level of the signal, but because of an improvement in the signal-to-noise ratio.

Visual training and auditory training may be helpful strategies. Modification of the environment to enhance visual information and reduce background noise is often an effective method to enhance communication. Management techniques for most types of hearing problems are described in Chapters 7 through 11 and may be useful with central auditory dysfunction (see Chapter 13).

REFERENCES

American National Standards Institute (1973). American national standard psychoacoustical terminology. ANSI S3.20-1973. New York: American National Standards Institute.

American National Standards Institute (1986). Methods for manual pure-tone threshold audiometry. ANSI S3.21-1978. New York: American National Standards Institute.

American National Standards Institute (1989). American national standards for audiometers. ANSI S3.6-1989. New York: American National Standards Institute.

American Speech-Language-Hearing Association (1978). Guidelines for acoustic immittance screening of middle-ear effusion. *Asha, 20,* 550-555.

American Speech-Language-Hearing Association (1988). Guidelines for determining threshold level for speech. *Asha, 20,* 88-89.

American Speech-Language-Hearing Association (1990a). Guidelines for audiometric symbols. *Asha, 32 (Suppl. 2)*, 25-30.

American Speech-Language-Hearing Association (1990b). Guidelines for screening for hearing impairments and middle ear disorders. *Asha, 32 (Suppl. 2)*, 17-24.

Bocca, E. (1958). Clinical aspects of cortical deafness. *Laryngoscope, 68,* 301-311.

Bocca, E., Calearo, E., & Cassinari, V. (1954). A new method for testing hearing in temporal lobe tumors. *Acta Otolaryngologica (Stockholm), 44,* 219-221.

Borg, E. (1973). On the neuronal organization of the acoustic middle ear reflex: A physiological and anatomical study. *Brain Research, 49,* 101-123.

Carhart, R. (1971). Observations of relations between thresholds for pure tones and for speech. *Journal of Speech and Hearing Disorders, 36,* 476-483.

Chaiklin, J. (1959). The relation among three selected auditory speech thresholds. *Journal of Speech and Hearing Research, 2,* 237-243.

Chaiklin, J. B. (1967). Interaural attenuation and cross-hearing in air-conditioned audiometry. *Journal of Auditory Research, 7,* 413-424.

Clark, J. (1981). Uses and abuses of hearing loss classification. *Asha, 23,* 493-500.

Davis, H., & Silverman, S. R. (1978). *Hearing and deafness* (4th ed.). New York: Holt, Rinehart & Winston.

Dirks, D. D. (1964a). Bone-conduction measurements. *Archives of Otolaryngology, 79,* 594-599.

Dirks, D. D. (1964b). Perception of dichotic and monaural verbal material and cerebral dominance for speech. *Acta Otolaryngologica (Stockholm), 58,* 773-80.

Egan, J. P. (1948). Articulation testing methods. *Laryngoscope, 58,* 855-991.

Eldert, M. A., & Davis, H. (1951). The articulation function of patients with conductive deafness. *Laryngoscope, 61,* 891-909.

Feldman, A. S. (1976). Tympanometry: Procedures, interpretation and variables. In A. S. Feldman & L. A. Wilber (Eds.), *Acoustic impedance and admittance: The measurement of middle ear function* (pp. 103-155). Baltimore: Williams & Wilkins.

Fifer, R. C., & Sierra-Irizarry, B. (1988). Clinical applications of the auditory middle latency response. *American Journal of Otology, 9,* 47-56.

Fowler, E. P. (1937). The diagnosis of diseases of the neural mechanism of hearing by the aid of sounds well above threshold. *Transactions of the American Otology Society, 27,* 207-219.

Goldstein, B. A., & Newman, C. W. (1985). Clinical masking: A decision-making process. In J. Katz (Ed.), *Handbook of clinical audiology* (3rd ed.) (pp. 170-201). Baltimore: Williams & Wilkins.

Goodman, A. (1965). Reference zero levels for pure-tone audiometer. *Asha, 7,* 262-263.

Green, D. S. (1985). Tone decay. In J. Katz (Ed.), *Handbook of clinical audiology* (3rd ed.) (pp. 304-318). Baltimore: Williams & Wilkins.

Griffiths, J. D. (1967). Rhyming minimal contrasts: A simplified diagnostic articulation test. *Journal of Acoustical Society of America, 42,* 236-241.

Haskins, H. A. (1949). A phonetically balanced test of speech discrimination for children. Evanston: Northwestern University. Thesis.

Hirsh, I. J. (1952). *The measurement of hearing.* New York: McGraw-Hill.

Hirsh, I. J., Davis, H., Silverman, S. R., Reynolds, E. G., Eldert, E., & Benson, R. W. (1952). Development of materials for speech audiometry. *Journal of Speech and Hearing Disorders, 17,* 321-337.

Ivey, R. G. (1969). Tests of CNS auditory function. Fort Collins: Colorado State University. Thesis.

Jacobson J. T., & Hyde, M. L. (1985). An introduction to auditory evoked potentials. In J. Katz (Ed.), *Handbook of clinical audiology* (3rd ed.) (pp. 496-533). Baltimore· Williams & Wilkins.

Jerger, J. (1962). The SISI test. *International Audiology, 1,* 246-247.

Jerger, J. F., Harford, E., Clemis, J., & Alford, B. (1974). The acoustic reflex in VIIIth nerve disorders. *Archives of Otolaryngology, 99,* 409-413.

Jerger, J. F., & Hayes, D. (1980). Diagnostic applications of impedance audiometry: Middle ear disorder, sensorineural disorder. In J. F. Jerger & J. L. Northern (Eds.). *Clinical impedance audiometry.* Acton: American Electromedics.

Jerger, J., & Jerger, S. (1971). Diagnostic significance of PB words functions. *Archives of Otolaryngology, 93,* 573-580.

Jerger, J. F., Jerger, S., & Neely, J. G. (1983). The neurological evaluation. *Seminars in Hearing, 4,* 81-178.

Jerger, S. (1980). Diagnostic application of impedance audiometry in central auditory disorders. In J. F. Jerger & J. L. Northern (Eds.), *Clinical impedance audiometry* (2nd ed.). Acton: American Electromedics.

Jerger, S., & Jerger, J. (1983). The evaluation of diagnostic audiometric tests. *Audiology, 33,* 93-98.

Jewett, D. L., & Williston, J. S. (1971). Auditory-evoked far fields averaged from the scalp of humans. *Brain, 94,* 681-696.

Johnson, J. J., Bagi, P., & Elberling, C. (1983). Evoked emission from the human ear. III. Findings in neonates. *Scandinavian Audiology, 12,* 17-24.

Kalikow, D. N., Stevens, K. N., & Elliot, L. L. (1977). Development of a test of speech intelligibility in noise using sentence materials with controlled word predictability. *Journal of Acoustical Society of America, 61,* 1337-1351.

Kaplan, H., Gladstone, V., & Lloyd, L. (1993). *Audiometric interpretation: A manual of basic audiometry.* Needham Heights: Allyn and Bacon.

Katz, J. (1962). The use of staggered spondaic words for assessing the integrity of the central auditory nervous system. *Journal of Auditory Research, 2,* 327-337.

Kemp, D. T. (1978). Stimulated acoustic emissions from within the human auditory system. *Journal of the Acoustical Society of America, 64,* 1386-1391.

Kibbe-Michel, K., Verkest, S. B., Gollegly, K. M., & Musiek, F. E. (1986). Late auditory potentials and the P300. *Hearing Instruments, 37,* 22-24.

Kopra, L. L., & Blosser, D. (1968). Effects of method of measurement on most comfortable loudness for speech. *Journal of Speech and Hearing Research, 11,* 497-508.

Margolis, R. H., & Shanks, J. E. (1985). Tympanometry. In J. Katz (Ed.), *Handbook of clinical audiology* (3rd ed.) (pp. 438-475). Baltimore: Williams & Wilkins.

Martin, F. (1994). *Introduction to audiology* (5th ed.). Englewood Cliffs: Prentice Hall.

Martin, F. (1991). *Introduction to audiology* (4th ed.). Englewood Cliffs: Prentice Hall.

Martin, F. N., & Dowdy, L, K. (1986). A modified spondee threshold procedure. *Journal of Auditory Research, 26,* 115-119.

Matzger, J. (1959). Two methods for the assessment of central auditory function in cases of brain disease. *Annals of Otology, Rhinology and Laryngology, 68,* 1155-1197.

Metz, O. (1946). The acoustic impedance measured on normal and pathological ears. *Acta Otolaryngologica (Suppl), 63,* 397-405.

Metz, O. (1952). Threshold of reflex contractions of muscles of middle ear and recruitment of loudness. *Archives of Otolaryngology, 55,* 536-543.

Moller, A. R., Jannetta, P. J., & Moller, M. B. (1981). Neural generators of the brainstem evoked responses: Results for human intracranial recordings. *Annals of Otology, Rhinology and Laryngology, 90,* 591-596.

Naatanen, R., & Picton, T. (1987). The N1 wave of the human electric and magnetic response to sound. *Psychophysiology, 24,* 375-425.

Owens, E., & Schubert, E. D. (1977). Development of the California Consonant Test. *Journal of Speech and Hearing Research, 30,* 463-474.

Reger, S. N. (1936). Differences in loudness response of normal and hard-of-hearing ears at intensity levels slightly above threshold. *Annals of Otology, Rhinology and Laryngology, 45,* 1029-1039.

Rintelmann, W. (Ed.) (1991). *Hearing assessment* (2nd ed.). Austin: Pro-Ed.

Ross, M., & Lerman, J. (1970). A picture identification test for hearing impaired child. *Journal of Speech and Hearing Research, 13,* 44-53.

Speaks, C., & Jerger, J. (1965). Method for measurement of speech identification. *Journal of Speech and Hearing Research, 8,* 185-194.

Tillman, T. W., & Carhart, R. (1966). An expanded test for speech discrimination utilizing CNC monosyllabic words: Northwestern University Auditory Test No. 6. (Technical Report No. SAM-TR-66-55). Brooks Air Force Base: USAF School of Aerospace Medicine.

Tonndorf, J. (1972). Bone conduction. In J. V. Tobias (Ed.), *Foundation of modern auditory theory.* New York: Academic Press.

Yantis, P. (1985). Pure tone air-conduction testing. In J. Katz (Ed.), *Handbook of clinical audiology* (3rd ed.) (pp. 153-169). Baltimore: Williams & Wilkins.

SUGGESTED READING

Bess, F., & Humes, L. (1990). *Audiology: The fundamentals.* Baltimore: Williams & Wilkins.

Jacobson, J., & Northern, J. (1991). *Diagnostic audiology.* Austin: Pro-Ed.

Jerger, J., & Jerger, S. (1981). *Auditory disorders: A manual for clinical intervention.* Boston: Little, Brown.

Katz, J. (ed.) (1994). *Handbook of clinical audiology* (4th ed.). Baltimore: Williams & Wilkins.

Newby, H., & Popelka, G. (1992). *Audiology* (6th ed.). Englewood Cliffs: Prentice Hall.

Northern, J. (1984). *Hearing disorders* (2nd ed.). Boston: Little, Brown.

Rose, D. (Ed.) (1978). *Audiological assessment* (2nd ed.). Englewood Cliffs: Prentice Hall.

Silman, S., & Silverman, C. (1991). *Auditory diagnosis: Principles and applications.* San Diego: Academic Press.

GLOSSARY

Adaptation   The gradual fading away of the perception of a signal.

Air-conduction testing   Tests that measurement the integrity of the entire auditory pathway. The stimuli are presented under headphones.

Air-bone gap   The arithmetical difference between air-conduction and bone-conduction thresholds with air-conduction thresholds at higher levels.

Audiogram   A graph of auditory threshold versus frequency. Threshold level (in dB) is the Y axis. Frequency (in Hz) is the X axis.

Auditory brainstem response (ABR)   An averaged electrical wave generated from auditory structures form the acoustic nerve, through the brainstem, to the midbrain. An extremely sensitive test for brainstem abnormalities and acoustic nerve dysfunction.

Bone-conduction testing   Testing of auditory function that bypasses the outer and middle ear and indicates the status of the cochlea and the acoustic nerve.

Cochlear implants   Medical devices that consist of very fine wires that are surgically implanted into the spiral ganglion. Used for a person with a severe to profound sensory hearing loss that is not remedied by ear-level amplification.

Compliance   The ease of energy transmission through the auditory system.

Conductive hearing loss   An auditory disorder caused by dysfunction in the outer or middle ear.

Difference limen   The smallest change in a stimulus that can be detected.

Electrocochleography (ECoG)   A test that measurements electrical activity in the cochlea by means of a small electrode placed either in the ear canal or through the tympanic membrane and touching the promontory of the cochlea.

Evoked otoacoustic emissions   A technique under investigation for possible clinical use whereby sounds are presented to the ear and acoustic responses from the cochlea are measured and averaged.

Immittance   All measurements of energy transmission through the conductive mechanism of the ear, including admittance, impedance, and compliance.

Impedance   Resistance to the flow of acoustic energy through the auditory system.

Interaural attenuation   The decrease in the amplitude of the signal as it crosses across the head to the contralateral ear.

Mixed hearing loss   A coexistent conductive and sensorineural hearing loss.

Most comfortable loudness level (MCL)   The level that a listener prefers to listen to speech.

Occlusion effect   An increase in loudness of bone-conducted sounds associated with a conductive hearing loss.

Performance-intensity function   A graph of speech discrimination score and the presentation level (in dB).

Peripheral auditory pathway   The outer ear, middle ear, inner ear, or any combination of these three regions of the auditory system.

Phonemic balance   The proportion of sounds based on the occurrence of sounds in connected speech.

Phonetic balance (PB)   Occurrence of phonetic elements in stimulus words in a list in the same proportion as occurrence in a given language.

Phonetic balance maximum (PBmax)   The stimulus presentation level associated with maximum word identification performance.

Pure-tone average   The arithmetical average of the pure-tone thresholds at 500, 1000, and 2000 Hz.

Pure-tone average (two frequency)   The arithmetical average of the better two thresholds at 500, 1000, and 2000 Hz.

Rollover   A reduction in speech understanding with an increase in presentation level.

Sensorineural hearing loss   Hearing loss caused by damage in the inner ear or eighth cranial nerve.

Sensory hearing loss   A hearing loss caused by cochlear dysfunction.

Slope (audiogram)   A description of the relative magnitude of auditory impairment at various frequencies.

Speech detection threshold (SDT)   The lowest intensity level at which a person can detect the presence of speech a specified percentage of time.

Speech discrimination testing   Perception of the difference between two similar speech stimuli.

Speech recognition (identification) testing   Evaluation of the accuracy of speech identification, usually at a suprathreshold level.

Speech recognition threshold (SRT)   The lowest level that a listener can understand or identify speech stimuli 50 percent of the time.

Spondees   Two-syllable words with equal emphasis on both syllables.

Static compliance   An indication of the overall mobility of the tympanic membrane–ossicular chain.

Stapedial reflex testing   Small changes in the immitance of the conductive mechanism associated with reflexive contraction of a muscle in the middle ear when the listener is exposed to sound of moderate or high intensity.

Stenger effect   The phenomenon that occurs when stimuli that are the same frequency and phase reach both cochleae but there is a difference in the amplitude of the stimuli. The stimulus is heard only on the side of the cochlea receiving the stimulus of higher amplitude.

Suprathreshold   Presentation levels above auditory threshold.

Threshold   The lowest intensity level at which a person can detect the presence of a stimulus a certain percentage of the time.

Tympanometry   Graphing of the transmission of energy through the ear at various air pressures.

Uncomfortable loudness level   The intensity at which speech is too loud to be tolerable for more than a short time.

7

Hearing Aids

Stephanie A. Davidson

Although speech-language pathologists, educators, and health care professionals are not directly involved in the selection and fitting of hearing aids, they routinely encounter people fit with hearing aids. Speech-language pathologists, in particular, need to be familiar with hearing aids because they are commonly regarded as the speech *and hearing* specialist in the school system or nursing home since an audiologist is rarely on staff. Even when an audiologist is available, speech-language pathologists, educators, and related health care professionals may be in a better position to spot a problem because of their ongoing relationship with the client, student, or patient. During a hearing aid fitting session, for example, the hearing aid user (or the hearing aid user's guardian) is given large amounts of information over a short period of time concerning hearing aid care, use, and maintenance. Many times the hearing aid user does not completely understand this information or simply cannot remember it all. Speech-language pathologists, educators, and health care professionals may be in a good position to review this information with the hearing aid user or to answer questions that the user has. Speech-language pathologists, health care professionals, and teachers may also be called on to assist in the selection of hearing aids. An audiologist may request input concerning a child's performance with hearing aids during daily activities because it often takes close observation by clinicians, parents, and teachers before final amplification decisions are made. Finally, and perhaps most common, speech-language pathologists, teachers, and health care professionals may be asked to perform hearing aid listening checks and basic troubleshooting of hearing aids.

This chapter is designed to acquaint the speech-language pathologist, teacher, and health care professional with general information concerning hearing aid candidacy, hearing aid and earmold style, electroacoustic characteristics of hearing aids, and the application of digital technology to hearing aids. Procedures used by dispensers in typical hearing aid evaluations to select appropriate amplification and to verify its benefit are described. In addition, this chapter discusses listener adjustment to hearing aids, as well as hearing aid checks, maintenance, and basic troubleshooting.

THE PURPOSE OF HEARING AIDS

The selection of appropriate amplification is central to the aural rehabilitation program for most people with a hearing loss. The purpose of a hearing aid for most people is to increase speech intelligibility by making as much of the speech spectrum as possible audible without making it so loud that it becomes uncomfortable. The hearing aids available today are highly sophisticated instruments. Problems that have plagued hearing aid users in the past (ie, problems understanding speech in background noise and the unpleasantness of loud sounds) have been lessened. Hearing aid users who complain of difficulty understanding speech in noise should be referred to an audiologist to discuss some of the newer circuitry available in hearing aids (described later in this chapter) or assistive listening devices (described in Chapter 8). Hearing aid users who complain that their hearing aid makes sound uncomfortably loud should also be referred to an audiologist; the hearing aids available today can be adjusted so that this does not occur.

Although many advances have been made in hearing aid performance, the hearing aid user must understand that hearing aids do not bring hearing sensitivity or speech understanding ability back to normal. Many newspaper, television, and radio advertisements suggest that a particular brand of hearing aid will remove background noise or make hearing normal again—such misleading advertising is simply not true. The application of advanced technologies has greatly improved the clarity and quality of the signal from today's hearing aids, but limitations still exist. Some limitations are imposed by the small size of the hearing aid (stereo quality sound is difficult to obtain in a device worn at ear level), but perhaps the biggest limitation is the impaired auditory system of the hearing aid user. Listeners with sensorineural hearing loss generally have reduced dynamic ranges (the range between the softest sound heard and the loudest sound tolerated) and also exhibit impaired frequency, intensity, and temporal resolving capabilities. These problems cannot be completely corrected with currently available hearing aids. Helping the potential hearing aid user have realistic expectations concerning hearing aid use is a crucial aspect of the rehabilitation process.

HEARING AID CANDIDACY

People with a hearing loss often ask how severe a hearing loss needs to become before a hearing aid should be considered. No standard audiometric criteria for hearing aid candidacy exist. A socially active person with a high reliance on oral communication may be troubled by a minimal hearing loss. On the other hand, a solitary person who does not rely on oral communication may not be bothered by even a moderate hearing loss. A host of other factors (eg, configuration of the loss; speech understanding ability; and the age, vocation, education, motivation, and financial resources of the client) also must be evaluated. Consequently, no simple audiometric rule can be applied to all people. A logical solution, then, is to involve the potential wearer in the decision-making process. The Vanderbilt Consensus Statement describes a hearing aid candidate as, "anyone who describes hearing difficulties in communicative situations" (Hawkins et al, 1991, p. 37).

Another question is, "Does there come a point when a hearing loss is so severe that a hearing aid would not be helpful?" As mentioned earlier, the selection and fitting of an appropriate amplification system is the most important component of the aural rehabilitation process for most people with a hearing loss. Most people, even with profound hearing losses, receive some auditory information when using amplification. Although hearing aids in these cases do not make speech intelligible in and of themselves, they may provide cues that aid in speechreading, resulting in greater ease of communication. Hearing aids may also assist in the detection of warning signals in cases of profound hearing loss. However, some people with severe to profound hearing losses, who technically might be able to make use of the information obtained from hearing aids, choose not to wear them. These people often make this choice because they identify themselves with the Deaf community and do not find auditory information necessary in their daily lives. Speech and hearing professionals should be respectful of these wishes. Of course, some people simply cannot benefit from auditory signals, no matter how intense. These people (as well as others who choose not to wear hearing aids) may be candidates for some of the assistive devices described in Chapter 8.

ELECTROACOUSTIC CHARACTERISTICS OF HEARING AIDS

Hearing aids are electroacoustic devices. The microphone of the hearing aid picks up an acoustic signal and changes it into an electrical signal analogous to the acoustic waveform. The resulting electrical signal is amplified and modified according to preset controls and sent to the hearing aid receiver. The receiver changes the amplified and modified electrical signal back into an acoustic signal, which is then delivered to the ear of the listener.

The electroacoustic characteristics of a hearing aid indicate the performance characteristics of that particular hearing aid. The electroacoustic characteristics of a hearing aid are measured during an electroacoustic analysis (EAA). The procedures used to perform an EAA are specified by the American National Standards Institute [ANSI] (1987) and are followed by manufacturers and hearing aid dispensers using specialized hearing aid analysis systems. In an EAA, the hearing aid is placed over a loudspeaker in a small sound-treated box and connected with a 2-cc coupler to a sound-measuring device. Precisely controlled signals are delivered to the hearing aid microphone through the loudspeaker, and the output from the hearing aid receiver is carefully measured and compared with the input. By comparing the difference between hearing aid input and hearing aid output, one can infer the hearing aid electroacoustic characteristics. An example of the results of an EAA is shown in Figure 7.1. An EAA is typically used to see if a hearing aid

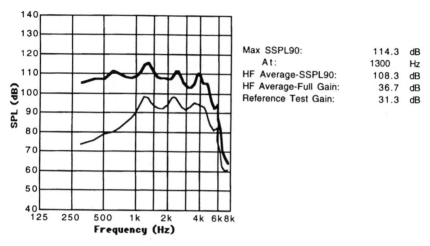

FIGURE 7.1 Results from an electroacoustic analysis of a hearing aid. The upper curve represents the saturation sound pressure level (SSPL90) of the hearing aid and the lower curve represents the frequency response of the hearing aid. The maximum output at a particular frequency can be determined by reading directly from the top curve. For example, the maximum output from the hearing aid at 1000 Hz is about 109 decibels sound pressure level (dB SPL). The gain of the hearing aid at a particular frequency can be calculated by determining the hearing aid output from the lower curve and subtracting 60 dB (the input level). For example, the gain at 1000 Hz for this hearing aid is 30 dB. The hearing aid analyzer calculates and numerically displays summary electroacoustic characteristics such as the maximum SSPL90, the high-frequency average (HFA) SSPL90, HFA full-on gain, and the reference test gain. These values are shown to the right of the graph.

is in proper working order. Hearing aids should be checked on a regular basis to determine if the measured electroacoustic characteristics match the manufacturer's specifications. Specifically, an EAA should be performed when a hearing aid is first fit, at regular hearing evaluations, or whenever a problem is suspected. Commonly measured electroacoustic characteristics and their relationship to hearing aid selection are as follows.

Gain and Frequency Response

The gain of a hearing aid represents the amount of amplification provided by the hearing aid and can be described in a number of ways. One way to describe the gain of the hearing aid is through a graphic representation of the gain across a range of frequencies. The resultant graph (the lower curve in Figure 7.l) is known as the *frequency response* of the hearing aid. Hearing aids amplify the frequency range between about 200 and 5000 Hz, although some newer hearing aids can amplify sounds through 7000 or 8000 Hz. Another way to describe gain is to define the gain at a particular frequency. In this case, gain is defined as the difference (in dB) between the input level and the output level at a particular frequency. Figure 7.1 shows the graph for a hearing aid with 30 dB of gain at 1000 Hz. This is the difference between the input level (60 dB SPL) and the output level (90 dB SPL) at 1000 Hz. Finally, gain can be described as the average amount of gain across a specified frequency range. ANSI standards call for the reporting of HFA gain. HFA gain is defined as the average of the gain at 1000, 1600, and 2500 Hz and allows for standardized comparisons in the amount of gain provided by different hearing aids or of the gain from the same hearing aid at different test times.

The amount of gain provided by a hearing aid depends on the volume control setting. Gain is measured with the volume control in two positions—a full-on position and a reference test position. The gain obtained with the volume wheel in the full-on position reflects the maximum amount of gain available from the hearing aid. The gain obtained with the volume wheel in the reference test position is a representation of the gain that can reasonably be expected from the hearing aid during actual use. Gain measurement obtained with the volume control in the full-on position is known as full-on gain. A measurement obtained with the volume control in the reference test position is known as reference test gain.

The amount of gain necessary for a particular client depends primarily on the degree of hearing loss; a greater hearing loss requires greater hearing aid gain. A general rule is that the amount of gain provided by the hearing aid should be approximately half of the degree of hearing loss (Lybarger, 1944). For example, a person with a 60 decibel hearing level (dB HL) threshold at 2000 Hz would require about 30 dB of gain at 2000 Hz. Adjustments to this rule are made to ensure that as much of the speech spectrum as possible becomes audible without becoming uncomfortably loud.

Saturation Sound Pressure Level

Hearing aids do not amplify sound in a linear manner indefinitely. All hearing aids reach a point where additional increases in input level do not result in additional increases in output level (ie, they are in saturation). This is a desirable feature; if hearing aids amplified all sounds equally, then loud sounds (eg, doors slamming, people shouting, and traffic noise) could become so intense that they would be uncomfortably loud to the client and could even potentially damage residual hearing. Consequently, all hearing aids have a method of limiting maximum output.

Currently available hearing aids use one of two methods to limit maximum output—either peak clipping or compression. Peak-clipping instruments (also known as linear instruments) amplify sound linearly until a preset level is reached. Above that level, the peaks of the acoustic waveform are clipped (ie, squared off), keeping the output below a predetermined level. Although this method is effective in limiting the output from the hearing aid, it adds unwanted distortion to the signal, which can be detrimental to speech understanding.

Compression instruments (also known as automatic gain control [AGC] instruments) use a different method to limit maximum output. In these instruments the gain of the hearing aid varies with input level. For low input levels, the gain of the hearing aid remains stable, but as input level increases, the gain decreases to keep the output level below a predetermined maximum output. Mueller et al (1984) suggested that compression instruments are preferable to peak-clipping instruments for most clients.

The SSPL90, also known as the maximum power output (MPO), is the highest SPL generated by a hearing aid, regardless of output limitation method. Because this measurement is made with a very high input level (90 dB SPL), it has come to be known as the SSPL90 of a hearing aid and can be defined in several ways. One definition is the maximum SSPL90, which is simply the maximum output level (at any frequency) from the hearing aid. In Figure 7.1, the maximum SSPL90 is 114 dB SPL. The SSPL90 curve (the upper curve in Figure 7.1) illustrates the maximum output throughout the operating range of the hearing aid. Finally, the HFA SSPL90 is the average of the SSPL90 values at 1000, 1600, and 2500 Hz.

The SSPL90 values appropriate for a particular client depend largely on the client's tolerance for loud sounds. Measurements of loudness discomfort levels (LDLs) should be obtained for each client before he or she is fit with a hearing aid. The LDLs can then be used to select and adjust a particular hearing aid so that the SSPL90 values obtained with the hearing aid are slightly below the levels reported as uncomfortably loud by the client.

Care should also be used in adjusting the SSPL90 setting to reduce the chance of further damage to the listener's auditory system. It is well known from experiments with humans and laboratory animals that prolonged exposure to high levels of sound can damage the inner ear. Consequently, one must consider the possibility that hearing aids that provide high output levels could cause noise-induced hearing loss.

Reviews of investigations with groups of clients suggest that hearing aid use is safe for most people (Mills, 1975; Ross & Lerman, 1967; Rintelmann & Bess, 1977), but several case reports of threshold deterioration directly related to hearing aid use have appeared in the literature (Rintelmann & Bess, 1977). Although dispensers and hearing aid users must put these isolated reports in perspective, because exaggerated concern could deprive children and adults of necessary amplification (Ross et al, 1991), the potential for damage does exist, and efforts to reduce the risk should be undertaken. Because high output levels may cause additional hearing loss in isolated instances, no hearing aid with a higher than necessary SSPL90 should be fit (Ross et al, 1991).

Rintelmann and Bess (1977) reported that some experts recommend limiting hearing aid output to 130 dB SPL. However, they also pointed out that the amount of hearing loss seems to be related to the potential for damage. People with mild to moderate hearing losses are at greater risk for threshold shift, and thus should be fit with hearing aids with a SSPL90 of less than 120 dB SPL. People with severe to profound hearing losses are at a lesser risk and may be able to tolerate output levels that approach the 130 dB SPL limit. In all cases, hearing reevaluations should be conducted on a regular basis; people fit with powerful hearing aids should undergo frequent reevaluations.

Other Electroacoustic Characteristics

A complete discussion of all the electroacoustic characteristics of hearing aids is beyond the scope of this chapter. However, a number of other characteristics are evaluated by the audiologist during an EAA. These features include measurements of harmonic distortion, equivalent input noise, telecoil strength; battery current drain; and compression characteristics. Further information on hearing aid electroacoustic characteristics and their measurement can be found in Staab and Lybarger (1994).

BATTERIES

All electronic hearing aids are powered by small, button-type batteries. If a hearing aid seems dead, the most likely cause is the battery—it may be dead, it may be the wrong size, or it may simply be placed in the hearing aid incorrectly. Hearing aid batteries are available in three different materials: mercury, zinc-oxide (commonly referred to as zinc-air), or silver-oxide. Silver-oxide batteries have a slightly higher voltage (resulting in slightly more gain and output from the hearing aid), but the high price of silver makes the cost of these batteries prohibitive for most people. Zinc-air and mercury batteries are relatively inexpensive and can be used interchangeably in most hearing aids. (Some hearing aid manufacturers still recommend mercury batteries for power hearing aids and hearing aids that will be used in humid weather [Shimon, 1992]). Although zinc-air and mercury batteries are equivalent in terms of powering the hearing aid, zinc-air batteries have several advantages over mercury batteries. First, each zinc-air battery lasts about twice as long as a mercury battery. This means increased convenience for the client because the battery does not have to be changed frequently. In addition, zinc-air batteries are not activated until the user pulls a piece of tape off the battery case, allowing air (which is an active ingredient) into the case. This means that the shelf life of zinc-air batteries is longer than that of mercury batteries, and the user is less likely to purchase a stale package. Finally, zinc-air batteries are safer for the environment than mercury batteries. Several states have legislation enacted or pending that bans mercury batteries or strictly regulates their disposal.

The life of a battery is highly variable, depending on a number of factors, including the power of the hearing aid, the hours of use per day, the type of battery, the size of the battery, and the type of circuitry incorporated into the hearing aid.

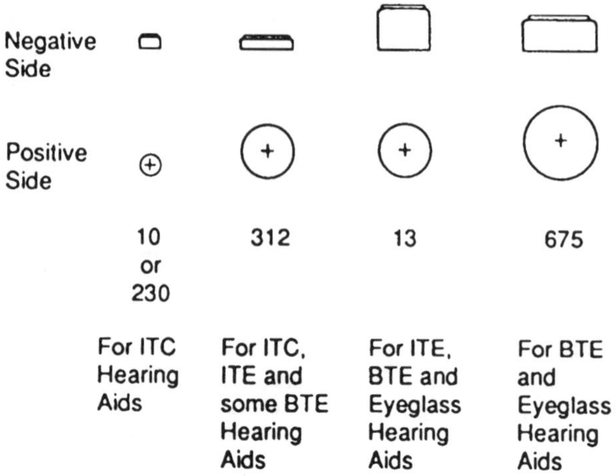

Negative Side	☐	▭	⬜	▭
Positive Side	⊕	⊕	⊕	⊕

FIGURE 7.2
The actual sizes and usual applications of commonly used hearing aid batteries. (ITC, in-the-canal; ITE, in-the-ear; BTE, behind-the-ear.)

(Reprinted with permission from Shimon, 1992.)

10 or 230	312	13	675
For ITC Hearing Aids	For ITC, ITE and some BTE Hearing Aids	For ITE, BTE and Eyeglass Hearing Aids	For BTE and Eyeglass Hearing Aids

An estimate of battery life for a particular hearing aid is shown on the hearing aid specification sheet. All hearing aid batteries are designed to produce a constant voltage and then die out relatively quickly. This design allows the gain of the hearing aid to remain constant throughout the life of the battery—a desirable feature. This means, however, that batteries can die with little warning. Consequently, hearing aid users should be told to have spare batteries handy at all times. Children should have spare batteries at school and adults should carry batteries with them. Any time a hearing aid seems to be malfunctioning, a fresh battery should be inserted as the first step in the troubleshooting process.

Hearing aid batteries are made by many different manufacturers and come in several different sizes. Although the manufacturer is not critical (batteries from any reputable manufacturer work with any hearing aid), the battery size is. Figure 7.2 shows the four commonly used battery sizes. As is the case with any electronic instrument, the hearing aid will not function unless an appropriately sized battery is inserted correctly (ie, the positive and negative poles are correctly aligned).

Batteries are easily obtained. They can be purchased in a variety of places, such as grocery stores, drug stores, or electronics stores, or through mail-order services (eg, group purchases through the American Association of Retired Persons [AARP]). Many hearing aid dispensers mail batteries to their clients on an as-needed basis. Battery safety must be emphasized to all hearing aid users and family members. Batteries that are swallowed or lodged in the ear canal or nasal passages are serious health hazards. Unfortunately, many cases of battery ingestion are reported each year. In some cases the batteries were mistaken for medication by older adults, but in most cases young children put the small batteries in their mouths. Adults must be instructed to keep the batteries separate from medications and out of the reach and view of children. Many hearing aids are available with child-resistant battery compartments. This option should be explained to all users and strongly recommended to the parents of children who wear hearing aids. In

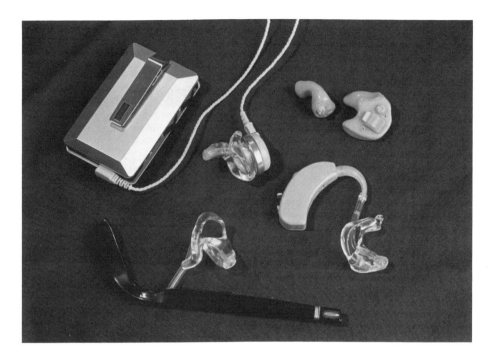

FIGURE 7.3 The five currently available hearing aid styles. Clockwise from upper left: body style, in-the-canal (ITC), in-the-ear (ITE), behind-the-ear (BTE), and eyeglass style.

the case of accidental ingestion of batteries (or the lodging of batteries in the ear canal or nasal passages), users should be instructed to proceed to an emergency room immediately. Recommended treatment procedures are available from the National Battery Hotline (202-625-3333).

HEARING AID STYLES

The following five styles of hearing aids are currently available: body, eyeglass, behind-the-ear (BTE), in-the-ear (ITE), and in-the-canal (ITC). Figure 7.3 illustrates each style of hearing aid, and Figure 7.4 depicts the percentage of 1992 market accounted for by each style of hearing aid (Kirkwood, 1992). ITE hearing aids are the most popular, accounting for about 56 percent of the United States market. ITC hearing aids are rapidly gaining in popularity and currently account for about 25 percent of sales. BTE hearing aids make up just under 20 percent of the market. Eyeglass and body-style hearing aids are used infrequently and account for only a small percentage of the market (less than 1 percent each).

Although the outer dimensions of these hearing aids differ dramatically from one another, the internal components are remarkably similar. All hearing aids contain a microphone to change acoustic energy into electrical energy, an amplifier

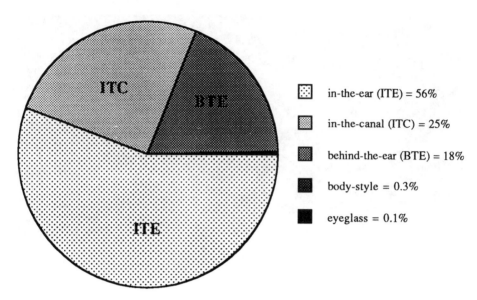

FIGURE 7.4 The percentage of the United States market accounted for by each style of hearing aid.

(Adapted from Newby and Popelka, 1992, and Kirkwood, 1992.)

to increase the amplitude of the electrical signal, and a receiver to change the electrical signal back into an acoustic signal, which is then delivered to the listener's ear. Hearing aids also require a small battery to power the instrument. Most hearing aids contain a user-adjustable volume control and many include other features that can be ordered and adjusted by the audiologist. As might be expected, the larger the instrument (ie, BTE vs ITE vs ITC), the greater the number of special features that can be ordered.

Body Aids

Body hearing aids are lightweight and about half the size of an audio cassette. They can be worn clipped onto clothing, in a shirt pocket, or in a special harness that can be worn over or under clothing. The microphone, amplifier, battery, and controls are located within the case of the body aid, and the receiver is snapped into a receiver-type earmold and worn at ear level. A wire connects the receiver to the case of the hearing aid.

Until recently, body aids provided considerably more gain and a broader frequency response than the other styles of hearing aids. Consequently, they were required for people with profound hearing losses. This is no longer true. BTE hearing aids now provide a large amount of gain over a broad range of frequencies;

most people with profound hearing losses choose the BTE style over the bulkier and more cumbersome body hearing aids.

Body hearing aids are helpful under some circumstances, however. One advantage of a body hearing aid is that it is less prone to feedback than the other hearing aid styles. Feedback is the high-pitched whistling that occurs when amplified sound from the hearing aid receiver is picked up by the hearing aid microphone and reamplified. In general, the higher the gain and the smaller the distance between the hearing aid receiver and the hearing aid microphone, the more likely is feedback to occur. Because the receiver of a body hearing aid is located at the ear and the microphone is located at the chest, feedback is highly unlikely. This can be especially useful for clients who must stay in bed. People in bed often experience feedback because the pillow surrounds the hearing aid, capturing amplified sound that is escaping from the ear canal and directing it back into the microphone. A body hearing aid prevents this problem.

Body hearing aids may also be helpful for people with visual or dexterity problems. The larger size of device makes it easier to control (ie, switch on and off or change the volume) and also makes changing batteries easier. An elderly person with dexterity problems, for example, may be able to operate a body aid independently, but would require help to cope with the small size of an ear-level hearing aid.

Some dispensers still recommend body hearing aids for infants and toddlers. This recommendation is based on the observation that body aids are sturdier than ear-level aids and are more likely to tolerate the abuse of a toddler. Proponents of body aids on infants point out that the pinnae of young children may be too soft and too small to support a BTE hearing aid. Even though supporting BTE hearing aids on small pinnae can be troublesome, the disadvantages of body hearing aids far outweigh the advantages. A disadvantage of body hearing aids is microphone location. Because the microphone is worn on the body, it is subject to clothing noise. Clothing noise is caused by fabric rubbing against the microphone of the hearing aid and can occur whether the hearing aid is worn above or underneath clothing. An additional problem encountered when wearing the microphone at chest level is the body-baffle effect (Skinner, 1988). Body baffle enhances sound energy in the low-frequency region while reducing sound energy in the high-frequency region—generally not a desirable effect. With ear-level aids, the microphone is in a more natural location. This allows for the normal head shadow and pinna effects that are used for localization. Consequently, most infants and young children should be considered candidates for ear-level hearing aids.

Eyeglass Hearing Aids

With eyeglass hearing aids, the microphone, amplifier, receiver, batteries, and controls are located within hollowed-out bows of eyeglass frames. The sound is delivered to the ear through a tube from the frame to an earmold. Eyeglass hearing aids were quite popular in the 1960s for cosmetic reasons (the BTE hearing aids available at that time were large, and body hearing aids were still common). Eyeglass hearing aids were also thought to be convenient for people who wore both glasses and a hearing aid. Today, however, eyeglass hearing aids make up a very small percentage of the market (less than 1 percent). The BTE, ITE, and ITC hearing aids available today are considered more cosmetically appealing because the frames necessary with eyeglass hearing aids are bulky and unattractive. In addition, the coupling of hearing aids and glasses is more of a problem than a convenience if one or the other is in need of repair. Most clinicians try to discourage clients from selecting eyeglass hearing aids unless the client is a candidate for a wired contralateral routing of signals (CROS) hearing aid (see section on CROS hearing aids).

Behind-the-Ear Hearing Aids

In BTE hearing aids the microphone, amplifier, battery, and receiver are all contained in a small plastic case that fits on top of and behind the pinna. Sound is delivered to the ear through a tube connected to an earmold. Figure 7.5 shows the location of the components on a typical BTE hearing aid. The BTE hearing aid style is the most versatile. BTE hearing aids are highly adjustable, rugged, and easily serviced (Lybarger, 1985). There is enough room in the case of a BTE hearing aid for a variety of hearing aid options and fitting adjustments. Consequently, these aids are appropriate for any degree of hearing loss and for any age of client. BTE hearing aids are considered, perhaps unjustly, less cosmetically appealing than ITE and ITC hearing aids, which accounts for the fact that they make up less than 20 percent of the hearing aid market in the United States. Although ITE and ITC hearing aids are a good option for a number of clients, some users, such as children, people with severe to profound hearing losses, and people with precipitously sloping hearing losses, are best served with BTE hearing aids.

In-the-Ear Hearing Aids

All of the components of an ITE hearing aid (the microphone, amplifier, receiver, and battery) are located in a small plastic case made from an impression of the wearer's concha and ear canal. Figure 7.6 illustrates the location of the components on a typical ITE hearing aid. ITE hearing aids come in a variety of case styles, ranging from those that completely fill the concha and canal (full-shell ITE) to those that approach the size of an ITC hearing aid (mini-ITE). Figure 7.7 illustrates the variety of sizes available in the ITE style. It should be noted, however, that the relatively small size of ITE hearing aid case restricts the number of options and fitting controls that can be incorporated. And, the smaller the ITE case, the fewer the options.

The ITE hearing aid is currently the most popular style on the market, accounting for 56 percent of sales in the United States. The popularity of the ITE

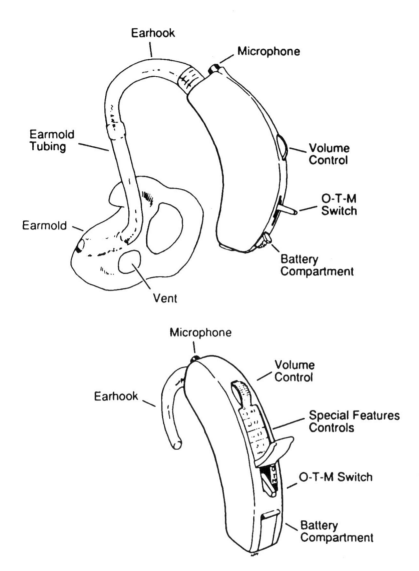

FIGURE 7.5 A behind-the-ear hearing aid and earmold, side and back views. (OTM, off-telephone-microphone.)

(Reprinted with permission from Shimon, 1992.)

hearing aid is presumably due to its perceived cosmetic appeal and perhaps to consumers' mistaken notion that ITE hearing aids are newer and more sophisticated than BTE hearing aids. ITE hearing aids are suitable for a wide variety of hearing losses. People with mild to moderate hearing losses are candidates for ITE

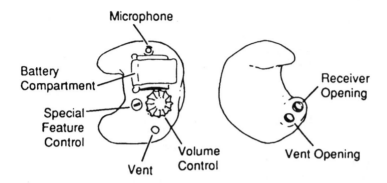

FIGURE 7.6 An in-the-ear (ITE) hearing aid, front (left) and back (right) views.

(Reprinted with permission from Shimon, 1992.)

hearing aids, and, with the increasing sophistication of ITE hearing aids over the past several years, even people with moderately-severe hearing losses can success-fully use them. However, the feedback limitations imposed by the proximity of the microphone and receiver within the relatively small case prevent the use of ITE hearing aids in people with severe to profound hearing losses and in many people with steeply sloping high-frequency hearing losses.

In-the-Canal Hearing Aids

ITC hearing aids, also known as canal hearing aids, are the smallest and most cosmetically appealing of all of the hearing aid styles. The microphone, amplifier, receiver, and battery are fit within a small plastic case made from an impression of the user's ear canal. The result is an instrument that fills the ear canal and protrudes, only slightly, into the concha area. Figure 7.8 on page 234 shows an example of a typical ITC style hearing aid. ITC hearing aids currently account for about 25 percent of the United States market. This percentage is likely to increase because of the increasing sophistication of electronic devices and the public's growing demand for unobtrusive hearing aids.

Fewer people can be fit with ITC hearing aids than with ITE or BTE hearing aids. Only moderate amounts of gain can be obtained from ITC hearing aids because of limitations imposed by feedback. Many people with normal hearing sensitivity in the low-frequency range find the sound from ITC hearing aids objectionable. People with relatively normal low-frequency hearing sensitivity are best fit with hearing aids (or earmolds) that occlude the ear canal as little as possible (Wernick, 1985). This configuration allows sound to enter the ear canal naturally and prevents excessive amplification of low-frequency sounds. ITC hearing aids,

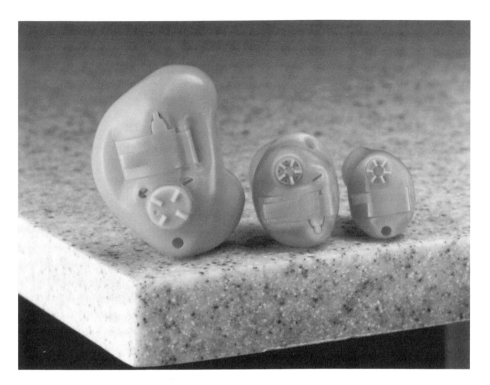

FIGURE 7.7   In-the-ear (ITE) hearing aid shells vary in size from a full-shell ITE hearing aid (left) to a mini-ITE hearing aid (center). An in-the-canal (ITC) hearing aid is shown on the right for comparison.

(Photo reprinted courtesy Starkey Laboratories, Inc., Minneapolis, Minn.)

on the other hand, tend to occlude the ear canal, which results in an unnatural sound quality. The best candidates for ITC hearing aids, then, are people with mild to moderate, flat, or gently sloping hearing losses.

SELECTING HEARING AID STYLE

Body hearing aids and eyeglass hearing aids are used only under special circumstances (eg, CROS fittings, need to stay in bed). Consequently, most people choose between the remaining three styles—BTE, ITE, and ITC. As alluded to in previous sections, the degree of hearing loss is a factor in the decision-making process. People with profound hearing losses are best fit with BTE hearing aids. Although people with severe hearing losses can be fit with ITE hearing aids, the likelihood of feedback increases as the severity of the loss increases, decreasing the likelihood of a successful fit. People with mild to moderately-severe hearing losses

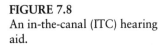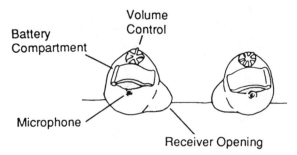

FIGURE 7.8
An in-the-canal (ITC) hearing aid.

(Reprinted with permission from Shimon, 1992.)

can be fit with either ITE or BTE hearing aids, and decisions regarding hearing aid style can be based on individual preference or special needs rather than the degree of loss.

When given a choice, most people with hearing impairments choose ITE over BTE aids and ITC over ITE aids, presumably because of the cosmetic appeal of smaller devices. ITC and ITE hearing aids have advantages over BTE beyond simple cosmetics. For example, the microphones of ITE and ITC hearing aids are located within the concha area rather than on top of the ear, as is the case with BTE hearing aids. This microphone placement preserves the natural pinna and concha resonances, enhancing high-frequency amplification. Another potential advantage of ITE hearing aids is ease of insertion. Many hearing aid users find the single-piece ITE hearing aids easier to insert than the two-piece (hearing aid case and earmold) BTE hearing aids (Upfold et al, 1990; Parving & Boisen, 1991; Stephens & Meredith, 1991). This advantage in ease of insertion may, however, be offset by the difficulties that many users (especially elderly users) have in adjusting the volume control and changing the batteries. Many older people find the tiny ITC hearing aids extremely difficult to manipulate (Plath, 1991; May et al, 1990; Stephens & Meredith, 1991), making ITC hearing aids impractical for many elderly hearing aid users.

BTE hearing aids have many advantages of their own. A basic advantage of a BTE hearing aid is its flexibility. BTE hearing aids are large enough to house a number of special options (eg, directional microphones, strong telecoils, direct audio input), resulting in a more sophisticated instrument. BTE hearing aids are also equipped with a number of dispenser-adjustable controls (eg, tone controls, output controls, compression controls) which allow the audiologist to fine tune the hearing aid at the time of the fitting, as the listener adapts to the new hearing aid, or even if the listener's hearing changes slightly over time. ITE hearing aids (and ITC hearing aids to an even greater extent) are limited in the number of features that can be fit into the hearing aid case. This means that it is more likely that these hearing aids will need to be returned to the manufacturer for response modifications during the fitting process (Wernick, 1985) and that new hearing aids will need to be purchased on a more frequent basis as the hearing loss progresses.

Another advantage of BTE hearing aids is their durability. ITE hearing aids and, to an even greater extent, ITC hearing aids are more likely to malfunction than BTE hearing aids. Placing the electronic components of the hearing aid within the ear canal and pinna subjects them to cerumen and moisture, which leads to malfunction.

SPECIAL OPTIONS AVAILABLE IN HEARING AIDS

Many special options can be built into hearing aids. As mentioned earlier, the larger the hearing aid, the more space there is for special features. Consequently, BTE hearing aids can accommodate many features, whereas ITC hearing aids can accommodate only one or two. In general, the more features ordered, the more expensive is the hearing aid.

Dispenser-Adjustable Controls

Dispenser-adjustable controls are included on most models of ITE and BTE hearing aids. The hearing aid has several controls (commonly referred to as trimpots or potentiometers) (see Figures 7.5 and 7.6), and the dispenser uses a small screwdriver to vary the gain (gain control), SSPL90 (output control), frequency response (tone control), or compression characteristics (AGC control) of the hearing aid. These adjustments allow the dispenser to adjust the hearing aid to better fit the client's preferences and to modify the hearing aid if the hearing loss changes slightly over time. Although many controls are standard on BTE hearing aids, the small size of ITE and especially of ITC hearing aids prohibits placement of numerous controls. Consequently, the dispenser must choose among options, the maximum number depending on the size of the hearing aid.

Telecoil

The telecoil circuit was originally designed to increase speech understanding when listening through a telephone. The telecoil itself is a small induction coil, located in the case of the hearing aid, which changes electromagnetic energy to electrical energy. The receiver portion of a telephone radiates an electromagnetic field that varies in proportion to the speech signal. The telecoil changes this electromagnetic signal into an electrical signal which can then be shaped and amplified by the hearing aid. In other words, the telecoil replaces the microphone of the hearing aid as the input transducer for the hearing aid. In fact, on most hearing aids the telecoil is activated by a toggle switch that allows the user to change between *M* for microphone and *T* for telephone.

Hearing aids can be used in conjunction with a telephone without activating the telecoil. This is known as acoustic coupling. In the acoustic coupling method, the telephone receiver is simply held next to the microphone of the hearing aid. (In the case of BTE hearing aids, this means holding the receiver at the top of the ear rather than covering the ear canal. With ITE and ITC hearing aids, the positioning is normal.) Although acoustic coupling is workable for some hearing aid users, it can lead to problems. One common complaint is feedback. Placing the receiver of the telephone close to the case of the hearing aid often leads to feedback because the amplified sound from the hearing aid is reflected off the surface of the telephone receiver and back into the microphone of the hearing aid. Small cushions are available to prevent this problem (see Chapter 8).

Many hearing aid users prefer an inductive coupling method to the acoustic coupling method. To use inductive coupling, the hearing aid user activates the telecoil of the hearing aid and places the telephone receiver in contact with the hearing aid case. The hearing aid volume usually needs to be increased when the telecoil is activated. The hearing aid user needs to experiment to determine the position of the phone receiver that provides the loudest signal. Inductive coupling has two distinct advantages over acoustic coupling. First, feedback does not occur. This is because the microphone of the hearing aid is deactivated when the hearing aid is switched to the telecoil position. A second advantage of inductive coupling is that only sounds coming directly from the telephone are amplified by the hearing aid. Environmental sounds are not amplified because the microphone is not functioning. This can make a great difference when the hearing aid user is trying to have a telephone conversation in a noisy setting.

There are two requirements for telecoils to function properly. First, the telephone must emit a relatively strong electromagnetic field. Second, the telecoil within the hearing aid must be adequate to receive the electromagnetic signal. In the past, all telephone receivers generated a relatively strong electromagnetic field as a by-product of their operation. Over the years, however, the design of telephone receivers has been improved, resulting in receivers that are more efficient, more durable, and less expensive to manufacture (Lybarger, 1982). Unfortunately, the improvements also resulted in receivers that no longer emitted a strong electromagnetic field, and many telephones were no longer compatible with hearing aid telecoils. In 1982, federal legislation addressed the compatibility issue. The Telecommunications for the Disabled Act (Public Law 97-410) requires that essential telephones (public and pay telephones, emergency telephones, and telephones in the workplace) be hearing aid compatible. Since 1989 the Federal Communications Commission has required that all telephones sold for use in the United States be hearing aid compatible (Staab & Lybarger, 1994).

Even if the electromagnetic signal emitted from the telephone is strong enough, the process can break down if the telecoil within the hearing aid is inadequate to process the incoming electromagnetic signal. To be maximally effective, the telecoil in the hearing aid must be large enough and correctly oriented in the hearing aid case. This can be easily accomplished in BTE hearing aids. ITE hearing aids, however, pose a problem. Because all the components of an ITE hearing aid must fit into a small case, the size and positioning of the telecoil may be compromised, resulting in a weak signal. In some cases, the manufacturer can correct this problem through the use of a preamplifier or additional coils of wire if space allows (Compton, 1989). Careful evaluation of the hearing aid telecoil is necessary, however; one cannot simply assume that it is working properly. If the client complains that the signal from the hearing aid is not strong enough, evaluation of the telecoil by the dispenser is warranted.

Although telecoils were originally designed to improve speech reception through the telephone, they are also widely used to couple hearing aids to assistive listening devices (see Chapter 8). The enactment of the Americans with Disabilities Act (ADA) in 1990 ensures that assistive devices will become more common in places of public accommodation (eg, theaters, retail stores, restaurants, doctor's offices, convention centers) and public offices (eg, federal, state, and local government offices). Consequently, an adequate telecoil is an asset. If a person is likely to be using assistive listening devices, it will behoove them to purchase a BTE hearing aid from a manufacturer known to produce strong and reliable telecoils.

Direct Audio Input

Direct audio input (DAI) is a means of delivering an electrical signal directly to a hearing aid through the use of a cord and snap-on boot that establishes an electrical connection to the hearing aid. Figure 8.10 on page 284 illustrates the connection. DAI is useful for coupling assistive listening devices to the hearing aid for further processing before being delivered to the listener's ear. DAI is available on most BTE instruments. Some manufacturers can equip specially ordered ITE hearing aids with DAI if space allows, but DAI is not currently available for ITC hearing aids (Compton, 1989). These factors must be taken into consideration when selecting hearing aid style. If a client is likely to be using an assistive listening device, a BTE hearing aid with DAI is highly desirable.

Directional Microphones

Directional microphones are designed to improve speech understanding in a noisy environment by fully amplifying sounds that originate in front of the listener (presumably desirable signals) while slightly reducing the amplification of sounds that originate behind the listener (presumably competing signals). Standard, or omnidirectional microphones, on the other hand, are approximately equally sensitive to sound from all directions. Although directional microphones lose their effectiveness in highly reverberant environments (Hawkins & Yacullo, 1984), most studies demonstrate improvement in speech understanding in a noisy environment when directional microphones are used (Hawkins & Yacullo, 1984; Mueller et al, 1984).

Noise Reduction Circuits

Some hearing aids incorporate circuitry designed specifically to improve speech understanding in a noisy environment. Noise reduction is accomplished by a variety of methods, and the circuits are known by numerous names (eg, automatic signal processing [ASP]; adaptive compression; Zeta Noise Blocker). Although these systems have not been shown to increase speech understanding in background noise, they do seem to increase user comfort and perceived sound quality (Van Tassel et al, 1988). Clients should speak with their audiologist to determine the noise reduction system that would best fit their needs.

Special Amplifiers

Many hearing aids are available with special amplifiers and receivers. These circuits have unique properties, but in general they are designed to increase speech clarity and client comfort (K-Amp™) or to increase the power a hearing aid can produce while keeping sound clear and preserving battery life (class D amplifiers, push-pull circuits, and dual receivers). Again, clients need to speak with their audiologist to determine which, if any, system is appropriate for their needs.

HEARING AIDS WITH SPECIAL APPLICATIONS

Specialized hearing aid systems are available for people with unique needs. One such system is the CROS hearing aid system, which has been designed for people with unilateral hearing impairments. Another system is the bone-conduction hearing aid which has been designed for people with conductive hearing losses who are not candidates for standard air-conduction hearing aids. Finally, a new type of hearing aid, an analog–digital hybrid hearing aid, is available for people with demanding communication needs.

Contralateral Routing of Signals Hearing Aids

In the past, people with one normal ear and one unaidable ear have been overlooked as hearing aid candidates. Most clinicians assumed that the difficulties experienced by people with this pattern of hearing loss were relatively minor, and that these people would learn to cope with their deficit. It has become increasingly evident, however, that the problems faced by these people are serious and should be addressed (Bess et al, 1986; Bess, 1985). Specifically, people with one normal ear and one unaidable ear describe difficulty locating the source of a sound and difficulty hearing in noisy settings, especially when the sound is coming from the side of the poor ear. Children especially are at risk for problems because this pattern of hearing loss can affect educational progress. Bess (1986) reported that 35 percent of children with one normal ear and one unaidable ear failed at least one grade (a rate 10 times greater than children with normal hearing sensitivity in both ears), and an additional 13 percent needed resource assistance.

Fortunately, special amplification systems, CROS hearing aids, designed specifically for people with one unaidable ear have been developed (Harford & Barry, 1965). A CROS system consists of two hearing aid cases—one worn at each ear. The microphone of the system is mounted in the case worn on the poor (unaidable) ear. The signal is then routed through a wire in a wired system or through radio waves in a wireless system to the amplifier and receiver mounted in the case on the good ear. Here the signal is amplified slightly and delivered by a nonoccluding earmold to the good ear. In this way the person can hear sound from both sides of the head, but all sound is heard in the good ear. Sound from the poor side is heard through the hearing aid, and sound from the normal side is heard in the usual manner through the nonoccluding earmold.

BICROS hearing aids are an extension of the CROS system. This system is required when the better ear is not normal, that is, if the better ear needs amplification as well. In a BICROS system, the hearing aid case on the unaidable side is the same as with the CROS system, but the hearing aid case worn on the better ear functions as a complete hearing aid rather than just an amplifier and receiver. Thus, sound picked up from the microphones on each side of the head is amplified and delivered to the better ear.

Bone-Conduction Hearing Aids

Most people with conductive hearing losses never need hearing aids because their hearing losses are addressed through medical or surgical intervention. Medical treatments, however, are not always successful, so some people with conductive hearing losses become candidates for hearing aids. These people usually are satisfactorily fit with standard air-conduction hearing aids. In fact, people with conductive impairments often do better with hearing aids than people with sensorineural hearing losses because the inner ear in people with conductive hearing losses functions normally (ie, without distortion).

Unfortunately, some people with conductive hearing losses cannot be fit with standard hearing aids. People with chronically draining ears, for example, cannot be fit with standard hearing aids because these aids occlude the external ear. People with abnormalities of the external ear (eg, aural atresia, anotia, severe microtia) often cannot support any style of air-conduction hearing aid. A bone-conduction hearing aid may be useful for these people. With a bone-conduction hearing aid, the small receiver at the output of a standard air-conduction hearing aid is replaced by a bone-conduction oscillator—much like that used for bone-conduction audiometric testing. The bone-conduction oscillator can be held on the mastoid process by a narrow metal headband or may be built into eyeglass frames.

Unfortunately, both methods often result in patient discomfort (eg, pain, headache, and skin irritation) and relatively poor sound quality (Johnson et al, 1988; Hakansson et al, 1990). The U.S. Food and Drug Administration (FDA) recently approved implantable bone-conduction hearing aids (Newby & Popelka, 1992). With this device, the bone-conduction oscillator is permanently implanted in the temporal bone and coupled to an external sound-processing device, resulting in less discomfort and higher sound quality (Hakansson et al, 1990; Dunham & Friedman, 1990).

Hybrid Hearing Aids

Most hearing aids purchased today are analog instruments. In analog instruments, the signals that pass through the hearing aid are continuous electrical waveforms analogous in shape to the incoming acoustic waveform. Digital hearing aids have been developed and tested, primarily in research laboratories. In digital hearing aids, the continuous acoustic waveform is changed, by means of an analog-to-digital converter, into a series of binary digits. Digital coding of the signal allows advanced forms of signal processing that are not possible with conventional analog hearing aids (Hussung & Hamill, 1990). True digital hearing aids are not commercially available, and ear-level digital hearing aids are not feasible at this time primarily because of the hefty power requirements of the digital electronics (Hussung & Hamill, 1990). (One true digital hearing aid, the Nicolet Phoenix, was placed on the market in 1987. It was later withdrawn; consumers were reluctant to wear a BTE hearing aid coupled by a wire to a body-worn signal processor and power pack.) Many manufacturers currently market analog hearing aids that are digitally controlled (Hearing Instruments, 1992). These hearing aids are known as hybrid systems and are available in BTE, ITE, and ITC versions, although at a substantially higher cost than typical analog hearing aids.

Hybrid technology enhances hearing aids in a number of ways. It makes the hearing aid programmable, allows the hearing aid to have multiple sets of electroacoustic characteristics or memories, and improves the noise reduction capabilities of the hearing aid.

Programmability is the most commonly used hybrid technology. As the name suggests, specific electroacoustic characteristics are programmed into the hearing aid at the time of the hearing aid fitting. The programming occurs by means of an external computer or a programmer specific to the hearing aid manufacturer. Programmable hearing aids have several advantages over analog hearing aids. First, they are extremely versatile. A wide variety of electroacoustic characteristics can be programmed into a single hearing aid, regardless of its size. Thus, programmable ITC instruments are almost as versatile as BTE hearing aids. The added versatility also enables a dispenser to take a single hearing aid and program it to be appropriate for almost any hearing loss. Moreover, the hearing aid can be reprogrammed at any time. This can be a great advantage when fitting children; the hearing aid can be adjusted as more specific information regarding the child's hearing loss and appropriate hearing aid characteristics becomes available. A programmable hearing aid is also ideal for someone with a progressive hearing loss. As the hearing sensitivity deteriorates, the client can have the hearing aid reprogrammed instead of purchasing a new hearing aid.

Hybrid technology has been used to produce multiple memories within a single hearing aid. Conventional analog hearing aids have one set of electroacoustic characteristics that must be used in all listening environments. Hybrid hearing aids with multiple memories are programmed in such a way that each memory (currently available models contain anywhere from two to ten different memories) contains a unique set of electroacoustic characteristics (Hearing Instruments, 1992). This feature allows the user to select different electroacoustic characteristics depending on the listening environment. For example, the user might select one set of electroacoustic characteristics for understanding speech in background noise, but a different set of characteristics for listening to a symphony.

Still another use of hybrid technology is noise reduction. The Zeta Noise Blocker is an example of this technology. This chip is designed to recognize noise and automatically reduce the gain in the frequency band where the noise is occurring. Unfortunately the amplitude of both the speech and the noise in the band is reduced. Technologies, such as Zeta Noise Blocker, are useful because they seem to improve sound quality and listener comfort in background noise, but there is no evidence that speech understanding is improved (Van Tassel et al, 1988).

MONAURAL AS OPPOSED TO BINAURAL AMPLIFICATION

On an intuitive level, most people understand that two hearing aids should be better than one. Unfortunately, many of the early studies examining performance with binaural as opposed to monaural hearing aids did not demonstrate an advantage to binaural amplification. Given the lack of objective evidence to support an advantage to binaural instruments, many dispensers were hesitant to recommend the more expensive option of two hearing aids. With the advent of more sensitive evaluation techniques, however, it has become increasingly clear that subtle, but noticeable, advantages to binaural amplification do exist. Objectively demonstrated advantages include improved localization skills, better speech understanding in noisy environments, and binaural loudness summation (Ross, 1980). Equally important are the subjective impressions of hearing aid users. Reports from experienced hearing aid users verify the objective data and further indicate that binaural amplification provides less stressful listening and a more balanced, natural sound. As a consequence, the number of binaural fittings has increased steadily over the past 15 years. The Vanderbilt/Veterans Administration (VA) consensus statement (Hawkins et al, 1991) indicates that "unless clear contraindications exist, binaural hearing aids should be considered the preferred fitting for the prospective hearing aid user" (p. 37).

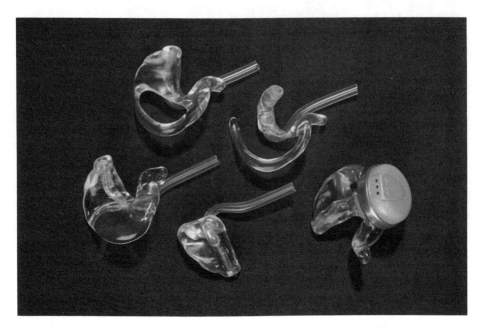

FIGURE 7.9 Commonly recommended earmold styles. Clockwise from lower right: standard (or receiver-type) with body aid receiver attached, canal, shell, skeleton, and CROS (or nonoccluding).

(Earmolds provided by Mid-States Laboratories, Inc., Wichita, Kan.)

EARMOLD CONSIDERATIONS

BTE, body, and eyeglass hearing aids require an earmold to couple the hearing aid to the ear. ITE and ITC hearing aids do not require an earmold; the custom molded case functions as an earmold. One important function of the earmold is to direct amplified sound toward the tympanic membrane in a way that prevents feedback. Feedback occurs when amplified sound of sufficient intensity escapes and travels back to the hearing aid microphone and is reamplified. Feedback can be prevented by obtaining a good seal between the earmold and the listener's ear. The more powerful the hearing aid, the more likely is feedback to occur and the better the fit must be. A second function of the earmold is to modify acoustically, or tune, the response of the hearing aid.

Earmold Style

Earmolds for BTE, body, and eyeglass hearing aids are available in several styles, which are illustrated in Figure 7.9. Earmold style refers to the shape of the exterior portion of the earmold. Except for the open mold style, acoustic performance is similar for each of the styles. It is the internal features of the earmold (eg, the length and diameter of the tubing, the length and diameter of the vents) rather than the external features that characterize the acoustic properties of an earmold.

Many of the styles shown in Figure 7.9 can be used interchangeably. The two exceptions are the standard (also known as the receiver-type) mold and the open (also known as the CROS) mold, which are designed for specific purposes. The standard mold is used with body hearing aids; the receiver portion of the hearing aid snaps into metal ring in the earmold. An open-style earmold is used for people with normal low- to mid-frequency hearing sensitivity or for people fit with CROS hearing aids. The selection of a particular earmold from the remaining styles is made on the basis of client comfort, cosmetic preference, and feedback reduction properties; feedback reduction being the most important consideration. Conventional wisdom is that the bulkier the earmold, the less likely it is that feedback will occur. Thus, shell earmolds should be more effective than skeleton earmolds in preventing feedback, and skeleton should be more effective than canal earmolds. As a consequence, most people with severe to profound hearing losses have been fit with shell earmolds to prevent feedback. A recent trend has been to fit people with severe to profound hearing losses with canal earmolds. This strategy has been effective in controlling feedback, and many of the clients prefer the less bulky feel of the canal-type earmold.

Earmold Materials

Earmolds can be ordered in a variety of materials and colors (clear, brown, pink, and flesh tone). The most commonly used material is a hard acrylic known as Lucite. Lucite is popular for a number of reasons. First, it is the most cosmetically appealing of the earmold materials. It is generally ordered in a clear color but can be tinted a pink or brown flesh tone. Lucite earmolds have a smooth, glossy finish that makes the earmold almost invisible when worn. A second advantage is that Lucite earmolds are easy to modify and are extremely durable; a Lucite earmold can maintain its shape and clarity indefinitely.

Although they can be used by most people with mild to moderate hearing losses, Lucite earmolds are not appropriate for people with severe to profound hearing losses. The smooth, hard material does not tightly seal the ear, allowing some amplified sound to travel from the ear canal back toward the microphone of the hearing aid. When the amplitude of the escaping sound is great enough, feedback occurs. Softer, more pliable materials form a better seal with the concha and ear canal and thus are used for people with severe to profound hearing losses. Soft materials are available in several different textures, ranging from almost as hard as Lucite to extremely pliable. The names and textures of the materials vary depending on the earmold laboratory from which they are ordered.

Soft materials are used primarily to prevent acoustic feedback in people with severe to profound hearing losses. They are also used for children, regardless of the severity of the loss, for two reasons. First, the softer materials do not have to be replaced as frequently as hard materials as the child grows. The seal between the earmold and the ear is lost as a child grows, resulting in feedback. Because a better bond between the earmold and ear occurs with soft materials, earmolds made from soft materials remain functional longer. Still, parents of young children must be told that new earmolds will be needed often. Northern and Downs (1984) suggest that children will need a new earmold every 3 to 6 months until the age of 5 and approximately once a year between the ages of 5 and 9 years. A second reason that soft materials are always used with children is that these materials are more comfortable when the child is bumped or hit in the ear.

A disadvantage of soft materials is their appearance. Soft materials are translucent rather than clear. To make matters worse, some of the soft materials can discolor over time. An additional disadvantage of some of the soft materials is that they can shrink slightly over time, resulting in feedback. Some of the softer materials are more resistant to shrinkage and discoloration than others. As new materials are developed this should become less of a problem.

Combination earmolds (earmolds that are made from two different materials) have been designed to incorporate the advantages of Lucite and soft materials into one earmold. A commonly used combination earmold has the concha portion of the earmold constructed of Lucite (for durability and cosmetic appeal) and the canal portion constructed of a soft material (for feedback prevention and comfort). This earmold works well for many clients with moderately-severe hearing losses, but earmolds constructed entirely from a soft material are still required for maximum feedback protection.

Some people with hearing impairments require silicone earmolds. This material is used for the small percentage of the population that has an allergic reaction to the more commonly used materials. Silicone earmolds are not cosmetically appealing—they are opaque, and in many cases the tubing does not adhere well to the earmold.

Earmold Acoustics

An important function of the earmold is to modify acoustically, or tune, the hearing aid response. When the length and diameter of the earmold tubing, bore, and vent are changed, the hearing aid response can be modified to better fit the needs of the particular user. Figure 7.10 illustrates the power of earmold modifications. All responses were obtained from the same hearing aid—only the earmold characteristics were changed. As can be seen, substantial changes in the hearing aid response can be obtained by simply modifying the earmold. A complete discussion of earmold acoustics is beyond the scope of this book, but earmold modifications can be used to vary almost any aspect of the response of the hearing aid. They can change the amount of gain and output provided by the hearing aid, extend the high-frequency response of the hearing aid, reduce the low-frequency response of the hearing aid, or smooth irregularities present in the response of the

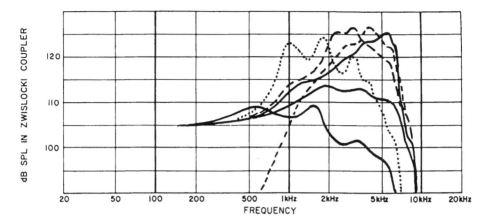

FIGURE 7.10 Frequency responses obtained from a single hearing aid using six distinctly different earmold configurations.

(Reprinted with permission from Killion, 1980.)

hearing aid. For a complete discussion of earmold acoustics the reader is referred to Lybarger (1985).

HEARING AID SELECTION AND FITTING

Hearing Aid Selection Approaches

Although it is widely acknowledged that the selection of appropriate amplification is a crucial first step in the rehabilitation of most listeners with a hearing loss, no agreement exists as to the most appropriate method of hearing aid selection. Hearing aid selection procedures have two different underlying philosophies—selection procedures based on the comparison of different hearing aids (comparative approaches) and selection procedures based on a client's audiometric profile (prescriptive approaches).

Carhart developed the comparative approach to hearing aid selection while working in a veterans' rehabilitation hospital after World War II (Carhart, 1946). Carhart's procedure was extremely comprehensive and included a wide range of aided and unaided assessments performed using many hearing aids over a period of several days.

Carhart's procedure was greatly abbreviated when adapted for routine clinical use. Dispensers who use a comparative approach today typically compare a small number of hearing aids using performance on a monosyllabic speech recognition test as the basis for comparison. Over the years, however, it has become increasingly evident that standard monosyllabic word recognition tests are not sensitive enough to detect differences among similar hearing aids (Shore et al, 1960; Walden et al, 1983). An additional difficulty was caused by the movement toward the use of ITE and ITC hearing aids; because these hearing aids are custom-made, comparison of several hearing aids is not feasible.

Discontent with the impracticalities of the comparative approach led many dispensers to a prescriptive approach. When using a prescriptive approach, the dispenser utilizes audiometric data (eg, thresholds, most comfortable loudness levels, LDLs) and a formula to determine the optimal electroacoustic characteristics for a particular person. Many prescriptive methods exist. In fact, during the 1970s and 1980s at least a dozen prescriptive approaches were developed (Bess & Humes, 1990). Although these approaches differ in detail, each method strives to make as much of the speech spectrum as possible audible without making it uncomfortably loud. Despite testimonials to the contrary, even prescriptive methods with different underlying philosophies tend to lead to the selection of hearing aids that are electroacoustically similar (Humes, 1986).

Although prescriptive approaches have been extremely popular for the past 10 years, limitations in their use are becoming increasingly apparent. Current prescriptive approaches prescribe only gain and SSPL90 characteristics, without providing guidance concerning the use of compression or other nonlinear processing strategies. Moreover, many of the digitally programmable hearing aids have multiple memories, necessitating multiple sets of electroacoustic characteristics for a single hearing aid. These observations have led dispensers to conclude that prescriptive approaches alone cannot provide all the necessary information.

Many dispensers have begun to use a combination of the prescriptive and the comparative approaches. The prescriptive approach is used as a starting point to select an initial set of electroacoustic characteristics. Once the hearing aid arrives, it can be modified with the comparative approach. For example, the client compares different hearing aid settings (eg, changes in compression, gain, and noise reduction) before final recommendations are made. Because standard monosyllabic word recognition tests are not sufficiently sensitive to differentiate among hearing aids (or among different settings on the same hearing aid), dispensers have turned to other measurements for comparison. A simple and effective procedure involves having the client make subjective judgments of the quality and clarity of connected discourse while listening through the hearing aid while it is adjusted in various ways. This procedure has been shown to be highly reliable (Studebaker et al, 1982) and can be used to examine any electroacoustic parameter.

Verification of Hearing Aid Characteristics

As mentioned previously, no agreement exists as to the most appropriate method of hearing aid selection. However, after the 1990 Vanderbilt/VA Hearing Aid Conference, a consensus statement outlining the recommended components of a hearing aid selection and evaluation procedure was published (Hawkins et al, 1991). Although the specific procedures used are left to the discretion of the dispenser, all dispensers are encouraged to include the following components: initial determination of desired electroacoustic characteristics, selection of hearing aids that contain the desired electroacoustic characteristics, verification of hearing aid characteristics on the user, and orientation and follow-up.

The initial determination of appropriate electroacoustic characteristics is usually made by means of a prescriptive method. This is followed by the selection of a hearing aid that meets the prescribed characteristics. If a BTE hearing aid is to be ordered, the dispenser examines specification sheets to find a hearing aid with the desired electroacoustic characteristics and options (eg, telecoil, directional microphone, direct audio input). If an ITE or an ITC aid is to be ordered, the prescribed values are sent to the manufacturer so that the aid can be manufactured to provide the desired electroacoustic characteristics and the desired options.

Once the hearing aid has been obtained, it is imperative that its performance (ie, its match to the prescriptive target) be verified on the user's ear. Although this may seem like an obvious statement, approximately 25 percent of the hearing aids dispensed in this country are never evaluated on the listener's ear at the time of the fitting (Grahl, 1993). Measuring the performance of a hearing aid in a hearing aid test box during an EAA is not adequate. Measurements made during an EAA provide an indication whether or not a hearing aid is functioning according to the manufacturer's specifications, but such measurements do not adequately represent the performance of the hearing aid while it is worn by the listener. This is because the physical properties of the ear canal and middle ear system differ substantially from person to person and from the properties of the 2-cc coupler that is used during an EAA. Consequently, a hearing aid performs differently on each person; the performance on a particular person cannot be inferred from the data obtained in the EAA.

Verification of the gain on the ear of the listener (real-ear gain) can be accomplished using either functional gain or insertion gain measurements. Functional gain is defined as the difference between aided soundfield thresholds and unaided soundfield thresholds. Figure 7.11 shows the results of a functional gain measurement. In this example, 40 dB of functional gain was obtained at 1000 Hz. Functional gain measurements are easy to obtain and require no special equipment. Because they require a behavioral response on the part of the listener, the practitioner can be sure that the gain provided by the hearing aid leads to a change in the listener's threshold.

Insertion gain measurements are obtained with a probe microphone measurement system, often called a real-ear measurement system. A probe microphone system consists of a speaker that presents signals across a wide range of frequencies, a probe microphone (a small microphone with a flexible silicone tube that is inserted into the ear canal of the listener), and a number of other components that serve to calibrate the system, compare the input signal with the level measured in the ear canal, and display the results in graphic form. Figure 7.12 illustrates a probe

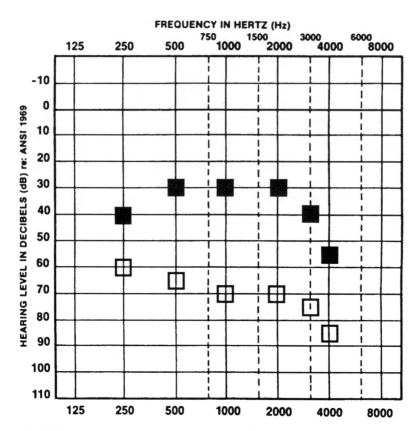

FIGURE 7.11 Functional gain measurement. The open squares represent the listener's unaided soundfield thresholds, and the filled squares represent the listener's soundfield thresholds while wearing a hearing aid. Functional gain from the hearing aid is defined as the difference between the listener's unaided and aided thresholds at a particular frequency.

microphone system. Insertion gain measurements are made by measuring the signal level in the ear canal first without the hearing aid in place and then with the hearing aid in place and turned on. Real-ear insertion gain (REIG) is defined as the difference, in dB, between these two measurements at a particular frequency. Real-ear insertion response (REIR) is the difference between the two measurements across the frequency range. Figure 7.13 illustrates a typical REIR. In this example, about 22 dB of real-ear gain was measured at 1000 Hz and a good match between target gain (gain suggested with a prescriptive approach) and the measured gain was obtained between 250 and 3000 Hz.

Insertion gain measurements are quick and easy to obtain (assuming a cooperative client), and they provide an indication of gain across the frequency

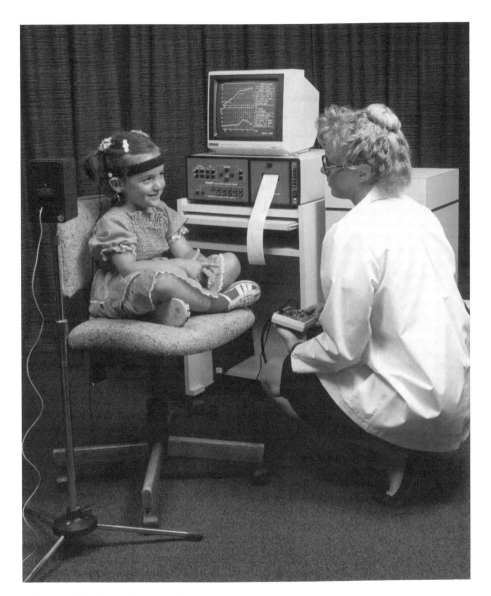

FIGURE 7.12 A probe microphone measurement system.

(Photo courtesy of Frye Electronics, Inc., Tigard, Ore.)

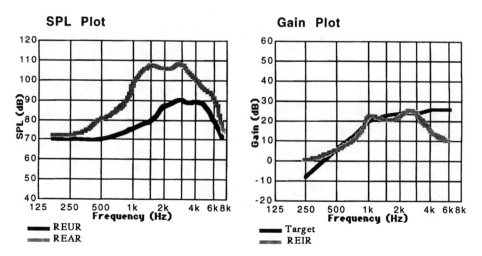

FIGURE 7.13 Measurements of hearing aid performance obtained with a probe microphone system and a 70 dB SPL input signal. The left plot shows signal amplification due to the natural resonance properties of the listener's ear canal (the real-ear unaided response, REUR) and the amplification provided by the combination of the hearing aid and the listener's ear canal resonance (the real-ear aided response, REAR). The right plot shows the gain suggested by a prescriptive approach (target) and the gain provided by the hearing aid across the frequency range (the real-ear insertion response, REIR). The REIR is the difference between the REAR and the REUR and represents the gain provided by the hearing aid on this patient.

range rather than just at discrete intervals. An additional advantage of insertion gain measurements is that they are generally obtained with a 60 to 70 dB SPL input signal, which is comparable to the level of normal conversational speech. Thus, the measured gain should reflect the gain provided by the hearing aid for conversational speech, even for instruments in which gain changes as a function of input level (ie, compression instruments). A potential disadvantage of insertion gain measurements is that they do not require a behavioral response. Consequently, a practitioner can only infer that the measured gain will improved aided performance. Although this is a safe assumption for most people with hearing impairments, people with severe to profound hearing losses are best assessed with functional gain measurements.

After verification and adjustment of real-ear gain, several other measurements of hearing aid performance should be obtained while the client is wearing the hearing aid. One often overlooked but vital component is a verification of hearing aid comfort for intense input signals. Initial SSPL90 settings are selected using measurements of the client's LDLs or by making inferences of the client's LDLs on the basis of his or her pure-tone thresholds. In either case, ear canal SPL or client reaction to intense sound should be measured with the hearing aid in place.

Measurement of the client's reaction to intense input signals cannot be overemphasized. A common reason for dissatisfaction with and rejection of hearing aids is an overamplification of loud sounds. If the hearing aid produces signals that are uncomfortably loud, the SSPL90 setting should be adjusted or a different hearing aid should be ordered. Ear canal SPL must be measured for all children and adults who wear hearing aids with high output levels in order to minimize the chance that further damage to the auditory system could occur (see earlier section concerning potential noise induced hearing loss from hearing aids).

Further measurements of aided performance should include an assessment of the listener's understanding of amplified speech as well as their subjective impressions concerning the quality of speech. Although speech recognition measurements are generally not useful for differentiating the performance of hearing aids with similar electroacoustic characteristics, these measurements do play a role in the verification of aided performance. As Mueller and Grimes (1983) point out, a comparison of aided with unaided speech recognition ability is useful for three reasons, "First, to demonstrate to the audiologist that a hearing aid provides significant improvement in speech recognition ability over the unaided condition; second to assist in demonstrating to the patient that use of amplification will improve his/her communication ability; and third to provide a framework for rehabilitation counseling" (p. 269).

HEARING AID ORIENTATION AND FOLLOW-UP

The final component of the hearing aid selection procedure outlined in the Vanderbilt/VA consensus statement involves client orientation and follow-up. Proper orientation to the care and use of hearing aids is necessary if they are to be used successfully. A complete orientation should include the following: a discussion of the components of the hearing aid and their function, information on the care and maintenance of the hearing aid, instruction concerning basic troubleshooting skills, and information concerning initial adjustment to the instrument. A complete hearing aid orientation should be done by the dispenser at the time of the hearing aid fitting. However, in some cases dispensers do a poor job presenting the information. In other cases, the hearing aid users forget what was said during the orientation. The unfortunate result is that many hearing aids are not worn or do not function optimally for the user. This problem becomes strikingly apparent in the examination of data on hearing aid function in schools and nursing homes.

According to Schow and Nerbonne (1980), the incidence of hearing loss among the institutionalized geriatric population is higher than 80 percent. Functional amplification would allow these patients to interact with family members, staff members, and other residents and to increase their enjoyment of television and radio. Unfortunately, a recent investigation by Bradley and Malloy (1991) indicated that more than 50 percent of the residents' hearing aids did not function properly. Moreover, they noted that more than half of the problems (eg, dead batteries, earmolds occluded with cerumen, improper switch positions) could have been easily corrected on site by anyone with training in basic troubleshooting skills.

The data on hearing aid performance in schools are no less appalling. Beginning with the Gaeth and Lounsbury investigation in 1966, numerous studies conducted in the 1960s and 1970s showed that, on any given day, approximately 50 percent of the children's hearing aids were not functioning appropriately. Moreover, interviews conducted with parents and teachers indicated that they were uncertain about many aspects of hearing aid use and function, and in many cases these caregivers were unable to tell if a hearing aid was functioning appropriately (Gaeth & Lounsbury, 1966; Bendet, 1980). As a result of these investigations, hearing aid monitoring programs were instituted in many school systems. Unfortunately, data collected during the late 1970s and early 1980s indicated that the problem still remained; 25 to 40 percent of children's hearing aids were found to be unsatisfactory, despite the reported use of routine hearing aid monitoring programs (Potts & Greenwood, 1983; Withrow, 1977; Robinson & Sterling, 1980). The disappointing results are most likely attributable to the quality of the hearing aid monitoring programs. In many cases the hearing aid check is perfunctory rather than thorough. As Hanners and Sitton (1974) noted, a common practice in a hearing aid check was to simply turn the volume control on the hearing aid up. If the hearing aid whistled, it was functioning. This clearly is not an adequate check of hearing aid performance.

Evidence does exist that consistently applied, high-quality maintenance programs do result in an improvement in hearing aid performance (Hanners & Sitton, 1974; Potts & Greenwood, 1983). Reichman and Healey (1989) established preferred practices for hearing aid monitoring programs. In brief, the preferred practices include daily visual and listening checks of hearing aids and auditory trainers; regular electroacoustic evaluation of hearing aids and auditory trainers; loaner hearing aids and auditory trainers available on the day the malfunction is noted; methods for replacing earmolds and other accessories; and instructions to parents, teachers, and students concerning hearing aid checks and maintenance.

Ideally, an audiologist would be on-site to supervise all hearing aid monitoring programs. Audiologists, however, assume direct responsibility for less than 30 percent of hearing aid monitoring programs (Reichman & Healey, 1989). More often, the classroom teacher or school nurse performs the daily monitoring and troubleshooting, relying on the school speech-language pathologist to oversee the program (including the training of personnel) and to assist with difficult cases. Consequently it is imperative that speech-language pathologists, educators, and school nurses become proficient at performing hearing aid checks and that they acquire basic troubleshooting skills.

Information on hearing aid orientation (including care and maintenance of the aid and adjustment of the aid), daily hearing aid checks, and troubleshooting hearing aid problems follows. This information is indispensable for practitioners who work with children with hearing losses or who are involved in school hearing aid monitoring programs. It is also useful for practitioners in contact with parents of children with hearing losses, nursing home personnel, or adults with hearing losses.

Hearing Aid Orientation

At the time of the hearing aid fitting, the hearing aid user (or the parents of a child) should be given basic information concerning the parts of the hearing aid and their function. The hearing aid microphone, receiver, on-off mechanism, and volume control should be identified and the functions described. It is also important to instruct the client on battery usage. The client needs to know the size of the battery to be used, where batteries can be purchased, and the correct insertion and removal technique. Because hearing aid batteries can die with little or no warning, the hearing aid user should be instructed to keep spare batteries handy. Spare batteries should always be kept at school or work. Small plastic battery cases that clip onto key chains are available, and many adult hearing aid users find this to be a convenient way to carry spare batteries. Clients should always be advised of issues related to battery safety. The function of the telecoil and other optional components (eg, a noise suppression switch, DAI, multiple memories) must be explained. If a BTE hearing aid is being fit, the earmold and tubing should be shown to the client. If a body aid is being fit, the hearing aid user needs to understand the function of the cord and the receiver portion of the hearing aid. Hearing aid insertion and removal should be practiced until the client is confident that he or she will be able to manage the process on his or her own.

It is also important for hearing aid users to be familiar with the routine care and maintenance of their instruments. Hearing aids are electronic devices and consequently can be harmed by extremes in temperature, by moisture, or by shocks. Consequently, people with hearing impairments should take care not to drop the hearing aid on hard surfaces and should be reminded not to leave their hearing aids in hot places (eg, in the car on a sunny day, near the radiator, near the stove) or cold places. They should also keep the hearing aid dry. Hearing aids must not be worn while swimming or bathing, but more subtle forms of moisture can also cause problems. For example, the client should not leave the hearing aid in areas of high humidity (ie, the bathroom) and should not apply hairspray while wearing the hearing aid. If the hearing aid user perspires heavily, he or she should consult with the dispenser concerning the purchase of moisture-resistant hearing aids or the use of protective hearing aid covers. People who live in humid climates should consider purchasing hearing aid dehumidifying kits for regular use. These kits can be obtained through hearing aid dispensers.

Hearing aids can be kept clean by simply wiping the case with a soft, dry cloth every evening. If the client has a BTE, body, or eyeglass hearing aid, the earmold can be detached periodically and washed in warm, soapy water. The earmold can then be dried (pipe cleaners or specially designed forced-air blowers work well for this purpose) and reattached to the hearing aid. If the client has an ITE or ITC hearing aid, the canal portion of the aid should be checked each evening for cerumen build-up. If cerumen is noted, it should be removed with the special tool provided by the hearing aid manufacturer. Each evening the battery compartment should be completely opened. This reduces the possibility of battery corrosion and extends battery life. If the hearing aid is not to be used for an extended period of time, the batteries should be removed.

Hearing Aid Adjustment Programs

Although a detailed account of hearing aid adjustment programs is beyond the scope of this book, it is important to note that new hearing aid users can become overwhelmed by amplification if they do not proceed through a hierarchy of listening experiences. New hearing aid users (and previous users fit with new hearing aids) are instructed to begin by wearing their hearing aid in quiet environments in which only one person is speaking and to gradually work up to noisy environments with multiple speakers. Thus, at first the hearing aid user may be instructed to wear the hearing aid in his or her living room while speaking to one person. As the listener becomes more comfortable with the hearing aid, he or she can move on to progressively more difficult situations, such as listening in the kitchen, speaking with more than one person at a time, conversing in the car, eating in a restaurant, and shopping. Listeners can also use this time to reacquaint themselves with environmental sounds, which may at first sound quite different than expected. The rate at which the hearing aid user progresses through the hierarchy is highly individualized. Some people can use their hearing aids in all situations within a few days. Others may take weeks to adjust. Moreover, most people find that the hearing aid is not helpful in some situations. These people may want to consider the use of assistive devices (see Chapter 8) for use in environments in which a hearing aid alone is inadequate. More detailed information related to hearing aid orientation for adults and additional considerations for children can be found in Hodgson (1986). Professionals who regularly treat people who are having trouble adjusting to their hearing aids should consult Wayner (1990).

Daily Check of Hearing Aid Performance

Hearing aid performance should be checked daily. Adolescents and adults can complete the daily check on their own. Younger children's hearing aids should be checked every day by the child's parents and again in the school monitoring program. The hearing aid check consists of two phases—a visual inspection of the hearing aid and earmold followed by a listening check of the system.

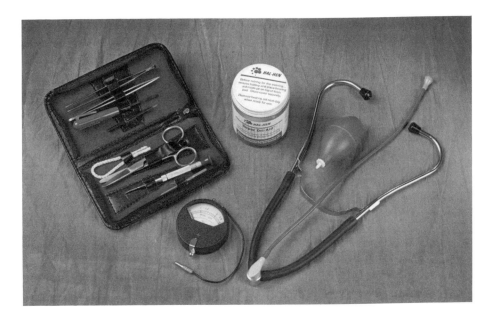

FIGURE 7.14 Equipment needed for hearing aid monitoring and troubleshooting. Clockwise from upper left: tool kit, dehumidifying kit, stethoscope, forced-air blower, and battery meter.

Equipment

Two pieces of equipment are needed to complete a hearing aid check, a hearing aid stethoscope (for listening to the hearing aid) and a battery meter (to indicate battery voltage). People who routinely deal with hearing aids (eg, speech-language pathologist, teachers, school nurses, nursing home personnel, parents of children with hearing aids, and hearing aid users themselves) often find several other items handy when troubleshooting hearing aid problems. These items include spare batteries, pipe cleaners, small screwdrivers, tweezers, forced-air blowers, dehumidifying kits, and wax removal tools. Figure 7.14 illustrates a hearing aid monitoring and troubleshooting kit. Kits containing similar equipment can be purchased from HARC Mercantile (800-445-9968 [United States] or 800-962-6634 [Michigan]).

To effectively check hearing aid function, the examiner must keep a file of pertinent information for each hearing aid to be checked. The file should include information concerning appropriate hearing aid settings, including the recommended volume setting. Information concerning battery size and earmold modifications (vents and filters) should be kept in the file. The person performing the check must be aware of the method used to couple the hearing aid to assistive devices in the classroom (eg, telecoil, silhouette inductor, DAI). Any changes in this coupling method or the types of cords or boots used can lead to changes in the electroacoustic characteristics of the hearing aid. Chapter 8 provides a more complete description of this topic.

Visual Check

Each hearing aid component should be visually inspected as follows:

1. *Earmold.* If the hearing aid has a separate earmold, the sound bore should be checked for cerumen. If cerumen is present, the bore should be cleaned with a pipe cleaner, or the earmold should be separated from the aid and washed in warm, soapy water. The earmold must be thoroughly dried before being recoupled to the hearing aid. The tubing and sound channel can be dried with a pipe cleaner or forced-air blower. The earmold should be examined for cracks (which can lead to feedback) or rough spots (which can cause discomfort in the listener). The tubing that connects the hearing aid to the earmold also should be examined. It should be soft and pliable. If it is hard and yellowed, it needs to be replaced by the dispenser. The tubing also should be checked for crimping and cracks. Crimping reduces the sound that reaches the earmold, and cracks can lead to feedback.

Some earmolds have vents, which are small channels or openings drilled next to the sound delivery canal in the earmold. The vent provides a connection between the air in the ear canal and the outside air. Vents are used to increase listener comfort and to acoustically modify the sound from the hearing aid. Many vents have small covers that are used to change the diameter of the vent. If the earmold has a vent cover, the cover should be checked to make sure it is in place. If the cover has fallen out, the quality of the sound coming from the hearing aid may be different, or feedback may occur.

ITE and ITC hearing aids do not have a separate earmold. The examiner should, however, carefully check the sound delivery channel to make sure it is not blocked by cerumen. Cerumen should be removed with a small brush or with the cerumen removal tool provided by the manufacturer. Care must be taken in this process because the receiver portion of the hearing aid lies near the opening and can be damaged if inappropriate tools are used. ITC and ITE hearing aids may have vents and vent covers. Again, the examiner should check to make sure the appropriate cover is in place.

2. *Hearing aid case.* The examiner should check the hearing aid case for dents, cracks, or separations. If the disfigurements are new, they could indicate hearing aid malfunction. The earhook (the plastic piece that lies over the pinna for BTE hearing aids) should be examined for cracks or separations from the hearing aid case because these problems can lead to feedback.

3. *Microphone.* The microphone should be checked to ensure that it is clean and free of visible damage. If it is dirty, it can be cleaned with a small brush.

4. *Battery compartment.* The examiner should open the battery compartment and remove the battery. The battery should be examined for corrosion, and its voltage should be tested with a voltage meter. If the battery voltage is less than 1.2 volts, the battery should be replaced. The battery contacts should be examined to make sure they

are not corroded, bent, or missing. If the contacts are corroded, they can be cleaned with a sharpened pencil eraser or a typewriter eraser. The examiner should make sure he or she removes the eraser particles when the cleaning is finished. In many cases, bent battery contacts can be straightened to improve the electrical connection. Hearing aids with missing battery contacts must be sent in for repair.

5. *Hearing aid controls.* The position of the hearing aid controls should be checked. For the listening check, the hearing aid microphone (not the telecoil) must be activated. The examiner checks to ensure the correct positioning of other external controls, such as a noise suppression switch or memory setting (only on some digitally programmable hearing aids). The correct settings should be listed in the information file.

6. *Body aid cords and receivers.* If the client uses a body hearing aid, the cords and receivers should be examined. The cords should be insulated throughout their entire length and should easily insert into the hearing aid and the receiver. The receiver should be examined for dents or cracks and should snap tightly into the earmold.

Listening Check

After the visual inspection, the hearing aid is connected to the hearing aid stethoscope for the listening check. Ideally, the listening check should be completed with the earmold in place. This allows the examiner to detect problems in the earmold as well as in the hearing aid. If the hearing aid stethoscope does not provide a tight seal around the earmold, feedback can occur. If feedback occurs, the earmold should be removed and the hearing aid should be coupled directly to the stethoscope.

Although listening checks can be conducted with any type of continuous discourse (eg, counting, the alphabet, simple sentences), repetition of the sounds used in Ling's five-sound test (Ling, 1975) is especially useful. By repeating the sounds /a/, /i/, /u/, /ʃ/, and /s/ (*ah, ee, oo, sh,* and *s*), the examiner will have a good representation of the amplification properties for low-frequency, mid-frequency, and high-frequency speech sounds.

1. *Volume.* Beginning with the hearing aid turned to its lowest setting, the examiner gradually increases the volume control while speaking. The volume should increase and decrease steadily with no jumping, scratchiness, or dead spots. If the volume range seems limited (ie, not enough gain), the listening check should be followed by a complete EAA. When possible, it is desirable to conduct the rest of the listening check at the volume setting used by the hearing aid user. High-gain hearing aids, however, may produce signals that are uncomfortably loud for a listener with normal hearing. The volume can be adjusted to a tolerable level when necessary.

2. *Sound quality.* Because the hearing aid has been adjusted for an impaired ear, the sound coming from the aid may sound hollow (high amounts of low-frequency amplification) or tinny (high amounts of high-frequency amplification). Nevertheless, the hearing aid should sound clear and free of obvious distortions. If changes from previous checks are noted, the listening check should be followed by a complete EAA.

3. *Intermittency*. Intermittent function indicates loose connections or broken cords. The examiner checks for intermittency by pressing on the case of the hearing aid, turning it in various positions, and gently shaking it. If a body aid is being evaluated, the examiner should also check for intermittency while moving the cords back and forth and pressing on the receiver. Broken cords and receivers are easily replaced on-site. Other problems require returning the hearing aid to the dispenser for repair.

4. *Feedback*. Feedback during a listening check most often results from an inadequate seal between the hearing aid stethoscope and the hearing aid. If the listening check is being done through the earmold, the earmold should be removed and the hearing aid directly coupled with the stethoscope. If feedback continues, the examiner should remove the hearing aid from the stethoscope and place his or her finger directly over the receiver of the hearing aid. If feedback is still audible, it may signal an internal problem and should be sent to the dispenser for repair.

Check on the User

The last step in the monitoring process occurs when the aid is replaced on the listener's ear. The examiner should make sure the earmold is seated correctly in the ear and that the switches are in the appropriate positions. The examiner should check to make sure the volume control setting is at the recommended level. He or she should listen for feedback that may occur when the hearing aid is placed on the listener. Feedback occurs when amplified sound reaches the hearing aid microphone and is reamplified. Most often the problem can be traced to the earmold. The examiner should check to ensure that the earmold is appropriately positioned in the ear and that it fits properly. A loosely fitting or improperly seated earmold allows amplified sound to escape from the ear canal. The volume setting should be checked. Many hearing aids produce feedback when the volume is adjusted near maximum. Feedback is a problem only if it occurs at recommended volume settings. The ear canal should be checked for excessive cerumen. If the canal is blocked by cerumen, amplified sound is reflected back toward the hearing aid microphone and can cause feedback. If cerumen occlusion is noted, the client should be referred to an audiologist or physician to have it removed. Finally, the earmold and tubing should be rechecked for cracks or missing vent covers.

Troubleshooting Hearing Aid Problems

Many problems noted during the listening check can be corrected on-site. Table 7.1 can be used as a guide to basic troubleshooting. If the cause cannot be identified on-site, the problem may be internal and the hearing aid should be returned to the dispenser for further evaluation and repair. Loaner hearing aids should be provided while the hearing aid is being repaired. Further information on hearing aid checks and hearing aid monitoring programs can be found in Ross et al (1991).

Table 7.1 Guide to Troubleshooting Hearing Aid Problems

Problem	Possible Causes	Possible Solutions
No sound	Hearing aid not turned on	Check on/off mechanism
	Dead battery	Insert new battery
	Wrong size battery	Use correct battery
	Battery inserted incorrectly	Insert battery correctly
	Battery compartment not closed	Close battery compartment
	Missing or corroded battery contacts	Clean contacts or send for repair
	Cerumen blockage	Clean cerumen from sound channel
	Hearing aid in *T* position	Change to *M* position
	Sound channel blocked with water	Dry sound channel
	Crimped tubing	Straighten or replace tubing
	Clogged damper	Return to dispenser for new damper
	Clogged microphone opening	Gently clean microphone cover
	Moisture in hearing aid	Use hearing aid dehumidifying kit
Intermittent sound	Weak battery	Replace battery
	Corroded or bent battery contacts	Clean and straighten contacts
	Dirty controls	Move all controls back and forth several times to loosen dirt; spray with contact cleaner if necessary
	Broken wire on body aid	Replace wire
	Poor connection to receiver	Replace wire or receiver or both
	Moisture in hearing aid	Use hearing aid dehumidifying kit
	Crimped tubing	Straighten or replace tubing
Weak sound	Weak battery	Replace battery
	Volume control at wrong setting	Set volume appropriately
	Missing vent cover	Insert new vent cover
	Paritally clogged sound channel	Clean sound channel
	Crimped tubing	Straighten or replace tubing
	Dirty microphone opening	Gently clean microphone cover
Poor or scratchy sound	Weak battery	Replace battery
	Dirty controls	Move all controls back and forth several times to loosen dirt; spray with contact cleaner if necessary
	Corroded battery contacts	Clean battery contacts
	Volume control set full-on	Adjust volume to appropriate level

continued

Table 7.1 *Continued*

Problem	Possible Causes	Possible Solutions
Poor or scratchy sound	Missing vent cover	Replace vent cover
	Dirty micorphone opening	Gently clean microphone cover
	Clothing noise (body aid)	Move microphone away from clothing if possible
	Wind noise	Stay out of wind if possible
Feedback	Incorrectly seated earmold*	Correctly seat earmold
	Incorrectly fitted earmold*	Order new earmold
	Missing vent cover	Replace vent cover
	Cracked or loosely fitting earhook	Replace earhook
	Cracked or loosely fitting tubing	Replace tubing
	Ear canal occluded with cerumen	Have cerumen removed
	Crimped tubing	Straighten or replace tubing
	Volume control set too high	Adjust volume to appropriate level
	Feedback inside case of hearing aid	Return aid for repair

*Earmold here refers to the separate ear piece used with BTE, body, and eyeglass hearing aids as well as to the case of ITE and ITC hearing aids.

REFERENCES

American National Standards Institute (1987). *American National Standard Specification of Hearing Aid Characteristics,* ANSI S3.22. New York: American National Standards Institute.

Bendet, R. (1980). A public school hearing aid maintenance program. *Volta Review, 82,* 149-153.

Bess, F. H. (1985). The minimally hearing-impaired child. *Ear and Hearing, 6,* 43-47.

Bess, F. H. (1986). The unilaterally hearing-impaired child: A final comment. *Ear and Hearing, 7,* 52-54.

Bess, F. H., & Humes, L.(1990). *Audiology: The fundamentals.* Baltimore: Williams & Wilkins.

Bess, F. H., Klee, T., & Culbertson, J. L. (1986). Identification, assessment, and management of children with unilateral sensorineural hearing loss. *Ear and Hearing, 7,* 43-54.

Bradley, S., & Malloy, P. (1991). Hearing aid malfunctions pose problems for nursing homes. *Hearing Journal, 44,* 24-26.

Carhart, R. (1946). Selection of hearing aids. *Archives of Otolaryngology, 44,* 1-18.

Compton, C. (1989). Assistive technology: Up close and personal. *Seminars in Hearing, 10,* 104-120.

Dunham, M., & Friedman, H. (1990). Audiologic management of bilateral external auditory canal atresia with the bone conducting implantable hearing device. *Cleft Palate Journal, 27,* 369-373.

Gaeth, J., & Lounsbury, E. (1966). Hearing aids and children in elementary schools. *Journal of Speech and Hearing Disorders, 31,* 283-289.

Grahl, C. (1993). A dispenser yardstick: How to measure your 1992 performance. *Hearing Instruments, 44,* 4-13.

Håkansson, B., Liden, G., Jacobsson, M., et al. (1990). Ten years of experience with the Swedish bone-anchored hearing system. *Annals of Otology, Rhinology, and Laryngology, 151,* 1-16.

Hanners, B. A., & Sitton, A. B. (1974). Ears to hear: A daily hearing aid monitor program. *Volta Review, 76,* 530-536.

Harford, E., & Barry, J. (1965). A rehabilitative approach to the problem of unilateral hearing impairment: The contralateral routing of signals (CROS). *Journal of Speech and Hearing Disorders, 30,* 121-138.

Hawkins, D., Beck, L., Bratt, G., Fabry, D., Mueller, H., & Stelmachowicz, P. (1991). The Vanderbilt/VA hearing aid conference 1990 consensus statement: Recommended components of a hearing aid selection procedure for adults. *Asha, 33,* 37-38.

Hawkins, D., & Yacullo, W. (1984). Signal-to-noise ratio advantage of binaural hearing aids and directional microphones under different levels of reverberation. *Journal of Speech and Hearing Disorders, 49,* 278-286.

Hearing Instruments (1992). Dispenser programmable hearing instruments update. *Hearing Instruments, 43,* 16-26.

Hodgson, W. (1986). Learning hearing aid use. In W. Hodgson (Ed.), *Hearing aid assessment and use in audiologic habilitation* (3rd ed.) (pp. 217-230). Baltimore: Williams & Wilkins.

Humes, L. (1986). An evaluation of several rationales for selecting hearing aid gain. *Journal of Speech and Hearing Disorders, 51,* 272-281.

Hussung, R., & Hamill, T. (1990). Recent advances in hearing aid technology: An introduction to digital terminology and concepts. *Seminars in Hearing, 11,* 1-15.

Johnson, R. J., Meikle, M., Vernon, J., & Schleuning, A. (1988). An implantable bone conduction hearing device. *American Journal of Otology, 9* (Suppl.), 93-100.

Killion, M. (1980). Problems in the application of broadband hearing aid earphones. In G. Studebaker & I. Hochberg (Eds.), *Acoustical factors affecting hearing aid performance* (pp. 219-266). Baltimore: University Park Press.

Kirkwood, D. H. (1992). 1992 U.S. hearing aid sales summary: Latest HIA reports show lull in market growth. *Hearing Journal, 45,* 7- 15.

Ling, D. (1975). Amplification for speech. In D. R. Calvert & S. R. Silverman (Eds.), *Speech and deafness.* Washington, DC: A. G. Bell Association for the Deaf.

Lybarger, S. (1944). U.S. Patent Application SN 543,278.

Lybarger, S. (1982). Telephone coupling. In G. Studebaker & F. Bess (Eds.), *The Vanderbilt hearing aid report* (pp. 91-93). Upper Darby: Monographs in Contemporary Audiology.

Lybarger, S. (1985). The physical and electroacoustic characteristics of hearing aids. In J. Katz (Ed.), *Handbook of clinical audiology* (3rd ed.) (pp. 849-884). Baltimore: Williams & Wilkins.

May, A. E., Upfold, L. J., & Battaglia, J. A. (1990). The advantages and disadvantages of ITC, ITE, and BTE hearing aids: Diary and interview reports from elderly users. *British Journal of Audiology, 24,* 301-309.

Mills, J. H. (1975). Noise and children: A review of literature. *Journal of the Acoustical Society of America, 58,* 767-779.

Mueller, H. G., & Grimes, A. M. (1983). Speech audiometry for hearing aid selection. *Seminars in Hearing, 4,* 255-272.

Mueller, H. G., Hawkins, D. B., & Sedge, R. K. (1984). Three important options in hearing aid selection. *Hearing Instruments, 35,* 14-17.

Newby, H. A., & Popelka, G. R. (1992). *Audiology* (6th ed.). Englewood Cliffs: Prentice Hall.

Northern, J. L., & Downs, M. P. (1984). *Hearing in children* (3rd ed.). Baltimore: Williams & Wilkins

Parving, A., & Boisen, G. (1990). In-the-canal hearing aids. *Scandinavian Audiology, 19,* 25-30.

Plath, P. (1991). Problems in fitting hearing aids in the elderly. *Acta Otolaryngolgica (Suppl. 476),* 278-280.

Potts, P. L., & Greenwood, J. (1983). Hearing aid monitoring: Are looking and listening enough? *Journal of Language, Speech, and Hearing Services in Schools, 14,* 157-163.

Reichman, J., & Healy, W. C. (1989). Amplification monitoring and maintenance in schools. *Asha, 31,* 43-45.

Rintelmann, W. F., & Bess, F. H. (1977). High-level amplification and potential hearing loss in children. In F. Bess (Ed.), *Childhood deafness: Causation, assessment and management* (pp. 267-294). New York: Grune & Stratton.

Robinson, D. O., & Sterling, G. R. (1980). Hearing aids and children in school: A follow-up study. *Volta Review, 82,* 229-235.

Ross, M. (1980). Binaural versus monaural hearing aid amplification for hearing impaired individuals. In E. R. Libby (Ed.), *Binaural hearing and amplification* (Vol. II) (pp. 1-21). Chicago: Zenetron.

Ross, M., Brackett, D., & Maxon, A. B. (1991). *Assessment and management of main-streamed hearing-impaired children: Principles and practices.* Austin: Pro-Ed.

Ross, M., & Lerman, J. (1967). Hearing-aid usage and its effect upon residual hearing. *Archives of Otolaryngology, 86,* 57-62.

Schow, R. L., & Nerbonne, M. A. (1980). Hearing levels among elderly nursing home residents. *Journal of Speech and Hearing Disorders, 45,* 124-132.

Shimon, D. (1992). *Coping with hearing loss and hearing aids.* San Diego: Singular.

Shore, I., Bilger, R., & Hirsh, I. (1960). Hearing aid evaluation: Reliability of repeated measurements. *Journal of Speech and Hearing Disorders, 25,* 152-167.

Skinner, M. W. (1988). *Hearing aid evaluation.* Englewood Cliffs: Prentice Hall.

Staab, W., & Lybarger, S. (1994). Characteristics and use of hearing aids. In J. Katz (Ed.), *Handbook of clinical audiology* (4th ed.) (pp. 657-722). Baltimore: Williams & Wilkins.

Stephens, S., & Meredith, R. (1991). Physical handling of hearing aids by the elderly. *Acta Otolaryngologica (Suppl. 476)*, 281-285.

Studebaker, G., Bisset, J., Van Ort, D., & Hoffnung, S. (1982). Paired comparison judgements of relative intelligibility in noise. *Journal of the Acoustical Society of America, 72,* 80-92.

Upfold, L. J., May, A. E., & Battaglia, J. A. (1990). Hearing aid manipulation skills in an elderly population: A comparison of ITE, BTE, and ITC aids. *British Journal of Audiology, 24,* 311- 318.

Van Tasell, D., Larson, S., & Fabry, D. (1988). Effects of an adaptive filter hearing aid on speech recognition in noise by hearing-impaired subjects. *Ear and Hearing, 9,* 15-21.

Walden, B.E., Schwartz, D.M., Williams, D. L., Holum-Hardegen, L. L., & Crowley, J. M. (1983). Test of the assumptions underlying comparative hearing aid evaluations. *Journal of Speech and Hearing Disorders, 48,* 264-273.

Wayner, D. (1990). *The hearing aid handbook: Clinician's guide to client orientation.* Washington, DC: Gallaudet University Press.

Wernick, J. (1985). Use of hearing aids. In J. Katz (Ed.), *Handbook of clinical audiology* (3rd ed.) (pp. 911-935). Baltimore: Williams & Wilkins.

Withrow, F. B. (1977). The condition of hearing aids worn by children in a public school. HEW Publication No. OE 77-05002. Washington, DC: Bureau of Education for the Handicapped.

SUGGESTED READING

Bentler, R. (1993). Amplification for the hearing-impaired child. In J. Alpiner & P. McCarthy (Eds.), *Rehabilitative audiology: Children and adults* (pp. 72-105). Baltimore: Williams & Wilkins.

How to buy a hearing aid (1992). *Consumer Reports,* November, pp. 716-721.

Hodgsen, W. (1986). *Hearing aid assessment and use in audiologic habilitation* (3rd ed.). Baltimore: Williams & Wilkins.

Katz, J. (1994) *Handbook of clinical audiology* (4th ed.). Baltimore: Williams & Wilkins.

Mueller, H., Hawkins, D., & Northern, J. (1992). *Probe microphone measurements: Hearing aid selection and assessment.* San Diego: Singular.

8

Assistive Devices

Stephanie A. Davidson

Assistive devices are becoming increasingly popular among people with hearing losses, and it is likely that speech-language pathologists, educators, and health care professionals will encounter these devices in their work settings. Speech-language pathologists in the school system find group amplification systems being used in classrooms for children with hearing losses. Personal assistive listening devices (ALDs) may be used by children with hearing losses who are mainstreamed into classrooms of children with normal hearing. Speech-language pathologists and health care professionals who work with adults are also likely to encounter these devices because adults with hearing losses are realizing that assistive devices can improve their ability to communicate in a variety of listening conditions.

Assistive devices are being used to supplement hearing aids in situations in which hearing aids alone are inadequate (ie, listening in background noise or listening on the telephone); and, in some cases, they are being used in place of a traditional hearing aid. Some speech-language pathologists and health care professionals keep on hand a portable ALD that can be used by clients or patients with hearing losses who are physically or mentally unable to operate a personal hearing aid.

Besides encountering assistive devices in the work setting, speech-language pathologists, educators, and health care professionals may be in a position to recognize the need for an assistive device when one has not been previously suggested. Although some assistive devices have been available for years, older technology has been greatly improved and new devices have been introduced. Consequently, many people with hearing losses who could benefit from the new technology need to be educated concerning its application. This chapter is designed to acquaint speech-language pathologists, educators, and health care professionals with assistive devices and how they can be used to assist communication.

DEFINITIONS

Assistive devices include a broad range of equipment designed to improve the communication abilities of people with hearing losses. Historically, all devices other than hearing aids designed to help people with hearing losses have been referred to as ALDs. However, as Leavitt (1989) correctly pointed out, this terminology is misleading because many of the devices do not involve listening. Rather, many of these devices provide a visual or tactile cue to indicate the presence of sound. Consequently, this chapter follows the categorization scheme used by Compton (1989, 1990) and divides assistive devices into three categories—ALDs, telecommunication devices, and alerting devices. Compton reserves the term *ALD* for systems designed specifically to help a person with a hearing loss to understand speech under less than ideal listening conditions (ie, those in which distance, noise, and reverberation are present). Telecommunication devices are designed to aid in communicating on the telephone and in watching television by providing either an enhanced auditory signal (eg, a telephone amplifier) or a visual signal (eg, a telecommunication device for the deaf [TDD] for the telephone or a closed-caption system for the television). Alerting devices are most commonly used by people with severe to profound hearing losses to alert them to acoustic stimuli that they might otherwise miss such as an alarm clock, a smoke detector, or the ring from a telephone.

ASSISTIVE LISTENING DEVICES

As noted above, ALDs are devices available to listeners with hearing losses to improve their ability to understand speech under less than ideal listening conditions. As described in Chapter 10, the foundation of any aural rehabilitation program is the selection and fitting of appropriate personal hearing aids. Hearing aids do serve people with hearing losses well under good listening conditions (ie, one-on-one communication with relatively little background noise). Unfortunately, many listening activities do not occur under such ideal conditions, and even the most technically advanced and carefully selected hearing aids have limitations. Hearing aid users often describe difficulty understanding speech any time they try to listen from a distance, amid background noise, or under reverberant conditions. Such situations are difficult because the desired signal arrives at the hearing aid microphone at a reduced intensity because of the distance it has traveled, is mixed with the background noise present in the environment, and is degraded by reverberation (Nabelek & Donahue, 1986). A hearing aid alone indiscriminately amplifies all these sounds, presenting both speech and noise to the ear of the listener. Simply turning up the volume of the hearing aid cannot solve the problem because both the speech and the noise become louder.

To further complicate the problem, it is well known that background noise and reverberation are especially troublesome for listeners with sensorineural hearing losses (Finitzo-Hieber & Tillman, 1978; Nabelek, 1980; Nabelek & Pickett, 1974; Olsen & Tillman, 1968), and recent research has indicated it might also be troublesome for elderly people—even those with relatively normal hearing sensitivity (Bergman, 1983; CHABA, 1988) and people with central auditory processing disorders (Stach et al, 1987). Consequently, levels of noise and reverberation that may be only mildly annoying to people with normal hearing can render a message incomprehensible to listeners with hearing losses, making a hearing aid inadequate in poor listening conditions.

ALDs solve the problem of listening under adverse conditions by placing the microphone of the system close to the signal of interest (eg, the speaker's mouth or the public address system) and then transmitting that signal, without a decrement in intensity and without additional background noise, directly to the ear of the listener. The signal can be transmitted to the listener by means of a variety of technologies (hardwired, induction loop, infrared, or frequency modulation [FM]), and the ALD can be used with or without a personal hearing aid. Regardless of the technology used, the result is the same—speech understanding is improved because the signal is delivered to the ear with an enhanced signal-to-noise ratio (S/N). Because the sound is picked up at its source and delivered directly to the ear of the listener, it is comparable to having the ear of the listener located within inches of the speaker. The improvements in speech understanding have been repeatedly verified for listeners in auditoriums (Nabelek & Donahue, 1986), in classrooms (Flexer et al, 1987; Hawkins, 1984; Noe, 1994), and through the comments of the many satisfied ALD users.

ALDs can be broadly divided into two categories—hardwired and wireless. Hardwired systems require a direct electrical connection between the microphone of the device and the ear of the listener with the hearing impairment. Wireless technologies transmit the signal from the microphone to the ear of the listener without a direct electrical connection. The wireless technologies commonly in use today can be divided into the following three types—induction loop, infrared, and FM. ALDs can stand alone or can be coupled to the listener's personal hearing aid. If the ALD stands alone, the listener usually receives the signal through a lightweight headset or earphone. As an alternative, the ALD can be coupled to the listener's own hearing aid to personalize the acoustics of the signal to better match the hearing loss of the listener.

Hardwired Systems

The first systems used were hardwired systems. These devices use a direct electrical connection (a wire) to connect the sound source with the listener. A hardwired system usually consists of a microphone that is placed close to the source of the sound and changes the acoustic energy into an electrical signal. This electrical signal is then sent through a wire to an amplifier and then again through a wired connection to the listener. The listener receives the signal either by wearing a lightweight headset that changes the electrical signal back into an acoustic signal to be delivered to the ear or through coupling to a personal hearing aid.

Large-Area Hardwired Systems

Hardwired systems have been used in public facilities such as places of worship, auditoriums, and theaters to assist listeners with hearing losses. The microphones for the system can be placed on the podium in front of the speaker, as in the case of a single speaker such as in a church or at a lecture; placed at several strategic locations around the stage, as in the case of a theatrical performance; or can be tied directly into an existing public address system. The amplified signal can then be routed through cables concealed within the structure or under the carpet to specific listening areas. The listeners plug in lightweight headsets to receive the signal or couple the system to their personal hearing aid.

Personal Hardwired Systems

Hardwired systems designed for use by one person at a time are known as personal amplification systems (PASs). These systems consist of a microphone, a small battery-powered amplifier (generally just slightly larger than the case of a body hearing aid), and a means of coupling the system to the listener's ear. A popular version of this device, the Williams Sound PockeTalker, is shown in Figure 8.1. The microphone of the system can be worn on the listener's body (this is known as self-wiring), placed on a table in front of the listener, or placed close to the source of the sound (ie, near the mouth of the talker or the speaker of a radio or television). The signal is then sent to the amplifier where the volume can be varied using a volume control wheel and then sent to the ear of the listener, most commonly using a lightweight earpiece.

PASs are becoming increasingly popular as an alternative to hearing aids for people who do not own a personal hearing aid. Because of its relatively low cost, its portability, its excellent sound quality, and its ease of operation (these systems are designed with large, easily accessible controls), a PAS is a logical alternative for people who are physically or mentally unable to operate a conventional hearing aid. Some elderly people who find the miniature components and day-to-day use of a hearing aid disconcerting adapt readily to the size, simplicity, and sound quality of the PAS.

PASs are also useful for professionals (eg, speech-language pathologists, nurses, physicians, emergency room personnel, lawyers, bankers, chaplains, psychologists) who interact with people with hearing losses who do not own personal hearing aids. One system, the PockeTalker (Williams Sound, Eden Prairie, Minn.) was designed for this purpose. These systems can be purchased for the office and used to facilitate communication with people with hearing losses or even elderly people with normal hearing if the listening conditions are less than ideal.

Strengths and Weaknesses of Hardwired Systems

Hardwired systems are relatively inexpensive to purchase and maintain and are free from interference from electrical signals, radio signals, and light. Mobility

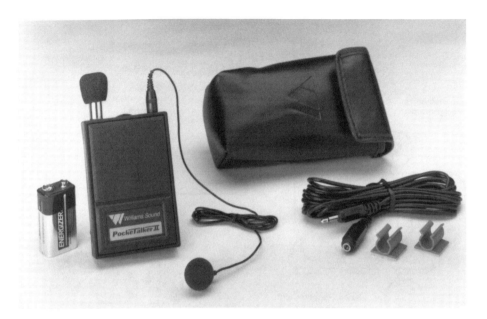

FIGURE 8.1 A hardwired personal amplification system, the Williams Sound PockeTalker.

(Photo courtesy Williams Sound Corporation, Eden Prairie, Minn.)

is, of course, limited by the need for a wired connection between the sound source and the listener. Listeners with hearing losses must sit in predetermined locations in the audience. Consequently, hardwired systems are generally not suitable for group use. However, they offer an option for personal use. Because these systems are portable, affordable, and easy to use, a PAS is often an ideal choice for personal use during stationary activities such as seated conversation (eg, in the car, during professional consultation, while playing cards) or television viewing.

Induction Loop Systems

Induction loop systems are based on the principle of magnetic induction. When an electrical current is amplified and passed through a loop of coiled wire, an electromagnetic field is generated in the vicinity of the loop, and this electromagnetic field varies in direct proportion to the electrical current flowing through the loop. When another coil of wire is placed in the vicinity of the electromagnetic field surrounding the loop, an electrical current, identical to the one flowing through the original loop, is induced in the coil. As discussed in Chapter 7, this is the method by which the telecoil in a hearing aid picks up the electromagnetic signal from the receiver of a telephone.

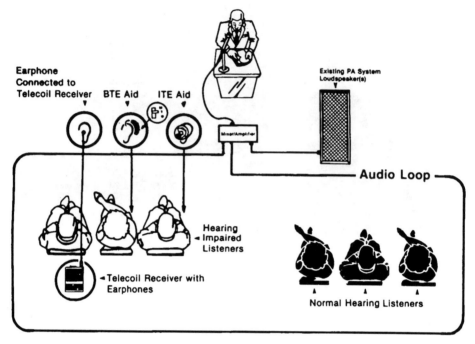

FIGURE 8.2 Schematic of a large-area induction loop system. BTE, behind-the-ear; ITE, in-the-ear.

(Reprinted with permission from Compton, 1989.)

This principle has been used to produce ALDs that transmit a signal from a sound source to a listener without a hardwired connection. A typical induction loop system consists of a microphone to pick up the signal close to the source of the sound and then to convert the acoustic energy into an electrical signal. The electrical signal is boosted by an amplifier and sent through a coil of wire (or loop) placed around the floor or ceiling of a room. This configuration produces an electromagnetic field within the room that induces a proportional electrical current in coils of wire placed in the vicinity of the electromagnetic field. Listeners with a hearing aid equipped with a telecoil can receive the signal simply by activating the telecoil in the hearing aid. Listeners without a hearing aid or with a hearing aid not equipped with a telecoil can use a special receiver with headphones.

Large-Area Loop Systems

Induction loop systems were very popular as classroom ALDs in the 1960s. For classroom use, the teacher places the microphone within inches of his or her mouth by wearing it around the neck or clipping it to his or her collar. The signal from the microphone is then amplified and sent through a loop that circles the classroom. To receive the signal, the children simply activate the telecoils of their hearing aids and are then free to move anywhere within the looped area. Although this system does substantially improve the signal-to-noise ratio at the ear of the student, numerous technical difficulties can exist with an induction loop system. Today, most classroom induction loop systems have been replaced by group FM systems (also known as FM auditory trainers), which are extremely versatile and less prone to technical difficulties.

Induction loop systems also have been used in auditoriums, theaters, and places of worship to improve speech understanding for listeners with hearing losses. The group systems can range in size from very large systems permanently installed in theaters to small, portable versions that can be used for smaller groups of listeners at meetings. In all cases, the signal is picked up by placing a microphone close to the source of the sound or is accessed electrically through an existing public address system. The entire audience area can be looped, allowing people with hearing losses to sit anywhere in the facility, or a section of the audience area can be looped, which necessitates that people with hearing losses sit within the looped area to receive the signal. A diagram of a large-area induction loop system is shown in Figure 8.2. As with classroom induction loop systems, loop systems in public facilities are declining in popularity because of technical difficulties. Many public facilities are choosing the newer FM or infrared assistive listening systems.

Personal Loop Systems

Small, commercially available induction loop systems are available for personal use. Figure 8.3 illustrates one such system used for television viewing. The microphone of the system is placed near the speaker of the television (or the signal can be obtained from an audio output jack on the television), and the signal is sent through a looped viewing area. The hearing-impaired listener simply sits within the looped area and activates the telecoil on his or her hearing aids. These personal systems can be used for a variety of other purposes such as small business meetings or social events such as card playing.

Strengths and Weaknesses of Induction Loop Systems

Induction loop systems are the least expensive of the wireless systems (Compton, 1989) and are relatively easy to maintain once installed. No special receivers are needed by listeners who own hearing aids equipped with telecoils, and listeners can move about the looped area. However, these devices are subject to a number of technical difficulties. One major problem is that they are vulnerable to electrical interference from fluorescent lighting, computers, and other electronic equipment. Such interference can be heard as an annoying buzzing sound (60-cycle hum) mixed with the signal. Interference (cross-talk) also can come from other loop systems operating in the area. This has made the systems impractical for use in school buildings where adjoining classrooms contain children with hearing losses.

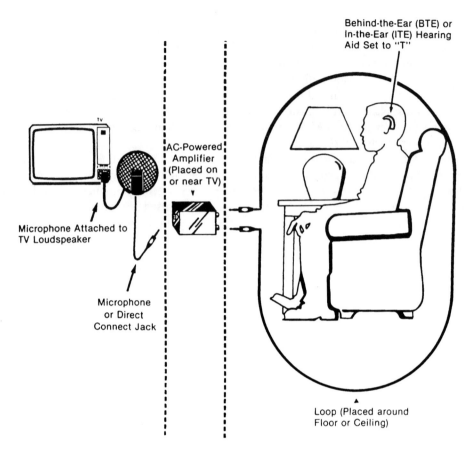

FIGURE 8.3 Schematic of personal induction loop system.

(Reprinted with permission from Compton, 1989.)

Students not only receive the signal from their own classroom but also may hear the voice of the teachers from adjoining classrooms. Recent advances in loop technology have reduced this problem. Another problem encountered with loop systems is that the strength of the electromagnetic field decreases sharply with distance from the loop. Consequently, systems for very large areas must be professionally installed, which greatly increases their cost. Finally, the orientation between the telecoil and the magnetic field generated by the loop is critical. Improperly positioned telecoils can substantially degrade the signal that reaches the listener's ear. This is of particular concern with in-the-ear (ITE) hearing aids. Because of the small size of these hearing aids, correct telecoil positioning may be sacrificed. More information on this topic is covered in the section. "Coupling an Assistive Listening Device with a Personal Hearing Aid."

Frequency Modulation Systems

Radio-frequency technology has been used in classrooms for the hearing impaired since the late 1960s. It was not until 1982, however, that the Federal Communications Commission (FCC) lifted the classroom-only restriction (Telecommunication for the Disabled Act, 1982), allowing the technology to be applied outside the classroom. Today, FM systems are extremely popular because they are the most versatile of the assistive listening technologies.

In general, FM ALDs can be considered scaled-down versions of a commercial radio station. The system consists of a microphone placed close to the source of the sound. The transmitter portion of the system uses the electrical signal from the microphone to modulate a designated carrier frequency in the 72 to 76 MHz band (the FCC has allocated frequencies in the 72 to 76 MHz band primarily for the use of FM technology to assist people with hearing losses). This signal is then transmitted through a broad area (usually several hundred feet) and can be picked up and demodulated by battery-powered FM receivers tuned to the same frequency. The signal from the FM receiver is delivered to the listener's ear through the use of earphones or is coupled to a personal hearing aid.

Large-Area Frequency Modulation Systems

Group FM systems have been used for years in classrooms for children with hearing losses, but these large-area systems are now coming into wider use in public facilities such as cinemas, theaters, places of worship, and auditoriums. A schematic of a large-area FM system is shown in Figure 8.4. The microphone of the system is placed near the source of the sound, or, commonly in public facilities, the electrical input to the FM transmitter is obtained from the existing public address system. Listeners who wish to use the system simply obtain an FM receiver when they enter the facility. The FM receivers are coupled to the listener's ears with headphones, earphones, or earbuds, or they can be coupled to a personal hearing aid. The receiver has a volume control that can be adjusted to suit the listener's needs. There is no limit to the number of FM receivers that can be used in the facility at the same time, and listeners have complete freedom in moving about the facility—they can even continue to receive the signal at the concession stand.

FM ALDs are extremely effective. Several investigators (Bankowski & Ross, 1984; Nabelek & Donahue, 1986; Nabelek et al, 1986; Noe, 1994) have demonstrated that listeners with hearing losses are better able to understand speech using an FM ALD than they can with the public address system alone or the public address system and a personal hearing aid.

Personal Frequency Modulation Systems

Many people with hearing losses are beginning to recognize the advantages provided by ALDs and are purchasing personal FM systems. An example of an FM system designed for personal use is the Easy Listener (Phonic Ear, Petaluma, Calif.),

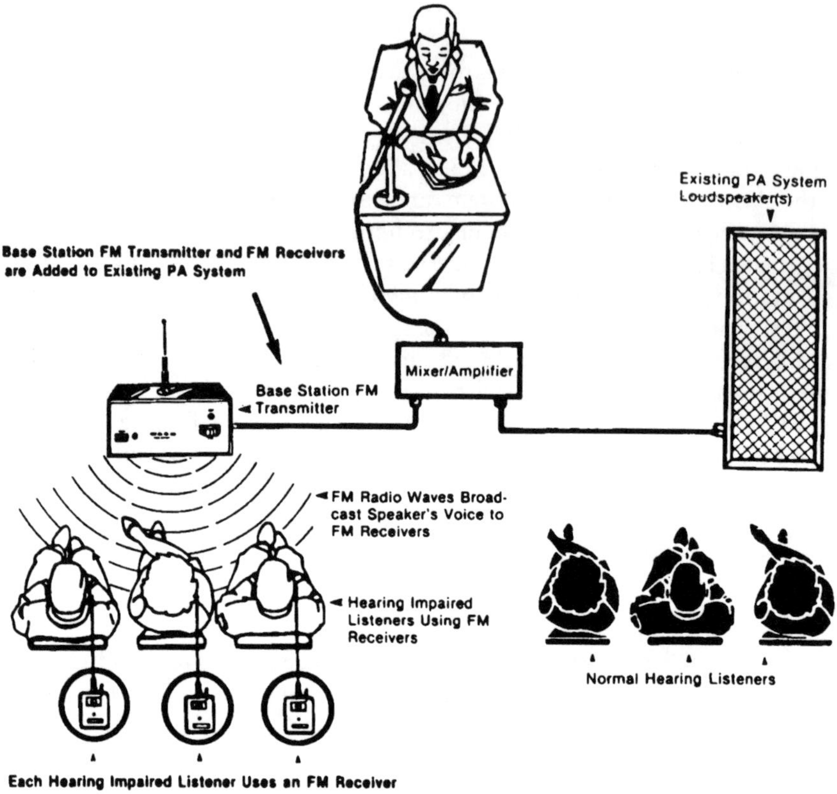

FIGURE 8.4 Schematic of a large-area FM system.

(Reprinted with permission from Compton, 1989.)

which is pictured in Figure 8.5. These systems generally consist of a microphone coupled to a battery-powered FM transmitter, which can be worn on the body of the person speaking or placed close to the sound's source (a wide variety of adapters are available to interface the FM transmitter with a variety of sound sources). The listener wears a battery-powered FM receiver, which delivers the signal to the listener's ear directly or through a hearing aid. Personal FM systems are portable and extremely versatile and thus can be used for a variety of applications. For example, they have become popular for use by children with hearing losses who are mainstreamed into classes with children with normal hearing, by adults with hearing losses who need an improved signal-to-noise ratio to understand speech, and by elderly adults and children with central auditory processing disorders, who can also benefit from an increased signal-to-noise ratio (Stach et al, 1987).

Personal FM systems provide an alternative (although a more expensive and slightly more complicated alternative) to the hardwired PASs described earlier.

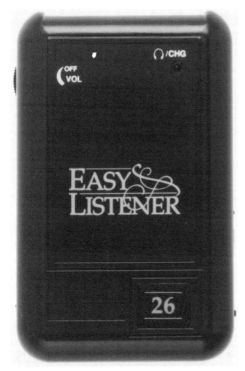

FIGURE 8.5
A receiver from a personal FM system, the Phonic Ear Easy Listener.

(Photo courtesy of Phonic Ear, Petaluma, Calif.)

They are ideal for use by speech-language pathologists, counselors, ministers, physicians, and nurses during communication with people with hearing impairments who do not own a hearing aid or who are not communicating effectively even with their hearing aids. The effect of both the FM and hardwired systems is the same: a clear speech signal is delivered to the ear of the listener regardless of background noise or room reverberation.

Strengths and Weaknesses of Frequency Modulation Systems

FM systems have excellent sound quality and are highly versatile. They can be used indoors and outdoors and transmit around corners, through obstructions, and over relatively large distances. Even though the signal can travel over several hundred feet, FM systems can easily be used in adjacent areas without cross-talk by simply using different carrier frequencies (the system generally has several frequency options). An additional advantage is that FM systems are not subject to the electrical interference that can plague loop systems or interference from other sources of infrared light, which limit the use of infrared systems.

Although the disadvantages of FM systems are few, there are some. FM systems are more expensive than hardwired or loop systems (although they are very simple and inexpensive to install). In addition, because the systems transmit through obstructions and over relatively long distances, they are not suitable for the presentation of confidential or copyrighted materials because eavesdropping and unauthorized recording are possible. A final problem is that FM systems are subject to interference from other FM signals in the area. Although the FCC has authorized the 72 to 76 MHz band primarily for use in technologies designed to assist people with hearing losses, the FCC has also authorized the use of a portion of this same frequency band for use by some other public communications (eg, city paging systems and emergency call boxes) (Compton, 1990). Consequently, in certain metropolitan areas, interference can be a problem for some frequencies, necessitating a change in the system carrier frequency.

Infrared Systems

Infrared systems were originally designed and operated in Europe, where laws prohibit the use of FM technology for hearing assistance. Infrared systems transmit sound through harmless light waves outside the boundaries of visible light (95 kHz has been designated the infrared light carrier frequency). These systems consist of a microphone placed near the source of the sound to change the acoustic signal into an electrical signal. The electrical signal is then sent to the alternating current (AC)-powered transmitter (or emitter), which uses the signal to modulate the invisible light wave. The light wave is then transmitted throughout the area by special light emitting diodes (LEDs) located on the front of the transmitter. The receiver for the system is a lightweight battery-powered headset. The receiver uses a photodiode to pick up the infrared signal, which is then demodulated into a high-quality audio signal and sent to headphones worn by the listener or coupled to the listener's personal hearing aid.

Large-Area Infrared Systems

Infrared systems are known for their excellent fidelity. This factor has made them increasingly popular in theaters and concert halls. They also are appropriate for use in places of worship and lecture halls. As with other assistive listening systems, the microphones for the system can be placed close to the mouth of the speaker, placed at several strategic locations around the stage, as would be required at a concert, or can be tied directly into an existing public address system. A single AC-powered transmitter, or several transmitters depending on the size and shape of the listening area, transmits the infrared signal throughout the listening area. The listeners with hearing impairments obtain battery-powered receivers and lightweight headphones to receive the signal. There is no limit to the number of infrared receivers that can be used in the audience at one time as long as a direct line of sight between the transmitter and receiver is maintained. A schematic of a large-area infrared system is shown in Figure 8.6.

An infrared system is the system of choice when confidentiality or copyright restrictions are a consideration. This is because, as is true of visible light, infrared light cannot penetrate walls or thick curtains. Consequently, the transmission of

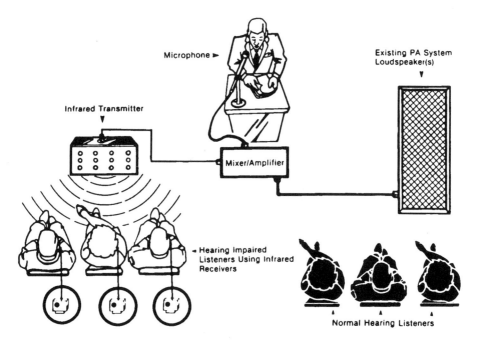

FIGURE 8.6 Schematic of a large-area infrared system.

(Reprinted with permission from Compton, 1989.)

the signal is completely confined to the room where the emitter is located, and eavesdropping from other locations is not possible. This makes an infrared system ideal for situations in which privacy or secrecy is imperative (eg, courtrooms or private boardrooms) or situations in which unauthorized recordings are prohibited (eg, concert or theater productions).

These systems add to the enjoyment of the audience. As with FM systems, evidence (Nabelek & Donahue, 1986; Nabelek et al, 1986; Noe, 1994) indicates that listeners are better able to understand speech when they use a large-area infrared system than they are when they use the public address system alone or the public address system and their personal hearing aid. No statistically significant difference between the listeners' performance with FM as opposed to infrared systems has been shown.

Personal Infrared Systems

Smaller versions of infrared systems are available for personal use. The most popular application of this technology is for television viewing. Several companies have developed personal infrared systems specifically for this purpose. Figure 8.7 shows one such device. The microphone for the system can be attached with Velcro fasteners to the speaker of the television (or the stereo), or the signal can be obtained

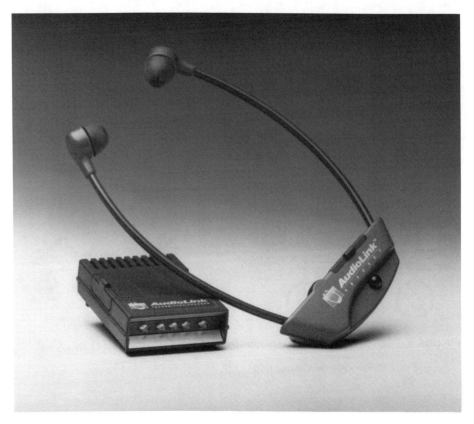

FIGURE 8.7 An infrared system designed for personal use, the NCI Audiolink Infrared System.

(Photo courtesy of the National Captioning Institute, Falls Church, Va.)

from the audio output jack if available. The AC-powered infrared transmitter is placed on top of the television and the listener wears the battery-powered receiver and stethoscope-style headphones. The system also can be coupled to the listener's hearing aid.

Personal infrared systems are appropriate for applications such as small-group conversations or meetings. As mentioned earlier, they are useful when confidentiality is a concern and are therefore ideal for private counseling sessions with psychologists, ministers, or attorneys.

Strengths and Weaknesses of Infrared Systems

Infrared technology is relatively expensive, but it provides excellent sound quality and is free from radio-frequency and electrical interference. Personal systems are easy to install; the user simply plugs the transmitter into an AC outlet, places the microphone near the source of the sound (or plugs the unit into the audio output jack of the television or stereo) and wears the receiver. An added advantage, as mentioned earlier, is that infrared light does not penetrate walls or other such barriers and thus can be used for adjoining classrooms without cross-talk and can be used in situations in which privacy is a concern. Although infrared technology is free from radio-frequency and electrical interference, it is subject to interference from other sources of infrared light, such as sunlight, fluorescent light, and even incandescent light to some extent. Consequently, infrared systems are most successfully used indoors in areas with few windows because any stray infrared light is picked up by the receivers and is heard as noise in the signal. An additional consideration is that obstructions between the transmitter and the receiver can decrease the quality of the infrared signal. A direct line of sight must exist between the two portions of the system, necessitating careful placement of multiple transmitters for large-area systems. A final disadvantage of the infrared systems is their lack of portability. Infrared transmitters are relatively bulky and have high power demands, necessitating that they be connected to an AC wall outlet. Thus, a speaker cannot wear a battery-powered transmitter and move freely around the room, as is possible with an FM system.

DELIVERING THE SIGNAL FROM THE ASSISTIVE LISTENING DEVICE TO THE LISTENER

Most ALDs deliver the signal to the listener in two different ways—directly to the ear of the listener (through the use of transducers that change the electrical signal from the ALD into an acoustic signal, which is then delivered to the ear) or by coupling the ALD to the listener's personal hearing aid (through the use of direct audio input [DAI] or inductive coupling). Whether or not the user chooses to couple the ALD to a personal hearing aid depends on several factors. One important factor is the degree of hearing loss. Most ALDs have a volume control that allows them to provide mild to moderate amounts of gain through a broad frequency range. Thus they can provide an adequate level of high-fidelity sound for listeners with mild to moderate degrees of hearing loss. However, for listeners with severe to profound hearing losses, or losses that require a tailored frequency response, the gain provided by an ALD alone is not sufficient. Coupling the ALD to the person's personal hearing aid can solve the problem for these listeners. The signal from the ALD is fed into a hearing aid that provides the gain and output appropriate for the person's hearing loss.

Another factor that determines whether or not the ALD is coupled to a personal hearing aid is, of course, whether or not the person has a hearing aid. All of the ALDs discussed in this chapter can be used as stand-alone listening systems, provided the person's amplification requirements do not exceed the output of the device. As mentioned earlier, this makes ALDs ideal as a substitute for hearing aids for people who because of physical or mental disabilities are not good candidates for conventional hearing aids or for temporary use for people who do not own a hearing aid.

Use of an Assistive Listening Device Without a Personal Hearing Aid

The signal from an ALD can be delivered to the ear of the listener through a wide variety of transducers (Figure 8.8). The transducers change the electrical signal from the ALD into an acoustic signal that can be delivered to the ear. These transducers often take the form of lightweight headsets (Figure 8.8, A) or earbuds (Figure 8.8, B). Another popular adaptation is to use a body hearing aid receiver coupled to a custom receiver-type earmold. Binaural delivery of the signal is usually preferable for enhanced speech understanding. These methods can be used to deliver a broadband high-quality signal with a mild to moderate amount of amplification to the listener.

Coupling an Assistive Listening Device with a Personal Hearing Aid

If a listener requires more than a moderate amount of gain or needs a precisely tailored frequency response, the ALD can be coupled to the person's personal hearing aid. This can be accomplished electrically, through DAI, or with an inductive system, through the use of a neckloop or a silhouette inductor and the telecoil of the hearing aid.

Inductive Coupling

The telecoil in a hearing aid was originally designed to convert the electro-magnetic signal near the receiver of a telephone into an electrical signal, which can then be amplified by the hearing aid. This same principle has been applied to bring a signal from an ALD to a hearing aid. The electrical signal from a sound source (a microphone or audio output jack on a television or radio) or from the receiver of an ALD is delivered to either a silhouette inductor (Figure 8.8, C) worn behind the ear or to a wire loop (neckloop or teleloop) worn around the neck (Figure 8.8, D). Inside the cord of the neckloop and inside the plastic case of the silhouette inductor are many small coils of wire. The electrical signal passing through these coils of wire generates an electromagnetic field in the vicinity of the neckloop or silhouette inductor. This signal is picked up by the telecoil in the listener's personal hearing aid. This signal is then amplified, changed into acoustic energy by the hearing aid receiver, and delivered to the listener's ear.

As discussed in Chapter 7, in reference to using a hearing aid with a telephone, the use of a telecoil in an ITE hearing aid can be a problem. Although they are standard on most behind-the-ear (BTE) hearing aids, telecoils are generally available

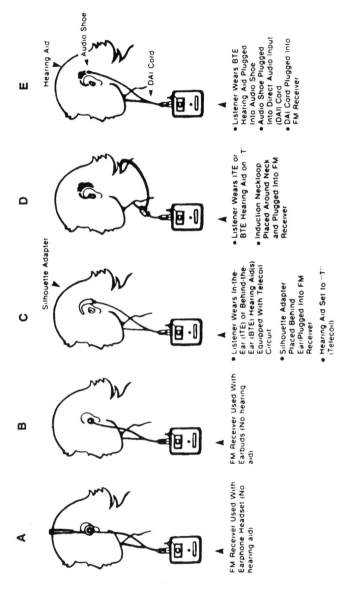

FIGURE 8.8 Methods for delivering the ALD signal to the listener's ear. A, lightweight headset for use without a hearing aid. B, earbuds for use without a hearing aid. C, silhouette inductor for use with a hearing aid with the telecoil activated. D, neckloop for use with a hearing aid with the telecoil activated. E, direct audio input (DAI) electrical connection between the ALD and the listener's hearing aid. BTE, behind-the-ear; ITE, in-the-ear.

(Adapted and reprinted with permission from Compton, 1989.)

only as an option on ITE hearing aids. Moreover, even when they are requested, the telecoil and associated amplifier often are not strong enough to adequately process the incoming signal (this is generally not a problem with BTE hearing aids). Manufacturers can, in some cases, increase the strength of the telecoil to solve the problem, but careful evaluation of the hearing aid is necessary—one cannot simply assume that the telecoil is working properly. If the client says the signal from the hearing aid is not strong enough, careful evaluation by the dispenser of the telecoil and its coupling to the ALD is warranted.

Care must be taken when using inductive coupling to deliver the signal from an ALD to the listener's ear. As is true for telephone use, the quality of the signal that reaches the listener's ear depends on several factors. These include the size of the telecoil within the hearing aid and its distance and orientation to the electromagnetic field generated by the neckloop or silhouette inductor. Hawkins and Van Tassel (1982) investigated the effects of head tilt and neck length on hearing aid output and found substantial effects when neckloops were used. They concluded that "the constantly fluctuating gain due to the child's head movements would at best be distracting and at worst reduce the child's ability to use the amplification system to perceive speech" (p. 359). Silhouette inductors are similarly subject to variable performance because of small movements between the hearing aid and the inductor and are also subject to higher levels of distortion and hearing aid internal noise (Hawkins & Schum, 1985). Consequently, at this time, silhouette inductors seem to be the least attractive of the ALD–hearing aid coupling methods.

Another important concern with the use of inductive coupling is the change in the frequency response of the hearing aid when the telecoil is activated. Hearing aids are most often selected on the basis of performance with the microphone activated. However, several studies (Davidson & Noe, 1994; Hawkins, 1984; Hawkins & Schum, 1985; Hawkins & Van Tassel, 1982) have shown that the electroacoustic characteristics of the hearing aid can change substantially when the hearing aid telecoil is activated and the hearing aid is coupled to an ALD. Moreover, these changes in gain and output are not predictable; they vary by coupling method (neckloop, silhouette inductor, or DAI), hearing aid, and even the brand of ALD.

Figure 8.9 shows an example of the change in frequency response that occurs when a hearing aid is coupled to an ALD with a neckloop compared with the frequency response of the hearing aid in the microphone mode. One cannot assume that the listener is receiving the same gain and output from the hearing aid when it is coupled to an ALD as when the hearing aid is operating independently. Thus, when coupled to an ALD, even the most carefully selected hearing aid may no longer be entirely appropriate for the hearing loss. The implication of this research is that it is necessary for the practitioner who dispenses the ALD to evaluate the performance characteristics of the system while it is coupled to the client's personal hearing aid. Hawkins (1987) described a probe measurement technique to provide this information. It behooves all users of ALDs to have such measurements made to assure that the system is appropriate.

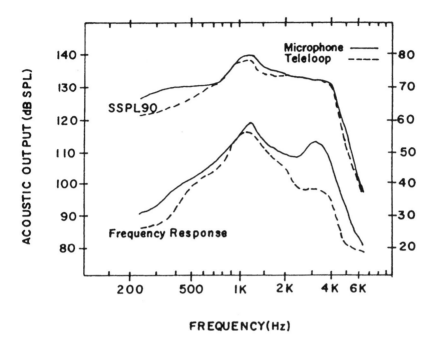

FREQUENCY(Hz)

FIGURE 8.9 Change in frequency response and output characteristics that can occur when the telecoil is activated. Solid line, gain and output characteristics when the microphone is activated. Dashed line, characteristics with the telecoil activated.

(Reprinted from Hawkins &. Van Tassel, 1982, with permission of the American Speech-Language-Hearing Association and D. Hawkins.)

Direct Audio Input

DAI is a means of delivering an electrical signal directly to a hearing aid. The electrical signal is delivered to the hearing aid through the use of a cord and snap-on boot that establishes an electrical connection to the hearing aid. Figures 8.10 and Figure 8.8, E illustrate the connection. The signal is then amplified according to the gain and frequency response characteristics of the hearing aid. The electrical signal fed into the hearing aid can come directly from a sound source (such as a microphone or audio output jack) or can come from the receiver of an infrared or FM ALD. As is true of inductive coupling, the electroacoustic characteristics of the hearing aid may change when DAI is used from those that occur for sounds that are input through the microphone of the hearing aid. Although Hawkins and Van Tassel (1982) demonstrated that coupling by means of DAI provided better agreement with the electroacoustic characteristics of the hearing aid alone than did inductive coupling, a more recent investigation by Hawkins and Schum (1985) found that no single coupling method (neckloop, silhouette inductor, or DAI) was

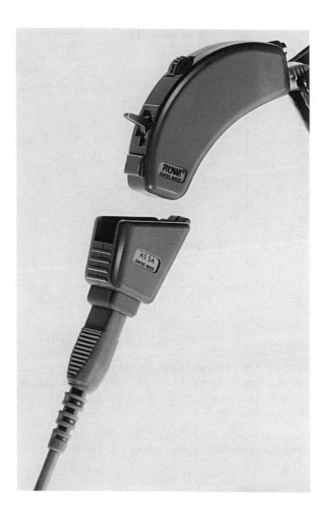

FIGURE 8.10
The audio shoe or boot
used to provide a direct
electrical connection
between the ALD and the
listener's hearing aid.

(Photo courtesy of Phonak,
Inc., Naperville, Ill.)

superior to the others in matching the electroacoustic characteristics of the hearing aid operating in the microphone mode. DAI, however, seems to have some advantage over inductive coupling in that the strength of the telecoil and its distance and orientation to the neckloop or silhouette inductor do not affect the performance of the hearing aid (Hawkins, 1984). DAI is widely available on BTE hearing aids and can sometimes be adapted to body hearing aids (Compton, 1989; 1990). Some manufacturers can equip specially ordered ITE hearing aids with DAI, if space allows, but DAI is not currently available for custom in-the-canal (ITC) hearing aids (Compton, 1989).

Behind-the-Ear Frequency Modulation Hearing Systems

Technologic advances have now made possible an integrated hearing aid and FM receiver system all enclosed in a single case the size and shape of a BTE hearing

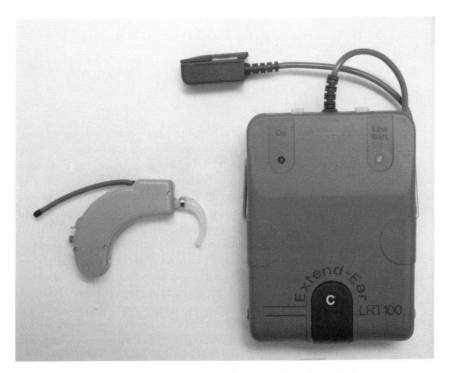

FIGURE 8.11 A BTE FM hearing system, the Extend-Ear from AVR Communications.

(Photo courtesy of Sonovation distributor for Ramat Yishai of Israel.)

aid. The listener simply wears what looks like a standard BTE hearing aid, but the system can function as a hearing aid, as an FM receiver, or as a combination hearing aid–FM receiver. Although these systems are new to the commercial market, they hold promise for everyone, but especially for listeners (eg, teenagers) who object to the bulkier and more noticeable FM receivers in current use. Figure 8.11 illustrates a BTE FM hearing system.

THE USE OF ASSISTIVE LISTENING DEVICES IN THE SCHOOL SYSTEM

Classrooms are poor acoustic environments for listeners with hearing impairments. The relatively long reverberation times, background noise (due to feet shuffling, chairs moving, and students talking), and distance between the student and the teacher make speech understanding a difficult task for students with hearing losses, even when they wear appropriately fit hearing aids. ALDs are ideally suited to this situation because they deliver the teacher's voice to the students' ears at an adequate signal-to-noise ratio regardless of the intervening distance. Research has indicated the effectiveness of ALDs in the classroom (Flexer et al, 1987; Nabelek et al, 1986; Noe, 1994; Ross & Giolas, 1971)

Auditory Trainers

Assistive listening systems used in the classroom have generally been referred to as auditory trainers. Four different types of auditory trainers—portable desk models (desk trainers), group hardwired units, induction loop units, and FM radio frequency units—have been used through the years (Berger & Millin, 1979). The portable desk models (which are simply individual hardwired units situated on the student's desk) and group hardwired units are not in general use. The induction loop units were popular in classrooms for children with hearing losses during the 1960s. In these systems, the electrical signal from the teacher's microphone is delivered to a loop around the classroom and the students can receive the signal simply by activating the telecoil in their hearing aids. Although induction loop systems do improve the speech understanding ability of the students in the classroom (Nabelek et al, 1986; Noe, 1994), problems exist. One problem is the lack of gain and poor sound quality that can exist if the hearing aid telecoil and its amplifier are not strong enough or if the telecoil is not situated in the hearing aid with the appropriate orientation to the electromagnetic field generated by the loop. This is especially prone to occur with ITE hearing aids. Another technical difficulty is the interference (cross-talk) that can occur when adjacent rooms are looped; children receive the signal from teachers in adjacent rooms as well as the signal from their own teacher. A final problem is that not all hearing aids come equipped with a telecoil.

These technical problems can be resolved when used in a classroom through the use of group FM systems, commonly referred to as FM auditory trainers. These systems have been used in the classroom since 1968 (Pehringer, 1989) and are the system of choice in most schools (Middleton & Ekhaml, 1987). FM auditory trainers are highly versatile. Because there are no connecting wires, the teacher and students are free to move throughout the classroom and can even go outdoors or to the lunchroom while maintaining contact. Cross-talk is not a problem with FM auditory trainers; adjacent classrooms simply use different carrier frequencies.

Personal FM Systems

In the past, all FM auditory training units used in the school systems were self-contained; that is, they were designed to function without the use of a personal hearing aid. In self-contained units, the receiver of the FM auditory trainer also functions as a hearing aid; it contains an environmental microphone and the gain, output, and frequency response of the system can be adjusted as appropriate for each student's hearing loss. The signal is then delivered to the student's ears through lightweight headsets or body hearing aid receivers coupled to custom receiver-type earmolds.

Another option, known as a personal FM system, has become available. This system incorporates the use of the student's personal hearing aid. The signal from the personal FM receiver is coupled to the student's hearing aid by means of DAI or through the use of a neckloop or silhouette inductor. The signal is further amplified and shaped by the hearing aid, converted to an acoustic signal at the hearing aid receiver, and delivered to the student's ear.

The advantage to the personal FM system is that students hear the classroom material through a personal hearing aid to which they are accustomed. However, Hawkins et al (Hawkins, 1984; Hawkins & Schum, 1985; Hawkins & Van Tassel, 1982) demonstrated that the electroacoustic characteristics of a personal hearing aid can change substantially when coupled to an ALD. Thus, it cannot be assumed that the signal to the student is appropriate simply because it is being processed through a hearing aid that has been fit to operate independently. If the student is to be assured of an optimal signal, it is important that the dispenser or educational audiologist evaluate the electroacoustic characteristics of the hearing aid when it is coupled to the FM system that is to be used in the classroom or therapy session.

The Use of Environmental Microphones

The receiver portion of a group auditory training system contains a microphone (known as the environmental microphone) that when activated allows the student to pick up sounds in the environment. Environmental microphones are included so that the child can monitor his or her own spoken communication and that of the other children in the classroom as well as hear the teacher's voice through FM transmission. The same option is generally available with personal FM systems. If the FM system is coupled to the hearing aid by means of an inductive system, activating the telecoil and microphone simultaneously (using the *M/T* switch position) is comparable with activating the environmental microphone on the FM auditory trainer. The hearing aid microphone can be selectively activated if DAI is used to couple the hearing aid to the FM system.

Although the advantages of activating the environmental microphone in the classroom are obvious, there are problems associated with its use. The environmental microphone indiscriminately picks up the background noise in the room and mixes it with the FM signal from the teacher's transmitter, reducing the signal-to-noise advantage that the FM system was designed to produce. Hawkins (1984) found that using an FM system, as compared with a hearing aid alone, resulted in an advantage equivalent to a 15-dB improvement in the signal-to-noise ratio. However, he also noted that activating the environmental microphone caused most of that advantage to disappear—and that was with optimal seating in the classroom. Hawkins (1984) concluded that the environmental microphone should not be activated unless it is necessary that the child self-monitor or listen to the others in the classroom. When it is necessary to use the environmental microphone, Hawkins suggests reducing the level of the environmental sounds relative to the FM signal coming from the teacher's transmitter. In a personal FM system, this can be accomplished by turning down the volume control on the hearing aid. Although this step reduces the level of the FM signal as well as the level of the environmental sounds, the level of the FM signal can be boosted by increasing the volume control on the FM receiver. In group FM auditory trainers, some manufacturers have added a separate volume control specifically for the FM signal so that it can be increased relative to the input from the environmental microphone.

Other Uses of FM Systems in the Classroom

FM systems have many uses in the educational setting beyond their traditional place in classrooms for children with hearing losses. Many children with hearing losses are being mainstreamed into regular classrooms. Even using appropriately fit binaural hearing aids and preferential seating, these students struggle to understand the teacher because of the adverse listening conditions in the typical classroom. Personal FM systems are ideally suited to this task. The student simply asks the classroom teacher to wear the microphone and transmitter during class. Because of its portability, the system can easily be moved from room to room as the student moves throughout the day. This type of system works well for students of all ages, preschoolers as well as college students.

Personal FM systems are beginning to be used with other populations of children in the classroom. It has been suggested that children with fluctuating hearing losses, unilateral hearing losses, or central auditory processing problems can benefit from the use of ALDs (Bess et al, 1986; Ferre, 1987; Flexer & Savage, 1992; Kenworthy et al, 1990; Stach et al, 1987). Although there is a lack of empiric evidence to verify these claims at the present time, the use of an ALD makes good sense. Children with fluctuating mild hearing losses, unilateral hearing losses, or central auditory processing disorders are more susceptible to difficulty under adverse listening conditions than are children with normal hearing. A personal FM system can provide a high-quality auditory signal at an improved signal-to-noise ratio for these students. Personal FM systems can be used without a hearing aid, and the volume can be adjusted to provide minimal gain for students with normal or near-normal hearing sensitivity.

THE USE OF ASSISTIVE LISTENING DEVICES BY THE ELDERLY
As an Alternative to a Personal Hearing Aid

ALDs are becoming increasingly popular among elderly listeners. Hardwired PASs are a practical alternative to conventional hearing aids. Because of the excellent sound quality, simple design, and large, easy to operate controls, some elderly listeners actually prefer PASs to hearing aids, which they may find too sophisticated or troublesome to operate. The large size also makes a PAS useful for people with physical or mental impairments who are unable to use conventional amplification.

As a Means of Improving the Signal-to-Noise Ratio

Both the peripheral and central components of the auditory system degenerate with age. In some people, degeneration of the central auditory system is marked, leading to increased difficulty in perceiving speech in background noise (Jerger & Hayes, 1977). Central auditory processing disorders accompany peripheral hearing losses in a large number of listeners older than 60 years (Davidson & Wall, 1988; Hayes & Jerger, 1979; Kricos et al, 1987; Shirinian & Arnst, 1982), and this fact has implications for successful hearing aid use. Although elderly listeners with central auditory processing disorders report benefit from conventional hearing aids (Kricos et al, 1987), the benefit would be expected to decrease, in some cases substantially, under adverse listening conditions. For these people, ALDs provide a means of increasing the signal-to-noise ratio so that the listener is better able to understand speech even under less than ideal listening conditions.

In a Nursing Home

Schow and Nerbonne (1980) found that more than 80 percent of residents of a nursing home had a clinically significant hearing loss, but only 11 percent were using hearing aids. According to Thibodeau (1989), the use of personal hearing aids in nursing homes is difficult for the following reasons: the limited number of staff members who are familiar with hearing aid operation and who are able to monitor the performance of the residents' hearing aids; the fear by the staff, the resident, or the resident's family that the hearing aid will be lost; and a lack of motivation on the part of the resident to wear the hearing aid. When the residents do not wear hearing aids, however, their quality of life is diminished. ALDs provide an alternative to full-time conventional hearing aid use.

Thibodeau (1989) suggests having an array of ALDs available for all residents. Residents can then borrow the systems as needed for television viewing, group activities, family visits, and telephone conversations. This system simplifies staff training (they have fewer amplification systems with which to become familiar) and in many cases is less intimidating to the residents. Specific suggestions on the most practical ALDs for nursing home use are discussed in detail by Thibodeau (1989). For residents who must stay in bed, a good choice is a hardwired PAS. This inexpensive system can remain at the bedside of these patients to facilitate communication with family and health care personnel and can even be used for television viewing.

THE USE OF ASSISTIVE LISTENING DEVICES IN THE HEALTH CARE SYSTEM

Hardwired PASs are being used in many emergency departments, hospitals, and clinics to facilitate communication with patients who are not wearing or who do not possess a hearing aid. In fact, as previously mentioned, the PockeTalker was designed specifically for this purpose. The broad frequency response, high fidelity, and variable volume control make the system (and others like it) appropriate for people with a mild to moderate degree of hearing loss. The low cost and ease of operation of such systems allow health care facilities to keep one or more of the units on hand to be used as the need arises.

Speech-language pathologists, nurses, psychologists, and other health care professionals may keep a PAS available to use with clients who do not wear a conventional hearing aid. Because of the small size and portability, these systems can easily be carried from one facility to another to use as needed. Clinicians should keep in mind that these systems do more than simply amplify the signal; they substantially improve the singal-to-noise ratio. Because of this feature, the devices are useful for clients with central auditory processing disorders. As discussed in Chapters 11 and 13, central auditory processing disorders can accompany stroke, head injury, or the aging process itself. Therapy sessions with these clients should be more effective when the client receives a clear auditory signal without the distraction of background noise.

Although hardwired PASs are used most frequently in the health care system, personal FM systems can provide the same benefit. Hardwired systems are, of course, much less expensive and slightly easier to operate. FM systems, on the other hand, give the client and clinician greater flexibility of movement.

TELECOMMUNICATION DEVICES

Devices designed to assist a person with a hearing loss to communicate with a telephone and to follow television programs are broadly categorized as telecommunication devices. Assistive devices for a telephone include those that amplify the signal from a telephone or serve to make a telephone more compatible with an personal hearing aid. For people who cannot communicate orally with a telephone, there are TDDs, also known as text telephones (TT), which are also considered in this category. Assistive devices for televisions include ALDs used specifically for television viewing as well as closed-caption devices.

Telephone

Telephone conversations are frequently difficult for people with hearing losses for a number of reasons. One reason is that the signal from a telephone has

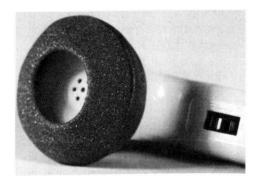

FIGURE 8.12 A Tel-EZE foam cushion used to prevent feedback during acoustic coupling of a telephone and hearing aid.

(Photo courtesy of HARC Mercantile, Ltd., Kalamazoo, Mich.)

a limited bandwidth (about 300 to 3000 Hz). Another is that the clarity and loudness of the signal vary according to the characteristics of a telephone line and a particular telephone. These problems are compounded when the listener is trying to follow conversation in a noisy room. Moreover, listeners are not able to use speechreading cues while using a telephone, and, to make matters worse, the signal is heard in only one ear. Consequently, it is not surprising that people with hearing losses often need assistance to successfully use a telephone.

In some cases, personal hearing aids alone solve the problem. Personal hearing aids can be acoustically or inductively coupled to a telephone. In the acoustic coupling method, a telephone receiver is simply held next to the microphone of the hearing aid. (In the case of BTE hearing aids, this generally means holding the receiver at the top of the ear rather than covering the ear canal. With ITE hearing aids, the positioning is normal.) Although acoustic coupling is feasible for some hearing aid users, it can lead to problems. One common complaint is that feedback occurs. Feedback is the high-pitched whistling sound that occurs when sound already amplified by the hearing aid is picked up by the microphone of the hearing aid and reamplified. Placing the receiver of a telephone close to the case of the hearing aid often leads to feedback because the amplified sound from the hearing aid reflects off the surface of the telephone receiver and back into the microphone of the hearing aid. The chances of feedback occurring can be reduced by holding the receiver of a telephone a small distance away from the hearing aid microphone. Special foam cushions (Figure 8.12) have been developed for this purpose. These inexpensive cushions are placed on a telephone receiver to keep it a constant distance away from the microphone of the hearing aid.

Hearing aid users with a telecoil switch on their hearing aids may prefer inductive coupling to acoustic coupling. As described in Chapter 7, the telecoil is an inductive coil located in the case of the hearing aid. When activated, this coil picks up the electromagnetic signal leaking from the receiver of a telephone and changes it into an electrical signal that is shaped and amplified by the hearing aid. To use inductive coupling, the hearing aid user activates the telecoil of the hearing aid and places the telephone receiver in contact with the hearing aid case. The hearing aid user needs to experiment to determine the position of the telephone receiver that results in the loudest signal. The hearing aid volume usually must be increased when the telecoil is activated.

Using inductive coupling has two distinct advantages over acoustic coupling. First, feedback does not occur. This is because the microphone of the hearing aid is deactivated when the hearing aid is switched to the telecoil position. A second advantage of using the telecoil is that only sounds coming through the telephone are amplified by the hearing aid. Environmental sounds are not amplified because the microphone is not functioning. This can make a considerable difference when a person is trying to converse in a noisy setting.

Although inductive coupling has advantages over acoustic coupling, problems also exist with this method. First, not all telephones are compatible with hearing aid telecoils. In the past, all telephone receivers generated a relatively strong electromagnetic field that had nothing to do with the performance of the telephone—it was simply a by-product. Over the years, however, the design of telephone receivers has been improved, resulting in receivers that are more efficient, durable, and less expensive to manufacture (Lybarger, 1982). Unfortunately, the improvements also resulted in receivers that no longer emitted a strong electromagnetic field; thus, many telephones were no longer compatible with hearing aid telecoils. Federal legislation has addressed this problem. Since 1989 the FCC has required that all telephones sold for use in the United States must be hearing aid compatible. Since 1993 the FCC has also required that telephones in the workplace, hotels and motels, health care facilities, and prisons be compatible with hearing aids (Staab & Lybarger, 1994). Public telephones that are hearing aid compatible are identified by a blue grommet at the base of the receiver (Figure 8.13). If a hearing aid-compatible telephone is not available, portable acoustic to magnetic couplers can be strapped over the receiver of a telephone to change the acoustic signal into a strong electromagnetic signal. These devices are described in more detail in the following section.

Using a hearing aid-compatible telephone does not guarantee that the listener receives an adequate signal. To be maximally efficient, the telecoil in the hearing aid must be large enough and must be correctly oriented in the hearing aid case. This can be easily accomplished in BTE hearing aids. ITE hearing aids, however, pose a problem. Because all the components of an ITE hearing aid must fit into a small case, the size and positioning of the telecoil may be compromised, resulting in a weak signal. If space allows, the manufacturer can correct this problem through the use of a preamplifier or additional coils of wire. However, if a hearing aid user relies on the hearing aid telecoil for telephone or ALD use, it may behoove the user to purchase a BTE hearing aid from a manufacturer known to produce strong and reliable telecoils.

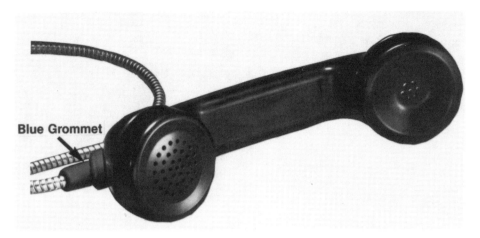

FIGURE 8.13 Blue grommet located at the base of the receiver indicates a public telephone is hearing aid-compatible.

(Photo courtesy of HARC Mercantile, Ltd., Kalamazoo, Mich.)

Telephone Amplifiers

For listeners who do not own personal hearing aids, who own hearing aids without a telecoil, or who have continued difficulty despite using hearing aid-compatible telephones and functional telecoils, telephone amplifiers may be necessary. Telephone amplifiers boost the intensity of the signal and can be used with or without a personal hearing aid (for people with more than a moderate degree of hearing loss, a hearing aid still is necessary for added gain). Telephone amplifiers can be grouped into four basic categories—built-in amplifiers, amplified replacement handsets, in-line amplifiers, and portable amplifiers.

Built-in amplifiers are built into the body of a telephone and purchased as an entire unit. The signal intensity is varied with an adjustable volume control. Until recently, these amplifiers were available only on large, desk-type telephones. Now, however, they are available for Trimline and similar telephones (Slager, 1989).

Amplifying replacement handsets (also known as handset amplifiers or volume control handsets) can be purchased to replace the standard handset on a telephone. The replacement handset contains an amplifier and an adjustable volume control. Figure 8.14 shows an example of such a handset. Amplifying handsets provide an easy and efficient means of amplifying the signal from a telephone receiver and are widely used. Unfortunately, these handsets can only be used with modular telephones (ie, those with a detachable receiver) and do not work on telephones in which the dials are in the handset (Slager, 1989). Slager pointed out that some inexpensive electronic telephones may not have enough power to the handset to power a replacement handset. Another problem is an

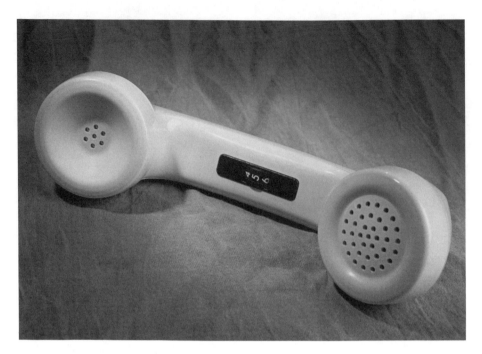

FIGURE 8.14 Amplifying handset, the StarTone GCR-01. The listener can adjust the volume level by rotating the numbered dial.

impedance mismatch between the new handset and the rest of the telephone. Purchasing amplifying handsets made by the same manufacturer as the telephone prevents these problems. Amplifying handsets are currently being installed in some public telephones. Users can identify these telephones by noting a telephone access symbol (Figure 8.15).

In-line amplifiers (also known as modular amplifiers) can be inserted between a telephone base and the handset. Like amplifying replacement handsets, these devices can be connected only to modular telephones.

The final category of telephone amplifier is the portable amplifier. Portable amplifiers are lightweight battery-powered amplifiers that strap over the receiver portion of a telephone handset. These devices are small and can easily be carried from place to place in a purse or a pocket. Two types of portable amplifiers can be purchased. One type is acoustically coupled to a telephone, and the other is inductively coupled. Portable amplifiers that are inductively coupled to a telephone can only be used on hearing aid-compatible telephones (ie, those that emit a relatively strong electromagnetic field). Consequently, Compton (1990) suggested that it is best to recommend portable amplifiers that couple acoustically to a telephone.

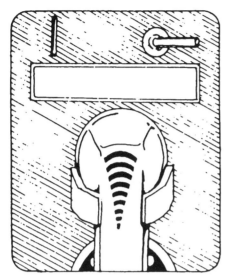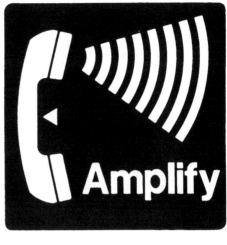

FIGURE 8.15 Symbols that denote amplified public telephones.

(Photos courtesy of HARC Mercantile, Ltd., Kalamazoo, Mich.)

A special category of portable telephone amplifier is the acoustic to magnetic adapter. An example of such a device is shown in Figure 8.16. Acoustic to magnetic adapters are designed to pick up an acoustic signal (such as that from a telephone receiver), amplify it, and convert it into a strong electromagnetic signal which can then be picked up by a hearing aid telecoil. Thus, any telephone can become hearing aid-compatible when such an adapter is used. Acoustic to magnetic adapters can be ordered with a variety of accessories such as neckloops, silhouette inductors or DAI connections. These accessories can then be used to route a telephone signal to both ears simultaneously which makes telephone use easier for listeners with hearing impairments.

Acoustic to magnetic couplers are relatively inexpensive and are versatile in that they can also be used as portable hardwired ALDs. Instead of strapping the device to a telephone receiver, the user places the device close to a sound source (eg, the television or a passenger in the car) and uses accessory cords to route the signal to his or her hearing aid.

Telecommunication Devices for the Deaf (Text Telephones)

According to Slager (1989), several million people in the United States cannot converse on a telephone even with the most sophisticated hearing aid and telephone amplifier. Some of these people are deaf whereas others have severe speech understanding problems. Still others cannot use a telephone because of severe speech production problems. These people, as well as those who wish to communicate with

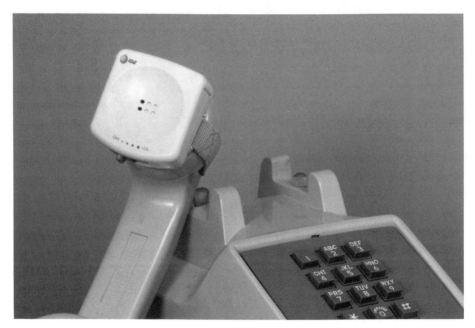

FIGURE 8.16 A portable acoustic to magnetic adapter, an AT&T telephone amplifier.

(Photo courtesy of HARC Mercantile, Ltd., Kalamazoo, Mich.)

them, can use a TDD. TDDs allow telephone conversations through print rather than voice. Modern TDDs consist of three basic parts—a keyboard for typing messages, a coupler (or modem) in which a telephone handset is placed to transmit and receive the message, and an LED display where the message is shown. Figure 8.17 shows an example of a TDD. As the message is typed into the device, the letters are converted into sequences of tones that are transmitted over telephone lines. At the other end of the line, a telephone receiver is coupled to another TDD, which decodes the message and displays it visually.

TDDs are available in portable or stationary models and can be purchased with a variety of options, including answering machines and printers. They are either acoustically coupled or directly connected to a telephone line. Acoustically coupled TDDs (those that use a coupler for a telephone receiver) have already been described. Acoustically coupled devices can produce garbled messages if the coupling is loose or if there is a great deal of background noise in the room. Direct-connect devices, on the other hand, plug directly into a telephone jack, completely replacing a standard telephone. Direct-connect TDDs reduce the number of garbled messages, but because these devices completely replace a telephone, they are not appropriate if others need access to a conventional telephone.

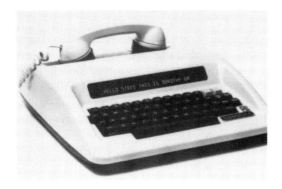

FIGURE 8.17
Example of a telecommunication
device for the deaf (TDD), the
Supercom TDD.

(Photo courtesy of HARC Mercantile,
Ltd., Kalamazoo, Mich.)

To communicate by means of a TDD, both parties to the conversation need a TDD. When a TDD user wants to call a person who does not have a TDD or TT, a message-relay system must be used. The message-relay system involves a third party, an operator at a message-relay service, who has both a TDD and a telephone. The message-relay operator acts as an intermediary between the two parties, typing the spoken message to the person with the hearing impairment and speaking the typed message to the hearing person. On July 26, 1993, Title IV of the Americans with Disabilities Act (ADA) went into effect. This portion of the act requires all telephone companies to provide relay services 24 hours a day, 7 days a week, for no additional charge, to relay users (Strauss, 1992). Information on TDD relay services can be obtained from one's local telephone company or from the Tele-Consumer Hotline (800-332-1124 [voice and TDD], 1910 K Street NW, Suite 610, Washington, DC 20006).

Training People with Hearing Losses to Use a Telephone

The treatment of specific telephone training techniques for people with hearing losses is beyond the scope of this chapter. Castle (1984) details a comprehensive telephone training program. Her text outlines two programs, one for people with severely limited speaking and listening skills and the other for people with some ability to talk and listen on a telephone. Developed specifically to train college students at the National Technical Institute for the Deaf (NTID), this program is appropriate for any adult client and with slight modification would even be appropriate for children. The text is a great source of information on telecommunications equipment in general, coupling telephones and personal hearing aids, and TDD use. It also includes information on the use of telephone codes and how to make emergency telephone calls. The training program can be obtained from the National Technical Institute for the Deaf, Rochester Institute of Technology, One Lomb Memorial Drive, P.O. Box 1887, Rochester, NY 14623.

Television

A common complaint of people with hearing losses is that they have difficulty following television programs. To solve this problem, many viewers simply increase the volume of the television until family members or neighbors complain. A more feasible solution is to apply one of the personal ALDs described earlier in this chapter. Hardwired, loop, infrared, and FM technologies all can be used to improve the listener's ability to hear the television without disturbing others in the household.

However, many people with severe to profound hearing losses cannot clearly understand television programs even with ALDs. For these people, closed captioning is available. Closed captioning uses a decoder to read a special code that accompanies the television signal and to translate the oral portion of television programming into a written message that appears across the bottom of the television screen. The effect is similar to watching a movie with subtitles (Figure 8.18). When closed captioning first became available in 1980, only 16 hours of programming per week were captioned (Jensema & Compton, 1989). Today, more than 450 hours of programming per week, including most of the top-rated shows, are closed captioned (National Captioning Institute, personal communication, 1992).

The Television Decoder Act requires built-in decoders on all televisions with 13-inch or larger screens produced after July 1, 1993 (Compton, 1989). Thus, new televisions with screens larger than 13 inches do not require separate decoders. Older televisions (and televisions with smaller screens) require a separate decoder. Several models of closed-captioning decoders have been developed since 1980. One currently available model, the Telecaption 4000, has been designed to be compatible with cable television and video cassette recorders. Telecaption decoders can be purchased for less than $200 from the National Captioning Institute (NCI) (see Appendix) or through a variety of dealers.

Closed-captioning systems have obvious applications for allowing deaf viewers to enjoy television programming and to keep abreast of current affairs by watching local and national newscasts. However, many people with less than severe hearing losses find them useful in filling in gaps of missing information during television viewing. Closed captioning can also be used as an educational tool (Jensema & Compton, 1989). According to research reported by the NCI, closed-captioned television programming can be an effective means of teaching reading and vocabulary to deaf students. NCI also reports that closed-captioned television programming is useful in teaching English to immigrants and foreign students.

ALERTING DEVICES

Alerting devices are used to alert people with hearing losses to the presence of environmental sounds they might otherwise miss. According to Larose et al (1989), the first alerting devices were developed to aid people with severe to profound hearing impairments in monitoring the important sounds in the environ-

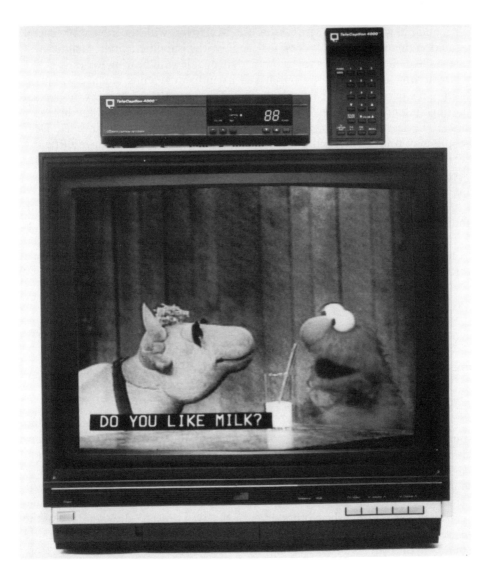

FIGURE 8.18 A closed-captioning device, the Telecaption 4000.

(Photo courtesy of the National Captioning Institute, Falls Church, Va.)

ment (eg, a smoke detector, a telephone, a crying baby). Even though most people who use alerting devices are deaf, the market is expanding. Many people with mild to moderate degrees of hearing loss have realized that they, too, find alerting devices helpful when trying to monitor acoustic signals under adverse listening conditions. For example, the ring of a doorbell or telephone may be audible in a quiet home but inaudible when the television is in use. Moreover, with the advent of federal regulations mandating equal access for people with disabilities, public facilities will be installing alerting devices to accommodate people with hearing losses.

Alerting devices can be purchased as individual units, each devoted to alerting the person to one particular sound. There are also a number of universal alerting systems that monitor a variety of acoustic signals around the home or office. The degree of hearing loss determines which kind of system is needed. Deaf people may find a universal system more efficient because they have difficulty hearing all sounds around the home or office. On the other hand, people who have difficulty with particular sounds may find it more economical to purchase a device devoted to detecting that particular sound.

Alerting devices work in three phases. In phase one, the sound is picked up and changed into an electrical signal. In phase two the electrical signal is transmitted, and in phase three, the electrical signal is changed into a cue that can be more easily perceived by the person. Each of these phases can be handled in a variety of ways.

Sound Pick-up

Acoustic signals in the environment can be monitored by microphone pick-up, direct electrical connection, and inductive pick-up.

Microphone Pick-up

In microphone pick-up, a microphone is placed in the vicinity of the sound source to be monitored. The microphone picks up the sound and changes it into an electrical signal ready for transmission. The advantage of this type of sound pick-up is that it can be used to monitor almost any sound. It can be used to monitor sounds that readily come to mind, such as the doorbell, a telephone, the alarm clock, the smoke detector, as well as less commonly thought of sounds, such as the signal from the clothes dryer or the oven timer. A disadvantage of the microphone pick-up method is that false signals can occur owing to other sound sources in the room. False signals can be avoided by placing the microphone close to the source of the sound and by adjusting the sensitivity of the microphone. Some devices are designed to respond only to frequencies within a certain bandwidth or to respond only when the signal is of a certain duration.

Direct Electrical Connection

Some sounds can be monitored by means of a direct electrical connection between the alerting device and the sound source. In this method, the alerting device detects the presence of a signal by monitoring the electrical system of the sound source in question. For instance, the ring of the doorbell or telephone can be monitored by detecting the electrical signal responsible for ringing the doorbell or telephone. An advantage of a direct electrical connection between the alerting device and the sound source is that other signals in the environment do not trigger false alarms, as can happen with microphone pick-up. A disadvantage of direct electrical connection, however, is that not all sound sources can be monitored. Crying babies, for example, do not lend themselves to the system.

Inductive Pick-up

Some sound sources (ie, the telephone and doorbell) generate an electromagnetic field when they ring. This electromagnetic field can be used to generate an electrical signal in an induction coil (in the same way the telecoil in a hearing aid works) placed close to the ringer. An advantage to this system is that it does not spuriously activate the alerting device because of extraneous noise in the room. However, a disadvantage is that is has a limited application; it can only be used with telephones and doorbells, and not all telephone rings produce an adequate electromagnetic signal to activate the device.

Signal Transmission

The electrical signal generated by the sound pick-up device can be transmitted to the alerting mechanism in three ways—hardwired transmission, FM line carrier, or FM airborne.

Hardwired Connection

In a hardwired connection, the alerting mechanism is physically tethered by a wire to the sound pick-up device. The advantage of this type of transmission is that it is relatively inexpensive and is portable. The disadvantage is that it can become expensive if many sounds in the house need to be monitored and if multiple alerting mechanisms are needed throughout the home. Figure 8.19 shows a hardwired device designed to produce a signal when a telephone rings. A telephone and the lamp are connected to the device. Whenever a telephone rings, the lamp flashes on and off.

FM Line Carrier

In FM line carrier transmission systems, the electrical signal from the sound pick-up device is transmitted through the electrical system of the entire home or office on an FM signal. Receivers can be plugged into any AC outlet to detect the presence of the signal. An advantage of the system is that many different sources of sound can be monitored in different areas of the home simultaneously. A disadvantage is that false electrical signals occasionally trigger the FM receivers. Figure 8.20 shows a device for FM line transmission. Microphone pick-ups are used to monitor several important signals in the home (a telephone ring and a baby's cry). Whenever one of these sounds occurs, a signal is sent through the electrical wiring in the home. Receivers plugged into AC outlets in various locations

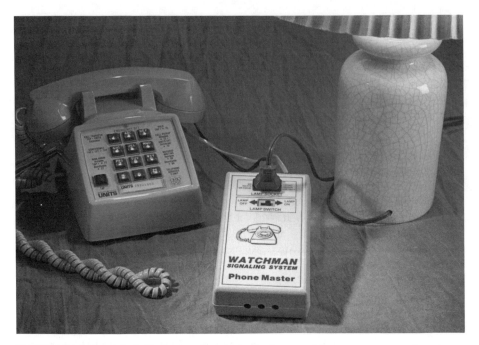

FIGURE 8.19 A hardwired alerting device. A telephone and lamp are connected to the device. The lamp flashes whenever the telephone rings.

throughout the home are attached to table lamps, which flash when a signal is detected. The flash patterns can be coded so that the person can determine which sound has occurred.

FM Airborne System

In the FM airborne system, the electrical signal from the sound pick-up device is used to modulate an FM radio signal that is sent through the air rather than through the electrical wiring of the home or office. Battery-powered receivers can then be worn to detect the presence of signals from up to 100 feet away (Compton, 1989). FM airborne systems have the same advantages as FM line transmission and the added advantage that only one receiver is needed for the entire house and the user can be anywhere in the building, even outside. A disadvantage is that spurious signals occasionally occur and that this system is more expensive than the others.

Figure 8.21 shows a device for FM airborne transmission of a signal. Microphone pick-ups are used to monitor a variety of acoustic signals throughout the home (eg, the smoke detector, the TDD, the doorbell, and the oven timer). If a sound is detected from any of these devices, a transmitter sends an airborne FM

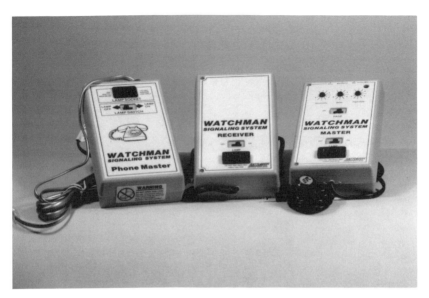

FIGURE 8.20 An FM line carrier system, the Watchman Signaling System (Ultra Tec, Madison, Wis.). The Watchman Master monitors auditory signals and transmits the signal to Watchman Receivers throughout the home.

(Photo courtesy of HARC Mercantile, Ltd., Kalamazoo, Mich.)

signal throughout the home. This signal is then detected by a receiver worn on the wrist. The receiver changes the signal into a coded vibrotactile cue that is felt on the wrist.

Cuing Mechanisms

The final job of an alerting device is to change the signal into a cue that can be easily perceived by a person with a hearing loss. Although many devices use a flashing light as the cue that a sound has occurred, the cue from the device can be auditory, visual, or tactile. Auditory signals from alerting devices are louder and lower pitched than the sounds the device is detecting. This may be all that is necessary for a person with a mild to moderate hearing loss. However, for people with severe to profound hearing losses, simply amplifying the sound or changing its pitch may not make it audible. For these people, the cue can be visual or tactile rather than auditory.

Visual cues can be obtained by using a lamp or a strobe light that flashes when a monitored sound occurs. As can be seen in the earlier examples, some alerting systems are coded so that different sound sources result in different patterns of light flashes.

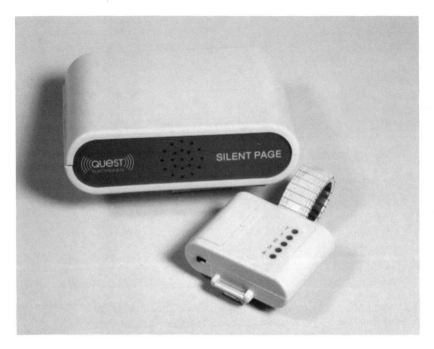

FIGURE 8.21 An FM airborne alerting system, the Quest Alerting System. Transmitters can be placed at various locations throughout the home and send an FM signal to a vibrotactile device worn on the wrist.

(Photo courtesy HARC Mercantile, Ltd., Kalamazoo, Mich.)

Alternatively, tactile cues (eg, vibrotactile signals delivered to the wrist, bed or pillow vibrators, or fans) can be used to alert a user that a sound has occurred.

Some devices allow people to choose the particular cuing device they find most effective. One simple device is an alarm clock with an electrical outlet in the side. The user can attach a lamp, pillow vibrator, strobe light, or fan, depending on personal preference.

REFERENCES

Bankowski, S., & Ross, M. (1984). FM systems effect on speech discrimination in an auditorium. *Hearing Instruments, 35*, 8-12.

Berger, K., & Millin, J. (1980). Amplification for the hearing impaired. In R. Schow & M. Nerbonne (Eds.), *Introduction to aural rehabilitation* (pp. 27-74). Baltimore: University Park Press.

Bergman, M. (1983). Assistive listening devices. Part I. New responsibilities. *Asha, 25,* 1923.

Bess, F., Klee, T., & Culbertson, J. L. (1986). Identification, assessment, and management of children with unilateral sensorineural hearing loss. *Ear and Hearing, 7,* 43-51.

Castle, D. (1984). Telephone training for hearing impaired persons: Amplified telephone, TDDs, codes. Rochester: Rochester Institute of Technology, National Technical Institute for the Deaf.

Committee on Hearing, Bioacoustics, and Biomechanics (CHABA) (1988). Speech understanding and aging. *Journal of the Acoustical Society of America, 83,* 859-894.

Compton, C. (1989). Assistive technology: Up close and personal. *Seminars in Hearing, 10,* 104-120.

Compton, C. (1990). *Assistive devices: Doorways to independence.* Washington, DC: Gallaudet University.

Davidson, S. & Noe, C. (1994). Digitally programmable telecoil responses: Potential advantages for assistive listening device fittings. *The American Journal of Audiology: A Journal of Clinical Practice, 3,* 59-64.

Davidson, S., & Wall, L. (1988). Hearing aid selection in the elderly: Consideration of central aging effects. *Folia Phoniatrica, 40,* 270-276.

Ferre, J. (1987). Pediatric central auditory processing disorder: Considerations for diagnosis, interpretation, and remediation. *Journal of the Academy of Rehabilitative Audiology, 20,* 73-81.

Finitzo-Hieber, T., & Tillman, T. (1978). Room acoustics effects on monosyllabic word discrimination ability for normal and hearing-impaired children. *Journal of Speech and Hearing Research, 21,* 440-458.

Flexer, C., & Savage, H. (1992). Using an ALD in speech-language assessment and training. *Hearing Journal, 45,* 26-35.

Flexer, C., Wray, D., Black, T., & Millin, J. (1987). Amplification devices: Evaluating classroom effectiveness for moderately hearing-impaired college students. *Volta Review, 89,* 347-357.

Hawkins, D. (1984). Comparisons of speech recognition in noise by mildly-to-moderately hearing-impaired children using hearing aids and FM systems. *Journal of Speech and Hearing Disorders, 49,* 409-418.

Hawkins, D. (1987). Assessment of FM systems with an ear canal probe tube microphone system. *Ear and Hearing, 8,* 301-303.

Hawkins, D., & Schum, D. (1985). Some effects of FM-system coupling on hearing aid characteristics. *Journal of Speech and Hearing Disorders, 50,* 132-141.

Hawkins, D., & Van Tassel, D. (1982). Electroacoustic characteristics of personal FM systems. *Journal of Speech and Hearing Disorders, 47,* 355-362.

Hayes, D., & Jerger, J. (1979). Aging and the use of hearing aids. *Scandinavian Audiology, 8,* 33-40.

Jensema, C., & Compton, C. (1989). Television for the hearing impaired. *Seminars in Hearing, 10,* 57-65.

Jerger, J., & Hayes, D. (1977). Diagnostic speech audiometry. *Archives of Otolaryngology, 103,* 216-222.

Kenworthy, O. T., Klee., T., & Tharpe, A. M. (1990). Speech recognition ability of children with unilateral sensorineural hearing loss as a function of amplification, speech stimuli and listening condition. *Ear and Hearing, 11,* 264-270.

Kricos, P., Lesner, S., Sandridge, S., & Yanke, R. (1987). Perceived benefit of amplification as a function of central auditory status in the elderly. *Ear and Hearing, 8,* 337-342.

Larose, G., Evans, M., & Larose, R. (1989). Alerting devices: Available options. *Seminars in Hearing, 10,* 66-77.

Leavitt, R. (1989). Considerations for the use of rehabilitation technology by hearing impaired persons. *Seminars in Hearing, 10,* 1-10.

Lybarger, S. (1982). Telephone coupling. In G. Studebaker & F. Bess (Eds.), *The Vanderbilt hearing aid report* (pp. 91-93). Upper Darby: Monographs in Contemporary Audiology.

Middleton, R., & Ekhaml, L. (1987). A selective study of the utilization of various assistive listening devices in schools, libraries, and hospitals. *Journal of Rehabilitation of the Deaf, 21,* 18-23.

Nabelek, A. (1980). Effects of room acoustics on speech perception through hearing aids by normal-hearing and hearing-impaired listeners. In G. A. Studebaker & I. Hochberg (Eds.), *Acoustical factors affecting hearing aid performance* (pp. 25-46). Baltimore: University Park Press.

Nabelek, A., & Donahue, A. (1986). Comparison of amplification systems in an auditorium. *Journal of the Acoustical Society of America, 79,* 2078-2082.

Nabelek, A., Donahue, A., & Letwoski, T. (1986). Comparison of amplification systems in a classroom. *Journal of Rehabilitation Research and Development, 23,* 41-52.

Nabelek, A., & Pickett, J. (1974). Monaural and binaural speech perception through hearing aids under noise and reverberation with normal and hearing impaired listeners. *Journal of Speech and Hearing Research, 17,* 724-739.

Noe, C. (1994). Comparison of large-group assistive listening devices in an adult classroom setting at the Veterans Affairs medical center. Unpublished doctoral dissertation. The Ohio State University.

Olsen, W., & Tillman, T., (1968). Hearing aids and sensorineural hearing loss. *Annals of Otology, Rhinology, and Laryngology, 77,* 717-726.

Pehringer, J. (1989). Assistive devices: Technology to improve communication. *Otolaryngologic Clinics of North America, 22,* 143-174.

Ross, M., & Giolas, T. (1971). The effects of three classroom listening conditions on speech intelligibility. *American Annals of the Deaf, 116,* 580-584.

Schow, R. L., & Nerbonne, M. A. (1980). Hearing levels among elderly nursing home residents. *Journal of Speech and Hearing Disorders, 45,* 124-132.

Shirinian, M., & Arnst, D. (1982). Patterns in the performance-intensity functions for phonetically balanced word lists and synthetic sentences in aged listeners. *Archives of Otolaryngology, 108,* 15-20.

Slager, R. (1989). Romancing the phone: The adventure continues. *Seminars in Hearing, 10,* 42-56.

Staab, W., & Lybarger, S. (1994). Characteristics and use of hearing aids. In J. Katz (Ed.), *Handbook of clinical audiology* (4th ed.) (pp. 657-722). Baltimore: Williams & Wilkins.

Stach, B., Loiselle, L., Jerger, J., Mintz, S., & Taylor, C. (1987). Clinical experience with personal FM assistive listening devices. *Hearing Journal, 40,* 24-30.

Strauss, K. (1992). Nationwide relay services. *Asha, 34,* 48-49.

Telecommunications for the Disabled Act of 1982 (Public Law 97-410).

Thibodeau, L. (1989). Facilitating communication in nursing homes through the use of assistive listening devices. *Nursing Homes, 38,* 25-28.

SUGGESTED READING

ASHA (1992). Guide to ADA Products. *Asha, 34,* 68-78.

Compton, C. L. (1989). Assistive devices. *Seminars in Hearing, 1-120.*

Compton, C. (1990). *Assistive devices: Doorways to independence.* Washington, DC: Gallaudet University.

Compton, C. L. (1993). Assistive technology for deaf and hard of hearing people. In J. Alpiner & P. McCarthy (Eds.), *Rehabilitative audiology: Children and adults* (2nd ed.) (pp. 441-469). Baltimore: Williams & Wilkins.

Montano, J. (1994). Rehabilitation technology for the hearing impaired. In J. Katz (Ed.), *Handbook of clinical audiology* (4th ed.) (pp. 638-654). Baltimore: Williams & Wilkins.

APPENDIX

Organizations

Alexander Graham Bell Association
1537 35th St. NW
Washington, DC 20007
202-337-5220 (voice and TDD)

American Speech-Language-Hearing Association (ASHA)
10801 Rockville Pike
Rockville, MD 20852
301-897-5700 (voice and TDD)

Gallaudet Assistive Devices Center
Gallaudet University
800 Florida Ave. NE
Washington, DC 20002
202-651-5328 (voice and TDD)

National Captioning Institute Inc. (NCI)
5203 Leesburg Pike
Falls Church, VA 22041
800-523-WORD (voice)
800-321-TDDS (TDD)

National Information Center on Deafness
800 Florida Ave. NE
Washington, DC 20002
202-651-5051 (voice and TDD)

Self Help for Hard of Hearing People (SHHH)
7800 Wisconsin Ave.
Bethesda, MD 20814
310-657-2248 (voice)
301-657-2249 (TDD)

Telecommunications for the Deaf, Inc. (TDI)
814 Thayer Ave.
Silver Spring, MD 20910
301-589-3006 (voice and TDD)

Distributors

Hal-Hen Co.
35-53 24th St.
Long Island City, NY 11106
718-392-6260

HARC Mercantile Ltd.
Division of HARC of America
3130 Portage Rd.
P.O. Box 3055
Kalamazoo, MI 49003-3055
800-445-9968 (US)
800-962-6634 (MI)

Sound Resources, Inc.
Mid-Audio Catalog of Assistive Devices for the Hearing Impaired
201 East Ogden
Hinsdale, IL 60521
312-323-6133

Williams Sound Corporation
10399 West 70th St.
Eden Prairie, MN 55344
800-328-6190 (voice and TDD)

9

Tactile Aids and Cochlear Implants

Janet M. Weisenberger

Advances in hearing aid technology in recent years have made it possible to fit the amplification requirements of a person with a hearing impairment with greater precision than ever before. Yet even with the advent of digital hearing aids, there remains a population of people with hearing impairments who do not derive measurable benefit from conventional amplification. For this group, an alternative means must be found for transmission of information about acoustic signals. The development of such alternative devices, called sensory aids, attempts to address this need. The two most typical sensory aids are tactile aids, which transmit acoustic information via the sense of touch, and cochlear implants, which supply electrical stimulation to fibers of the eighth cranial nerve in the cochlea to provide an auditory percept.

Most candidates for sensory aids have a hearing loss in the profound range. However, some people with severe hearing losses derive only minimal benefit from a hearing aid and thus also may be considered candidates for sensory aids (Hodgson, 1986). Some people whose audiometric configuration might suggest the use of a sensory aid may have no desire to use one. These people consider themselves part of the deaf community, which has not been receptive to the use of sensory aids, particularly cochlear implants. Nonetheless, many people who cannot perceive acoustic stimuli with a hearing aid do feel a need to understand spoken language and communicate with the hearing community, particularly if they interact regularly with people with normal hearing in family or other situations.

Sensory aids have been developed both as sensory substitute and as sensory supplement (Bach-y-Rita, 1974). Devices designed to be sensory substitutes attempt to provide all the functions typically performed by the auditory system. Sensory supplements are designed to provide some of the information normally transmitted by the auditory system, but they rely on residual auditory function or on visual information from speechreading to provide the remainder. Both tactile aids and cochlear implants can serve as either substitutes or supplements, depending on the complexity of the information to be conveyed, the processing strategy and output scheme of the device, and individual user characteristics. For example, a tactile aid or cochlear implant might provide effective substitution for the normal auditory channel in allowing the user to detect sound or to make discriminations based on envelope characteristics of the stimulus. However, these devices may not be a complete substitute for the auditory channel when the stimulus is running speech. In this case, a sensory aid might be used in conjunction with speechreading to provide the user with adequate information about the stimulus.

THE TEAM APPROACH TO SENSORY AIDS

Some familiarity with both tactile aids and cochlear implants may prove quite useful to the speech-language pathologist, who may encounter users of sensory aids in a variety of clinical environments. In nearly all cochlear implant programs, a team approach has been implemented in patient selection, assessment, surgical procedure, and training and rehabilitation (Fraser, 1991). This team typically includes an otolaryngologist, audiologist, psychologist, speech-language pathologist, and for children, a teacher from the child's education program.

The otolaryngologist is responsible for assessment of the medical fitness of the implant candidate and the viability of the auditory nerve for implantation and for the surgical procedure itself. The audiologist administers the extensive battery of audiologic and psychophysical tests that make up the evaluation for candidacy for a cochlear implant. In addition, the audiologist may be involved in the design of an effective rehabilitation program and in the actual implementation of the program. The psychologist is responsible for assessing psychological variables, including intelligence and emotional stability, that have been implicated in the success of the use of cochlear implants and may be called upon to participate in the rehabilitation process to provide support and counseling. The speech-language pathologist is part of both assessment and rehabilitation. The speech-language pathologist may administer tests of speech and language function before implantation and often has primary responsibility for both speech perception and speech production training. As Read (1989) pointed out, the speech production skills of people with profound hearing impairments are quite variable across individuals, although there is some relation between the length of time since the onset of hearing loss and the quality of the speech. For children, and for some adults, a substantial aspect of the rehabilitation program may involve speech production training. The educator participates as a member of the team by helping determine how the child's educational environment can be tailored to accommodate the new sensory aid and how aspects of the rehabilitation program can be incorporated into the educational environment.

A similar team approach is often used with the fitting and rehabilitation program for tactile aids, although the involvement of a surgeon is not usually necessary. The other members of the team (audiologist, speech-language pathologist, teacher) serve in a capacity similar to their roles on the cochlear implant team.

In fact, tactile aid programs often are administered by the same professionals who make up the cochlear implant team.

At present, cochlear implant and tactile aid centers are found primarily in larger cities, and a center may provide services to a large and geographically diverse regional population. For many patients, it is not possible to remain at the cochlear implant or tactile aid center for an extended period of time for a rehabilitation program that may last many months. These patients must rely on professionals in their home town for provision of training and rehabilitation. Often the bulk of this training is provided by speech-language pathologists, who in effect become remote-site members of the implant team.

COMMUNICATION OF THE ACOUSTIC ENVIRONMENT

For both the designers of sensory aids and for the professionals who are involved in training and rehabilitation, it is important to consider the functions performed by the normal auditory system and the degree to which these functions may be compensated by the addition of a sensory aid. Auditory processing ranges from an awareness of the auditory environment without specific attention to a stimulus (background acoustic stimulation) to the comprehension of long passages of connected speech (Cooper, 1991; Weisenberger, 1992). These levels vary in the complexity of processing of the input signal that is required as well as in the complexity of the response that is appropriate.

Background Acoustic Stimulation

Ramsdell (1978) argued that hearing provides a sense of connectedness to the world, on a very primitive level, typically in the absence of conscious attention by the listener. Ramsdell pointed out that the loss of this sense of connectedness can result in confusion or depression and that it constitutes an important component of the sense of security and well-being. Changes in the level or characteristics of the background stimulation signal the listener to focus attention on the acoustic environment, preparing the listener to make appropriate responses to the acoustic stimulus. In people with hearing impairments, this signaling function is not available. One possible function of a sensory aid could be to reestablish this feeling of connectedness to the world by conveying some sense of this background acoustic stimulation.

Detection

The simplest level on which the auditory system processes an actively-attended stimulus is detection. Detection of sound requires only minimal analysis of the waveform but is necessary for subsequent processing. It is essential that a sensory aid render a stimulus detectable to the user. However, it may not be necessary to provide detection of all the possible stimuli that might be detected by the normal auditory system. Rather, a useful sensory aid might concentrate on rendering detectable signals that occur above certain levels (eg, in the range occupied by speech and environmental sounds) and still be of considerable benefit to the user.

Localization

Once a sound is detected, the listener attempts to determine its source. The normal auditory system localizes sound with impressive accuracy, at least in the horizontal plane. It accomplishes this activity via the use of binaural time and intensity cues (Phillips & Brugge, 1985). A few sensory aids (Weisenberger et al, 1987; Richardson, 1982) have attempted to provide this binaural information to wearers, but usually only a single sensory aid, with a single microphone and display, is worn. Thus, localization must be accomplished by means of monaural cues, but the task can still be performed effectively if movement of the head or body is allowed, so that the user can perceive changes in stimulus level as he or she moves closer to or farther from the sound source.

Discrimination

With slightly more processing of an input acoustic waveform, it is possible for the auditory system to determine that one stimulus is different from another stimulus; that is, the two stimuli can be discriminated from one another. The two stimuli can differ in any of a number of dimensions, including spectral, temporal, and intensive. Thus, the task of discrimination of two stimuli can be relatively simple if the differences between stimuli are large, or quite difficult if only small differences between stimuli are present. Sensory aids can be characterized according to whether they provide relatively global information about the amplitude envelope of the stimulus or whether specific information about fine-structure spectral and temporal features is also provided. The amplitude envelope of a sound is a representation of the overall intensity of the stimulus over time. Fine-structure spectral information refers to the frequency content of the stimulus over time, and fine-structure temporal information refers to small timing differences within the stimulus.

Cues in the amplitude envelope allow discrimination of stimuli that are very different from one another in their envelope characteristics, such as environmental sounds. In addition, envelope differences signal suprasegmental aspects of speech sounds, such as syllable number and stress, allowing the user to distinguish the word *baseball* from *bat*. Although this may not seem to be a large amount of information in attempts to comprehend running speech, studies of auditory coding strategies have shown that an auditory signal that provides only the amplitude envelope of speech can provide substantial benefit to listeners when combined with speechreading (Grant et al, 1985).

For some discriminations, amplitude envelope information is not sufficient. For example, discriminating *bat* from *mat* requires an in-depth analysis of the stimulus that focuses on fine-structure spectral and temporal aspects of the waveform. Fine-structure temporal cues can provide information about such things as vowel duration, which is useful in discriminating vowels such as /i/ and /I/, and voice onset time (VOT), which is useful in discriminating consonants such as /b/ and /p/. Still other distinctions depend on information about the spectral content of the stimulus, such as the discrimination of /u/ from /i/. Thus, the ideal sensory aid, to serve as an effective substitute for the auditory system, provides information about the fine-structure spectral and temporal aspects of the acoustic stimulus in addition to envelope characteristics.

Identification and Recognition

Identification is defined as the ability to select a particular stimulus from among a limited set of stimuli. This task requires processing beyond that necessary for discrimination. Cooper (1991) differentiated identification from *recognition*, arguing that identification is a closed-set task, whereas recognition is an open-set task. That is, the patient is not given a response set to choose from but must identify the stimulus on the basis of an internal representation of its features. As the size of the closed set in the identification task increases, the task becomes more difficult and more closely approximates the recognition task. Each of these tasks depends on the transmission of information about the acoustic stimulus. When the stimuli are very different in envelope characteristics, such as a set of environmental sounds, a sensory aid that provides only amplitude envelope information allows a relatively high level of performance in a closed-set identification task. For most speech sounds, however, fine-structure spectral and temporal cues are required for identification or recognition. Thus, for this level of stimulus processing, a sensory aid that provides fine-structure information is required.

Comprehension

The ability to identify or recognize individual speech sounds does not guarantee that a listener will understand a spoken message. To ascertain the meaning of an utterance, the listener must comprehend the stimulus, which implies a higher level of stimulus processing than that required for the preceding tasks. In comprehension, higher cognitive processes of lexical access and interpretation of contextual cues must be accessed. Tasks that involve the presentation of sentence or text material require a degree of comprehension of the material for optimal performance. Although a sensory aid is not designed to provide this cognitive information, a useful device facilitates, rather than impedes, such processing. A sensory aid that functions as an effective substitute for normal auditory function on its own provides sufficient information about the input stimulus so higher-level processing can occur. A sensory supplement attempts to provide some of this information but relies on other modes of input, such as speechreading, for the remainder of the information. In either case, an effective sensory aid is one that can provide benefits to the user attempting to comprehend connected speech.

As discussed later in the chapter, training and rehabilitation with a sensory aid is designed around this hierarchy of stimulus processing. A program is implemented that takes into account the kind of information transmitted by the sensory aid and that builds user skills gradually from detection to comprehension. At all stages materials are used to maximize the usefulness of the cues provided by the sensory aid.

TACTILE AIDS

Investigations of the effectiveness of tactile devices to provide information about speech stimuli date back to the 1920s (Gault, 1927). Some of the earliest tactile aids were only minimally successful, in part because their design did not take into account the characteristics of the tactile sensory system. An in-depth discussion of tactile physiology and psychophysics is beyond the scope of this chapter, but excellent reviews are provided by Sherrick and Cholewiak (1986) and Verrillo and Gescheider (1992). The design of an effective tactile aid depends on an understanding of certain tactile psychophysical characteristics. For example, the frequency range to which the tactile system is sensitive to vibration is approximately 1 to 1000 Hz, which does not begin to approximate the 20,000-Hz auditory frequency range. More problematic is the fact that frequency resolution abilities in the tactile system are quite poor (Goff, 1967; Rothenberg et al, 1977) compared with those of the auditory system. These two facts suggest that presenting acoustic frequency as tactile vibration frequency would be a poor encoding strategy for a tactile aid. Consequently, the more successful multichannel tactile devices have used a dimension along which the tactile system shows good resolution ability (spatial location) (Weinstein, 1968) to code input acoustic frequency. Fortunately, intensity and temporal resolution for vibrotactile stimuli, although not as fine as those of the auditory system, are nonetheless sufficient for the transmission of information about speech and environmental sounds (Craig, 1972; Gescheider, 1974; Weisenberger, 1986). Thus, acoustic waveform intensitive and temporal features can be coded along intensive and temporal dimensions for vibrotactile stimuli. In the next section, tactile aid designs that take these psychophysical aspects of the tactile system into account are discussed.

Processing Strategies and Transducer Design

Tactile aids can be classified according to several schemes, including the number of transducer channels, the modality of stimulation (vibratory or electro-tactile), and acoustic encoding strategy. A thorough discussion of tactile aid classification can be found in Reed et al (1982). The first consideration in a tactile aid design is which aspects of the acoustic environment are to be encoded. The earliest wearable tactile aids employed relatively simple encoding strategies and directed output to a single vibratory transducer. Because wearable tactile aids have been available for only a relatively short time, many people still use these relatively simple single-channel devices. Thus it is possible that a speech-language pathologist might encounter a client for rehabilitation who wears a single-channel tactile aid. Successfully marketed, commercially available single-channel tactile aids include the Tactaid I (Audiological Engineering, Somerville, Mass., the Minivib (AB Special Instrument, Stockholm, Sweden), and the TAM (Summit, Exeter, United Kingdom). All of these devices are relatively small and lightweight, wearable even by young children. The tactile transducer is worn on the wrist by adults and on the wrist or sternum by children. Each of these devices employs a microphone to pick up an acoustic stimulus and a processor that extracts the amplitude envelope of the stimulus. In the case of the TAM, the temporal characteristics of the envelope are conveyed by using the envelope to turn on and off a fixed-frequency, fixed-intensity 220-Hz vibration. The Tactaid I and Minivib use the amplitude envelope to modulate the amplitude of a fixed-frequency vibration of approximately 250 Hz. Thus, they provide intensity cues as well as temporal cues from the waveform envelope.

Although these devices have provided useful benefits to wearers for a variety of acoustic stimuli, their benefits are restricted to tasks that can be performed using envelope characteristics alone. As discussed earlier, more complex stimulus identification and recognition tasks require information about the fine-structure spectral and temporal aspects of the acoustic stimulus. This need has led to the development of tactile devices with more than a single channel. Initially, these were primarily two-channel devices, the most successful of which has been the Tactaid II (Audiological Engineering). The Tactaid II splits the incoming acoustic waveform into two parts by filtering portions of the input between 100 Hz and 1.8 kHz into one channel and portions of the input between 1.5 and 8.1 kHz into another channel. An envelope extraction is then performed in both the low-frequency and the high-frequency channels, and the resulting envelopes are used to modulate the amplitude of two fixed-frequency 250-Hz signals delivered to two different tactile transducers. Again, the transducers are fitted to a wrist strap for adults and older children and to a sternum harness for younger children.

This device is compatible with frequency modulation (FM) amplification systems by means of an external input and thus can be used with classroom-based FM systems. The low-frequency channel of the Tactaid II preserves cues from the waveform envelope, and the high-frequency channel provides information about high-frequency spectral components, as might signal the presence of frication or voiceless stop consonants.

More ambitious multichannel tactile aids have employed anywhere from 5 to 32 channels of stimulation (Weisenberger, 1992). Most of these devices have been laboratory-based prototypes rather than commercially available, wearable tactile aids. With many channels, the options available for conveying information about the acoustic waveform are expanded, and thus a larger range of processing strategies is possible. Researchers have investigated the effectiveness of providing information about voice fundamental frequency, or F0 (Boothroyd & Hnath-Chisholm, 1988); a vocoder-style output (Brooks et al, 1986; Weisenberger et al, 1989); waveform principal components (Abbott et al, 1989); and first or second formant frequency, or F1 and F2 (Blamey & Clark, 1985).

At the time of this writing, only one multichannel tactile aid is commercially available in the United States. The Tactaid VII (Audiological Engineering) is a seven-channel vibrotactile device that employs a flexible array of transducers that can be worn on a number of body sites, including sternum, neck, arm, or abdomen, depending on user preference (Figure 9.1). The processor of the device extracts information about F1 and F2 and displays this information on the tactile array by using channels 1 to 4 to signify the value of F1 and channels 4 to 7 to signify the value of F2. Within these ranges, the location of stimulation on the array indicates the frequency of the formant. Thus, each channel covers a limited frequency range, transforming input acoustic energy into location on the skin surface. The vibratory stimulus delivered to each transducer is a fixed-frequency 250-Hz signal, the intensity of which corresponds to the amplitude of the formant. The user of the Tactaid VII perceives a vibratory signal that moves along the array as input formant frequencies vary; he or she must learn to associate specific patterns of vibration with specific speech sounds.

Performance of Tactile Aids

In considering the aforedescribed hierarchy of listening tasks performed by the auditory system, the potential benefits of tactile aids can be assessed by determining the degree to which each of the tasks in the hierarchy can be performed by a client with a hearing impairment more successfully with a tactile aid than without. First, all tactile devices provide some degree of connectedness to the acoustic environment, although the distance at which sound sources are picked up depends on the microphone gain of the system. Most tactile aids have adjustable microphone gain, because in many situations it is crucial to maximize the signal-to-noise ratio (S/N) for perceiving the speech of a nearby person who is talking, which may mean minimizing the impact of sounds in the surrounding environment, such as air conditioners.

With respect to sound detection, again, all tactile aids must provide sound detection to the user, so that further processing of the signal can occur. Weisenberger

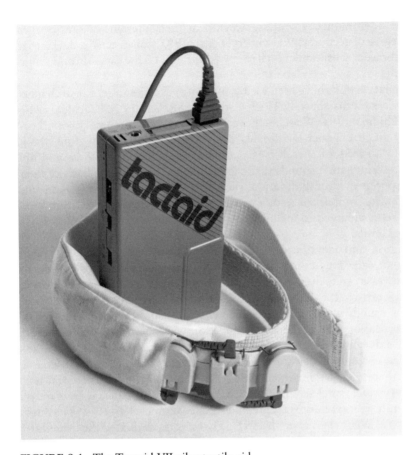

FIGURE 9.1   The Tactaid VII vibrotactile aid.

(Used with permission from Audiological Engineering, Somerville, Mass.)

and Russell (1989) measured the detection performance of two single-channel tactile devices—the Minivib and the Minifonator (Siemens Hearing Instruments, Piscataway, N.J.)—in a standard audiologic testing situation and derived "audiograms" for sound detection for wearers of each device. The results indicated that across frequencies (125 to 8000 Hz), thresholds ranged between 40 and 55 decibels hearing level (dB HL) for both devices. Thus, while very soft sounds would not likely be detectable, conversational levels of speech would be detectable and would not likely be contaminated by low-level sounds in the environment.

The ability to localize sound sources has been measured only in laboratory-based prototype binaural tactile aids. Richardson (1982) performed a series of experiments with a device that employed two head-mounted microphones and directed tactile stimulation to a finger on each hand. Richardson found that subjects could localize high-frequency sounds, which generated interaural intensity cues with a high degree of accuracy. Weisenberger et al (1987) constructed a device that produced a vibratory sensation in each ear by vibrating a Lucite earmold and found a similar result.

Discrimination tasks have been used in numerous evaluations of single-channel tactile aid devices (Bernstein et al, 1989; Carney, 1988; Carney & Beachler, 1986; Thornton & Phillips, 1992; Weisenberger & Russell, 1989). In general, the authors reported that single-channel tactile aids can provide useful information about suprasegmental aspects of speech, such as syllable number and stress, and are beneficial in discriminating sounds that can be differentiated on the basis of their amplitude envelope or overall duration, such as environmental sounds and some vowels. In pairwise comparisons, some consonants can be discriminated, but when the response set is enlarged to include even four alternatives, performance drops to near chance levels.

Recognition and identification tasks were investigated for single-channel tactile aids in the same studies in which discrimination was evaluated. The overall results for these tasks were disappointing. The results suggested that single-channel tactile aids do not by themselves provide sufficient information for closed-set recognition of sounds with similar envelope characteristics or for any degree of open-set identification. When used in conjunction with speechreading, however, single-channel aids can yield higher levels of performance than found for speechreading alone. Even in a comprehension task, such as tracking of connected discourse (DeFilippo & Scott, 1978), in which the user of the tactile aid must repeat text presented by a reader, single-channel devices improve performance by five to ten words per minute over rates for speechreading alone (Skinner et al, 1988; Thornton & Phillips, 1992; Weisenberger et al, 1991). Two studies evaluated the benefits of single-channel tactile aids for young children with prelingual deafness in an educational setting and found that the addition of the tactile aid appeared to facilitate the acquisition of both receptive and expressive vocabulary, with astonishing increases in the rate of acquisition of new words once the children began wearing the device (Geers, 1986; Proctor & Goldstein, 1983). Thus, it can be seen that the benefits of single-channel tactile devices, although limited, are nonetheless a substantial improvement over the non-aided situation.

For two-channel devices, some improvements over single-channel tactile aids have been reported. In general, the envelope cues provided by a single-channel device are preserved in a two-channel aid, and additional high-frequency cues are available. In tasks in which the detection of frication is beneficial, such as in some consonant discriminations, a two-channel tactile aid is superior to a single-channel device. Thornton and Phillips (1992) reported higher performance for the Tactaid II than for three single-channel aids in consonant recognition and connected discourse tracking tasks. Lynch et al (1989) found greater benefits to speechreading in the connected discourse tracking task for the Tactaid II than for a 16-channel tactile aid.

The foregoing result notwithstanding, evaluations of multichannel tactile aids have found that the multichannel devices far outpace single-channel devices in performance at all levels in the auditory task hierarchy. Specific comparisons (Weisenberger et al, 1991) indicate that highly accurate discrimination of vowels and consonants and substantial benefits to speechreading in large-set identification and connected discourse tracking tasks can be obtained with multichannel devices as compared with single-channel devices. Evaluations of a number of multichannel tactile aids report similarly encouraging levels of performance (Brooks et al, 1986; Bernstein et al, 1991; Cowan et al, 1990; Weisenberger et al, 1989; Weisenberger et al, 1991). Most of these studies were relatively short in duration and involved use of the tactile aid only during training sessions. Because multichannel tactile aids have only recently become available, it is too soon to determine whether even greater benefits can be obtained when the device can be worn during all waking hours. Studies in progress by Osberger et al (1991a) and Geers and Moog (1991) are evaluating the long-term benefits of multichannel tactile aids for children in clinical and educational settings.

COCHLEAR IMPLANTS

Processing Strategies and Transducer Design

The development of cochlear implants dates back to preliminary experiments such as those of Djourno and Eyrie (1957) and Simmons (1966), in which it was demonstrated that sound could be detected by means of electrical stimulation of the auditory nerve. In the 1960s, most activity in the development of cochlear implants was centered in the United States, specifically the House Ear Institute (House & Berliner, 1991). In 1961 several patients underwent cochlear implantation performed by House. While work proceeded through the 1960s and 1970s on improvements in basic design, cochlear implants were controversial in the audiologic community. Considerable opposition to cochlear implants focused on the relatively limited benefits observed with early designs (Bilger et al, 1977) and on the lack of knowledge about whether electrical stimulation of the cochlea would result in further deterioration of auditory structures. By the 1980s, however, reports of greater benefits and increased interest on the part of otolaryngologists and people with hearing impairments led to widespread activity in the United States, Europe, and Australia (Hochmair-Desoyer et al, 1981; Clark et al, 1977; Mecklenburg & Lehnhardt, 1991) as well as to activity by the United States Food and Drug Administration (FDA) to determine the safety and effectiveness of these devices. FDA approval for the 3M/House single-channel implant (3M, Minneapolis, Minn.) was granted in 1984 and for the Nucleus multichannel implant (Cochlear Corporation, Englewood, Colo.) in 1990. Both of these devices are approved for use by both adults and children. At present, cochlear implants are no longer considered controversial by the audiologic community; rather, they are an accepted treatment for patients who do not benefit from conventional hearing aids. Initial concerns about electrical stimulation and about possible difficulties in explanting a device should it become necessary, have proved to be unfounded (Brimacombe et al, 1988).

The basic concept of a cochlear implant begins with a microphone that picks up acoustic energy in the environment, which is sent as an analog electrical signal to an externally worn signal processor. The processor extracts features of interest from the signal, depending on the processing strategy employed, and sends this information to an external transmitter, from which it is transferred through the skin (percutaneously) or across the skin (transcutaneously, by means of radio-frequency link) to a surgically implanted electrode or electrodes in the cochlea. Cochlear implant designs can be characterized according to a number of different schemes on the basis of the number of channels (electrodes), processing strategy, type of electrodes (monopolar or bipolar), type of electrical signal (analog or pulsatile), or electrode placement (intracochlear or extracochlear). Excellent descriptions of the surgical procedures involved in the implantation of single-channel and multichannel cochlear implants can be found in Graham (1991) and Clark et al (1991).

The most commonly encountered single-channel cochlear implant in the United States is the 3M/House single-channel implant. In general, single-channel implants present an analog version of the acoustic signal, with circuitry for automatic gain control and some frequency-dependent amplification (eg, selective boosting of high frequency signal components), to a single electrode in the cochlea. All cochlear implants are limited in design by a fundamental characteristic of the psychophysics of electrical stimulation, ie, the extremely limited dynamic range available for electrical stimuli between the threshold for perception and the threshold for pain. Estimates of the usable dynamic range in patients with hearing disorders vary from 2 to 15 dB (Brown & Stevens, 1992), which does not begin to compare with the 120-dB dynamic range for the normal auditory system. Thus, only a limited range of intensities can be coded in a cochlear implant, and care must be taken to ensure that output stimulation does not exceed the dynamic range of the patient.

In multichannel implant designs, such as the Nucleus device (Cochlear Corporation), a feature-extraction strategy is used (Figure 9.2). In the case of the Nucleus implant, 22 electrodes arranged along a wire are inserted into the cochlea in such a way that different electrodes stimulate auditory nerve fibers at different locations along the cochlea. The processor extracts information about voice F0 and F1 and F2. F0 is encoded as the pulse rate of the electrical stimulation; some of the electrodes (the five most apical electrodes) code the frequency and level of F1; some of the remaining electrodes code F2. In recent versions of the speech processor, additional processing for three higher-frequency bands (2000 to 8000 Hz) is presented on three electrodes located more basally in the cochlea to provide information about high-frequency components of the acoustic signal. A more detailed description of this processing scheme, and others, can be found in Wilson (1993). Figure 9.3 shows the location of the various components of the Nucleus implant after implantation.

The processor for a cochlear implant fits into a relatively small package, similar in size to a body hearing aid, that can be placed in a pocket or clipped to

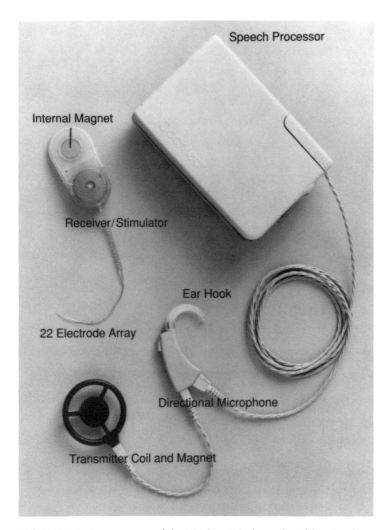

FIGURE 9.2 Components of the Nucleus 22-channel cochlear implant.

(Used with permission from Cochlear Corporation, Englewood, Colo.)

a belt. The microphone is mounted into a behind-the-ear (BTE) casing and connected by wire to the processor. The transmitter, for a transcutaneous device, is worn on the head above and slightly behind the ear and is held in place magnetically to an implanted receiver placed under the skin surface at that location. The receiver sends signals via wire to the electrode array. Rechargeable batteries power the entire device. As described later, the processing characteristics of the Nucleus implant are tailored for the particular user, to maximize the number of available electrodes, and to keep stimulation within comfortable parameters.

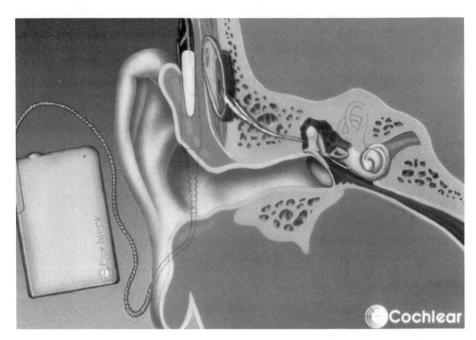

FIGURE 9.3   Location of components of the Nucleus cochlear implant after implantation.

(Used with permission from Cochlear Corporation, Englewood, Colo.)

Performance of Single-Channel and Multichannel Cochlear Implants

There is by now a considerable amount of literature evaluating the benefits of both single-channel and multichannel cochlear implants. Early studies of the effectiveness of cochlear implants were often plagued by a tendency to emphasize the performance of exceptionally successful users, rather than reporting average and variability measures. More recent studies take a more balanced approach. Stimulus detection is evaluated when the processor of the implant is customized for individual use, as described in the next section. Thielemeir et al (1985) reported on the audiologic abilities of patients with single-channel cochlear implants. They found that sounds in the range of conversational speech were rendered detectable by the device. Shannon and Muller (1990) noted that most users of single-channel implants can obtain at least temporal information that corresponds to amplitude envelope changes, whereas some users also perceive fundamental frequency information (Fourcin et al, 1979). Corresponding studies show that single-channel implant users can perform tasks that are based on amplitude envelope distinctions, such as the determination of syllable number and stress, and the discrimination of environmental sounds (Brimacombe et al, 1984; Tyler et al, 1989). The ability to follow F0 allows judgments about intonation contours of an utterance (ie, whether the utterance was a statement or a question) (Fourcin et al, 1979).

In discrimination and identification tasks that employ vowels and consonants, a wide range of performance on the part of users of single-channel cochlear implants has been observed (Tyler et al, 1989). The best users show a considerable ability to distinguish consonants and vowels but often do not show much ability to recognize items in open sets, such as word lists or words in sentences (Owens et al, 1983; Tyler et al, 1985). One surprising report on a group of children who had received 3M/House implants described abilities in phoneme discrimination, word identification, and sentence tasks that implied that these children were receiving some fine-structure spectral information from the device (Geers & Moog, 1988). It should be noted, however, that these children constituted the exception rather than the rule for users of single-channel implants.

Results for multichannel cochlear implants also show huge variability among users, but the mean performance, as well as the performance of the best users, far outreaches that achieved with a single-channel implant. Performance on tasks that require amplitude envelope information is generally superior for users of multichannel implants, as compared with users of single-channel implants (Tyler et al, 1989; Staller et al, 1990). Similarly, tasks that require fine-structure spectral and temporal information, such as vowel and consonant discrimination and identification, are performed poorly by users of single-channel implants, whereas many users of multichannel implants show impressive levels of accuracy on these tasks (Staller et al, 1990; Dowell et al, 1986; Tye-Murray & Tyler, 1989; Blamey et al, 1992). The most successful users of multichannel implants report some ability to recognize words in the absence of speechreading and even to use the telephone (Tyler et al, 1989). On average, improvements in speechreading performance can also be observed in many people who have received implants.

Overall, multichannel cochlear implants provide impressive benefits to speech perception abilities in people with hearing impairments. There is also some evidence of improvement in speech production skills in users of multichannel cochlear implants, both adults and children (Read, 1991; Perkell et al, 1992; Geers & Moog, 1991; Tobey et al, 1991). Particular improvements are noted in suprasegmental aspects of timing, maintenance of appropriate F0, and contrastive stress. However, improvements in segmental aspects of speech have been observed, particularly in children (Geers & Moog, 1991).

TRAINING AND REHABILITATION FOR SENSORY AIDS

The general philosophy and procedures that underlie aural rehabilitation programs for hearing aids can be applied to the use of tactile aids and cochlear implants. However, differences in the signal provided by these devices, as compared with that provided by a hearing aid, suggest that a simple adoption of hearing aid aural rehabilitation programs for use with a sensory aid may not meet with unqualified success. Training protocols for the Tactaid II (Plant, 1988) and the Tactaid VII have been developed (Robbins et al, 1993), as have general training protocols for sensory aids (Plant, 1984). The Tactaid II and Tactaid VII protocols emphasize the acquisition of extremely basic skills by children, whereas the Commtram program (Plant, 1984) was developed for adults. With these exceptions, however, there has been a lack of alternatives for training and rehabilitation for users of tactile aids.

Considerably more interest has been shown in the development of training and rehabilitation programs for users of cochlear implants. Cochlear Corporation provides a set of training materials with a recommended protocol for use with the Nucleus implant. Rehabilitation with the Nucleus implant follows, at least initially, a set of recommended steps outlined by Cochlear Corporation.

After the implant operation, a period of 4 to 6 weeks should elapse before the processor is activated, to allow adequate time for healing and to ensure that postoperative complications have not occurred. However, many patients find it difficult to undergo this waiting period, and the surgeon usually activates the processor for a short time soon after the operation to ascertain that it is working. This provides some encouragement to the patient. At the end of the waiting period, the patient returns to the implant center for the initial fitting of the processor. For the Nucleus implant, the processor is plugged directly into a computer, so that an individual program can be established for the user and downloaded directly to the processor.

The initial psychophysical fitting includes a determination of which electrodes are active in the cochlea (sometimes placement of the electrode array or localized loss of auditory nerve fibers renders an electrode nonviable). For each viable electrode, threshold and uncomfortable levels are measured to provide a range within which stimulation will be presented. Next, loudness balancing of adjacent electrodes and of a sweeping stimulus across the entire electrode array is performed, so that stimulus levels will not show large variation across channels. Finally, pitch perception across electrodes is assessed and the frequency response of individual channels is adjusted, if necessary, to provide maximal speech information to the user. This information is stored as a map for a particular patient in the memory of the computer as well as in the device itself, so that if the processor is damaged, the map can be reloaded. Patients return to the implant center for remapping 3 months after implantation, for fine-tuning of the map. Return visits at 6 months and 1 year after implantation for processor checks are often prescribed.

It should be emphasized that cochlear implants, even for patients who show considerable benefits, do not provide normal hearing. Nor, obviously, do tactile aids. In most cases, considerable training and rehabilitation are necessary for attainment of maximal benefits. For tactile aids, this training may cover a period of years (Sherrick, 1984), given the arbitrary nature of the tactile speech signal. A similar period may be necessary for training with cochlear implants, particularly for children with prelingual hearing impairments.

Training programs that begin with relatively simple auditory tasks (eg, sound detection) and move gradually up the hierarchy of listening tasks through discrimination, identification, recognition, and comprehension have been recommended by Cooper (1991), among others. The Cochlear Corporation training manual for the Nucleus implant follows this hierarchy. There is some dispute among researchers, however, about whether training and rehabilitation for tactile aids and cochlear implants should follow an analytic training strategy or a synthetic training strategy. Analytic training focuses on segmental distinctions at the phoneme level and on suprasegmental aspects such as syllable number and stress. Synthetic training focuses on connected speech and employs sentence identification, tracking of connected discourse, and interactive communication tasks.

The philosophy behind analytic training is that some degree of familiarity with the elements of speech is necessary for comprehension of connected discourse and that without such familiarity the amount of information in connected speech is uninterpretable. Proponents of synthetic training point out that the acoustic features of utterances presented in single-item, citation form are very different from the same utterances presented in connected speech (Bernstein, 1992). Thus, it is argued that analytic training may encourage users of sensory aids to focus on irrelevant or even misleading cues when attempting to understand connected speech. Comparative training studies (Weisenberger, 1991) have not found one method to be superior to the other in assessing the eventual performance of users of tactile aids in laboratory studies. Most rehabilitation and training protocols include a combination of analytic and synthetic training tasks.

Of crucial interest in speech perception training for users of cochlear implants and tactile aids is the role of speechreading in effective use. As mentioned earlier, multichannel tactile devices do not deliver sufficient speech information to allow the comprehension of connected speech or high levels of open-set word recognition without the addition of speechreading. Some users of multichannel cochlear implants do show a degree of open-set word recognition and connected-speech comprehension under implant-alone conditions, but most users rely on speechreading to provide additional information in connected-speech situations. Thus, it is important to consider how best to facilitate the integration of visual and implant or tactile cues. As discussed later, users with good speechreading skills tend to be successful users of sensory aids. For this reason, training of speechreading skills may be useful as part of the rehabilitation program. It is of interest to note that multichannel tactile aids provide substantial information about the manner of articulation of consonants but do not provide cues for place of articulation. Although this design aspect was not intentional, it is fortuitous in the sense that information on place of articulation is more easily available from speechreading than is manner of articulation. Thus, the two modalities serve a complementary function, to some degree.

An extended form of multimodality integration was studied by Lynch et al (1989). They evaluated the benefits provided by a tactile aid in conjunction with both speechreading and a hearing aid. The results suggested that performance in the three-modality (visual, auditory, and tactile) condition was superior to that for any single modality or any combination of two modalities. A similar approach has been taken by Geers and Moog (1991) and Osberger et al (1991b) in their longitudinal studies of the performance of children with tactile aids and cochlear implants. It is possible that a three-modality approach may be beneficial for some users of sensory aids. However, if substantial residual hearing is present, care must be taken to avoid a signal from the tactile aid that is audible, either by air or bone conduction, which might interfere with auditory input.

For a speech-language pathologist who is a member of a rehabilitation team, training and rehabilitation procedures for speech production improvements are of considerable importance. A knowledge of the cues delivered to the user by the tactile device or cochlear implant is essential to plan an effective course of speech therapy, particularly if the patient does not effectively use normal kinesthetic cues that accompany speech production. For example, if a device delivers only amplitude envelope information, it may be useful in improving speech timing, stress, and pitch maintenance but may not provide benefits in producing specific phonemes, because the information necessary for these distinctions is not perceptible in the speech of others, or in the patient's own speech. It is recommended that the speech-language pathologist assisting a user of a tactile aid with speech remediation become familiar with the device by actually wearing it and gaining firsthand knowledge of the signal provided by the aid. This is not possible in the case of cochlear implants, of course, but simulations of implant signals have been developed for auditory presentation that may shed some light on the patient's experience.

When the user of an implant or tactile aid is a child, additional factors must be addressed. If the child's hearing loss was congenital or was sustained very early in life, it is possible that oral language will not have developed before implantation. For these children, the rehabilitation program must be very carefully tailored to meet the child's communication level. The program may contain a substantial language training component, which may be administered by a speech-language pathologist. Many characteristics of such children correspond to those of language-delayed children with normal hearing. There is some evidence that similar therapeutic techniques may be helpful in stimulating language acquisition.

Who Will Be a Successful User of a Sensory Aid?

For cochlear implants, most centers follow established criteria for patient selection. To some degree, similar criteria are used to determine candidates for tactile aids. The candidate must have bilateral, profound, sensorineural hearing loss and must derive minimal benefit from a hearing aid. For cochlear implants, it is also important to assess the viability of the auditory nerve, if possible, and to evaluate psychological variables. For patients in whom the auditory nerve is not viable, a tactile aid is the recommended option. If hearing aids have not been tried previously by the candidate, a hearing aid fitting and trial is often performed.

Children who are candidates for implantation must not be younger than 2 years; elective surgical procedures may be risky for very young children. Candidates must show high levels of motivation and familial support and must have realistic expectations about the benefits of the device. Medical evaluation must show no evidence of conditions that might contraindicate either the operation or the potential for use of the device (for example, at one time it was thought that the presence of ossification of the cochlea would not allow implantation. However, more recent reports (Clark et al, 1991) suggest that this bone growth is relatively soft and can be removed from the cochlea before implantation of the electrode array). For children, evidence that the child's educational environment contains a substantial oral-aural component is often sought, both for facilitation of training and because this environment is likely to motivate the child to use the implant.

Much effort has been invested in determining characteristics of candidates for tactile aids and cochlear implants that might predict successful use. This is of particular interest for recipients of cochlear implants given the expense and effort involved in the surgical procedure and rehabilitation program. Numerous variables have been investigated, including preoperative response to extracochlear electrical stimulation and the cause of the hearing loss. At present, several factors appear to have a positive correlation with successful use of a cochlear implant. These include whether the hearing loss is prelingual or postlingual (people with postlingual deafness show higher levels of performance) (Somers, 1991); the primary communication mode of the patient (oral-aural communicators show greater benefits than people who primarily use sign language as their communication mode) (Somers, 1991); neuronal survival in the population of auditory nerve fibers of the candidate, which cannot be assessed directly but must be inferred from other measures (Otte et al, 1978); and length of time since the onset of hearing loss—patients who have been deaf for the least amount of time show greater benefits (Gantz et al, 1988). Correlations of speechreading ability with implant use have been found by some investigators (Cooper, 1991) but not by others (Gantz et al, 1988). A similar inconsistency of findings is true for measurements of electrical dynamic range (Gantz et al, 1988). Some studies showed that patients with larger dynamic ranges for electrical stimulation were more successful implant users.

CONCLUSIONS

Both cochlear implants and tactile aids, although accepted in the audiologic community as treatment of profound hearing loss that is not ameliorated by conventional hearing aids, are still in the early stages of development. Research efforts in both areas are concentrating on improving the processors and transducer arrays for these devices, and each successive development appears to yield higher levels of performance. New methods of signal delivery, such as the continuous interleaved sampling technique developed by Wilson (1993) for the Ineraid multichannel cochlear implant (Symbion/Richards, Salt Lake City, Utah), are just one example of the advances in the design of sensory aids. It is still too early to determine the level of benefit possible with multichannel tactile devices, given their relatively recent introduction into the commercial market. It is possible that with extended everyday use, levels of performance that exceed those previously measured in laboratory evaluations will be observed.

Blamey and Cowan (1992), in comparing the benefits provided by cochlear implants and tactile aids, emphasize that the word *potential* must be used in all discussions of sensory aid benefit. Because of the factors discussed herein and the constantly changing state of the technology of the field, the ultimate benefits of tactile aids and cochlear implants have not been observed. Blamey and Cowan argue, in addition, that it is difficult to predict the levels to be reached by subsequent generations of sensory aids. Involvement as a member of the rehabilitation team in this rapidly evolving field represents an exciting challenge for speech-language pathologists as well as for engineers, surgeons, audiologists, educators, and health care professionals.

REFERENCES

Abbott, G. D., Craig, J. C., & Weisenberger, J. M. (1989). The AKL representation in a tactile aid for the deaf. Presented at the 11th IEEE Engineering in Medicine and Biology Meeting, November 9-12, Seattle.

Bach-y-Rita, P. (1974). Visual information through the skin: A tactile vision substitution system. *Transactions of the American Academy of Ophthalmology and Otolaryngology, 78,* OP-729–OP-739.

Bernstein, L. E. (1992). The evaluation of tactile aids. In I. Summers (Ed.), *Tactile aids for the hearing impaired* (pp. 167-186). San Diego: Singular.

Bernstein, L. E., Eberhardt, S. P., & Demorest, M. E. (1989). Single-channel vibrotactile supplements to visual perception of intonation and stress. *Journal of the Acoustical Society of America, 85,* 397-405.

Bernstein, L. E., Demorest, M. E., Coulter, D. C., & O'Connell, M. P. (1991). Speechreading sentences with vibrotactile vocoders: Performance of normal-hearing and hearing-impaired subjects. *Journal of the Acoustical Society of America, 90,* 2971-2984.

Bilger, R. C., Black, F. O., & Hopkinson, N. T. (1977). Research plan for evaluating subjects presently fitted with implanted auditory prostheses. *Annals of Otology, Rhinology, & Laryngology, 86 (Suppl. 38),* 21-24.

Blamey, P. J., Brown, A. M., Busby, P. A., et al (1992). Cochlear implants in children, adolescents, and prelinguistically deafened adults: Speech perception. *Journal of Speech and Hearing Research, 35,* 401-417.

Acknowledgment: Preparation of this chapter was supported by grant DC00306 from the National Institutes of Health.

Blamey, P. J., & Clark, G. M. (1985). A wearable multiple-electrode electrotactile speech processor for the profoundly deaf. *Journal of the Acoustical Society of America, 77,* 1619-1620.

Blamey, P. J., & Cowan, R. S. C. (1992). The potential benefit and cost-effectiveness of tactile devices in comparison with cochlear implants. In I. Summers (Ed.), *Tactile aids for the hearing impaired* (pp. 187-217). San Diego: Singular.

Boothroyd, A. & Hnath-Chisholm, T. (1988). Spatial, tactile presentation of voice funda-mental frequency as a supplement to lipreading: Results of extended training with a single subject. *Journal of Rehabilitation Research and Development, 25,* 51-56.

Brimacombe, J. A., Edgerton, B. J., Doyle, K. J., Erratt, J. D., & Dannhauer, J. L. (1984). Auditory capabilities of patients implanted with the House single-channel cochlear implant. *Acta Oto-Laryngologica, 411 (Suppl.),* 204-216.

Brimacombe, J. A., Beiter, A. L., Barket, M. J., Mikami, K. A., & Staller, S. J. (1988). Comparative results of speech recognition testing with patients who have used both a single channel and multichannel cochlear implant system. *Proceedings of the American Auditory Society,* 17 November, Boston.

Brooks, P. L., Frost, B. J., Mason, J. L., & Gibson, D. M. (1986). Continuing evaluation of the Queen's University tactile vocoder. II. Identification of open-set sentences and tracking narrative. *Journal of Rehabilitation Research and Development, 23,* 129-138.

Brown, B. H., & Stevens, J. C. (1992). Electrical stimulation of the skin. In I. Summers (Ed.), *Tactile aids for the hearing impaired* (pp. 37-56). San Diego: Singular.

Carney, A. E. (1988). Vibrotactile perception of segmental features of speech: A comparison of single- and multichannel aids. *Journal of Speech and Hearing Research, 31,* 438-448.

Carney, A. E., & Beachler, C. R. (1986). Vibrotactile perception of suprasegmental features of speech: A comparison of single-channel and multichannel instruments. *Journal of the Acoustical Society of America, 79,* 131-140.

Clark, G., Franz, B., Pyman, B., & Webb, R. (1991). Surgery for multichannel cochlear implantation. In H. Cooper (Ed.), *Cochlear implants: A practical guide* (pp. 169-200). San Diego: Singular.

Clark, G. M., Tong, Y. C., Black, R., Forster, I. C., Patrick, J. F., & Dewhurst, D. J. (1977). A multiple electrode cochlear implant. *Journal of Laryngology and Otology, 91,* 935-945.

Cooper, H. (1991). Training and rehabilitation for cochlear implant users. In H. Cooper (Ed.), *Cochlear implants: A practical guide* (pp. 219-239). San Diego: Singular.

Cowan, R. S. C., Blamey, P. J., Galvin, K. L., Sarant, J. Z., Alcantara, J. I., & Clark, G. M. (1990). Perception of sentences, words, and speech features by profoundly hearing-impaired children using a multichannel electrotactile speech processor. *Journal of the Acoustical Society of America, 88,* 1374-1384.

Craig, J. C. (1972). Difference threshold for intensity of tactile stimuli. *Perception & Psychophysics, 11,* 150-152.

DeFilippo, C. L., & Scott, B. L. (1978). A method for training and evaluating the reception of ongoing speech. *Journal of the Acoustical Society of America, 63,* 1186-1192.

Djourno, A., & Eyries, C. (1957). Prosthèse auditive par excitation electrique à distance du nerf sensoriel à l'aide d'un bobinage inclus à demeure. *Presse Medicine, 35,* 14-17.

Dowell, R. C., Mecklenburg, D. J., & Clark, G. M. (1986). Speech recognition for 40 patients receiving multichannel cochlear implants. *Archives of Otolaryngology–Head and Neck Surgery, 112,* 1054-1059.

Fourcin, A. J., Rosen, S. M., Moore, B. C. J., Clarke, G. P., Dodson, H., & Bannister, L. H. (1979). External electrical stimulation of the cochlea: Clinical, psychophysical, speech perceptual and histological findings. *British Journal of Audiology, 13,* 85-107.

Fraser, G. (1991). The cochlear implant team. In H. Cooper (Ed.), *Cochlear implants: A practical guide* (pp. 84-92). San Diego: Singular.

Gantz, B. J., Tyler, R. S., Knutson, J. F., et al (1988). Evaluation of five different cochlear implant designs: Audiologic assessment and predictors of performance. *Laryngoscope, 98,* 1100-1106.

Gault, R. H. (1927). "Hearing" through the sense organs of touch and vibration. *Journal of the Franklin Institute, 204,* 329-358.

Geers, A. E. (1986). Vibrotactile stimulation: Case study with a profoundly deaf child. *Journal of Rehabilitation Research and Development, 23,* 111-117.

Geers, A. E., & Moog, J. S. (1988). Predicting long-term benefits of the single-channel cochlear implant in profoundly deaf children. *American Journal of Otolaryngology, 37,* 224-250.

Geers, A. E., & Moog, J. S. (1991). Evaluating the benefits of cochlear implants in an educational setting. *American Journal of Otology, 12 (Suppl.),* 116-125.

Gescheider, G. A.. (1974). Temporal relations in cutaneous stimulation. In F. A. Geldard (Ed.), *Cutaneous communication systems and devices* (pp. 33-37). Austin: Psychonomic Society.

Goff, G. D. (1967). Differential discrimination of frequency of cutaneous mechanical vibration. *Journal of Experimental Psychology, 74,* 158-165.

Graham, J. (1991). Surgery for single-channel cochlear implantation. In H. Cooper (Ed.), *Cochlear implants: A practical guide* (pp. 155-168). San Diego: Singular.

Grant, K. W., Ardell, L. H., Kuhl, P. K., & Sparks, D. W. (1985). The contribution of fundamental frequency, amplitude envelope, and voicing duration cues to speechreading in normal-hearing subjects. *Journal of the Acoustical Society of America, 77,* 671-677.

Hochmair-Desoyer, I. J., Hochmair, E. S., Burian, K., & Fischer, R. E. (1981). Four years of experience with cochlear prostheses. *Medical Program Technology, 8,* 107-119.

Hodgson, W. R. (1986). *Hearing aid assessment and use in audiologic habilitation.* Baltimore: Williams & Wilkins.

House, W. F., & Berliner, K. I. (1991). Cochlear implants: From idea to clinical practice. In H. Cooper (Ed.), *Cochlear implants: A practical guide* (pp. 9-33). San Diego: Singular.

Lynch, M. P., Eilers, R. E., Oller, D. K., Urbano, R. C., & Pero, P. J. (1989). Multisensory narrative tracking by a profoundly deaf subject using an electrocutaneous vocoder and a vibrotactile aid. *Journal of Speech and Hearing Research, 32,* 331-338.

Mecklenburg, D., & Lehnhardt, E. (1991). The development of cochlear implants in Europe, Asia, and Australia. In H. Cooper (Ed.), *Cochlear implants: A practical guide* (pp. 34-57). San Diego: Singular.

Osberger, M. J., Robbins, A. M., Miyamoto, R. T., et al (1991a). Speech perception abilities of children with cochlear implants, tactile aids, or hearing aids. *American Journal of Otology, 12 (Suppl.)*, 105-115.

Osberger, M. J., Robbins, A. M., Todd, S. L., & Brown, C. J. (1991b). Initial findings with a wearable multichannel vibrotactile aid. *American Journal of Otology, 12 (Suppl.)*, 179-182.

Otte, J., Schuknecht, H. F., & Kerr, A. G. (1978). Ganglion cell population in normal and pathological human cochleae: Implications for cochlear implantation. *Laryngoscope, 38*, 1231-1246.

Owens, E., Kessler, D., & Raggio, M. (1983). Results for some patients with cochlear implants on the Minimal Auditory Capabilities (MAC) battery. In C. W. Parkins & S. W. Anderson (Eds.), *Cochlear prostheses: An international symposium* (pp. 443-450). New York: New York Academy of Sciences.

Perkell, J., Lane, H., & Svirsky, M. (1992). Speech of cochlear implant patients: A longitudinal study of vowel production. *Journal of the Acoustical Society of America, 91*, 2962-2978.

Phillips, D. P., & Brugge, J. F. (1985). Progress in neurophysiology of sound localization. *Annual Review of Psychology, 36*, 245-274.

Plant, G. (1984). *Commtram: A communication training program for profoundly hearing impaired adults.* Sydney: National Acoustic Laboratories.

Plant, G. (1988). *Tactaid II training program.* Sydney: National Acoustic Laboratories.

Proctor, A., & Goldstein, M. H., Jr. (1983). Development of lexical comprehension in a profoundly deaf child using a wearable vibrotactile communication aid. *Language, Speech and Hearing Services in Schools, 14*, 138-149.

Ramsdell, S. A. (1978). The psychology of the hard-of-hearing and the deafened adult. In H. Davis & S. R. Silverman (Eds.), *Hearing and deafness* (pp. 435-446). New York: Holt, Rinehart, & Winston.

Read, T. (1989). Improvement in speech production following use of the UCH/RNID cochlear implant. *Journal of Laryngology and Otology, 18 (Suppl.)*, 45-49.

Read, T. (1991). Speech production in postlinguistically deafened adult cochlear implant users. In H. Cooper (Ed.), *Cochlear implants: A practical guide* (pp. 346-354). San Diego: Singular.

Reed, C. M., Durlach, N. I., & Braida, L. D. (1982). Research on tactile communication of speech: A review. *Asha, 20*.

Richardson, B. L. (1982). Using the skin for the purpose of sound localization. In R. W. Gatehouse (Ed.), *Localization of sound: Theory and applications* (pp. 155-168). Groton, CT: Amphora.

Robbins, A. M., Hesketh, L. J., & Bivins, C. (1993). *Targo: Tactaid 7 reference guide and orientation.* Somerville, MA: Audiological Engineering.

Rothenberg, M., Verrillo, R. T., Zahorian, S. A., Brachman, M. L., & Bolanowski, S. J., Jr. (1977). Vibrotactile frequency for encoding a speech parameter. *Journal of the Acoustical Society of America, 62*, 1003-1012.

Shannon, R. V., & Muller, C. (1990). Temporal modulation transfer functions in patients with cochlear implants. *Journal of the Acoustical Society of America, 88,* 741-744.

Sherrick, C. E. (1984). Basic and applied research on tactile aids for deaf people: Progress and prospects. *Journal of the Acoustical Society of America, 86,* 981-988.

Sherrick, C. E., & Cholewiak, R. W. (1986). Cutaneous sensitivity. In K. Boff, L. Kaufman, & J. L. Thomas (Eds.), *Handbook of perception and human performance* (pp. 12-1–12-58). New York: Wiley.

Simmons, F. B. (1966). Electrical stimulation of the auditory nerve in man. *Archives of Otolaryngology, 84,* 24-76.

Skinner, M. W., Binzer, S. M., Frederickson, J. M., et al (1988). Comparison of benefit from vibrotactile aid and cochlear implant for postlingually deaf adults. *Laryngoscope, 98,* 1092-1099.

Somers, M. N. (1991). Effects of cochlear implants in children: Implications for rehabilitation. In H. Cooper (Ed.), *Cochlear implants: A practical guide* (pp. 322-345). San Diego: Singular.

Staller, S. J., Beiter, A. L., Brimacombe, J. A., Mecklenburg, D. J., & Arndt, P. L. (1990). Pediatric performance with the Nucleus 22-channel cochlear implant system. *American Journal of Otology, 12 (Suppl.),* 126-136.

Thielemeir, M., Tonokawa, L., & Peterson, B. (1985). Audiological results in children with a cochlear implant. *Ear and Hearing, 6 (Suppl. 3),* 27-35.

Thornton, R. D., & Phillips, A. J. (1992). A comparative trial of four vibrotactile aids. In I. Summers (Ed.), *Tactile aids for the hearing impaired* (pp. 231-252). San Diego: Singular.

Tobey, E. A., Angelette, S., Murchison, C., et al (1991). Speech production performance in children with multichannel cochlear implants. *American Journal of Otology, 12 (Suppl.),* 165-173.

Tye-Murray, N., & Tyler, R.S. (1989). Auditory consonant and word recognition skills of cochlear implant users. *Ear and Hearing, 10,* 292-298.

Tyler, R. S., Gantz, B. J., McCabe, B. F., Lowder, M. W., Otto, S. R., & Preece, J. P. (1985). Audiological results with two single-channel cochlear implants. *Annals of Otology, Rhinology, and Laryngology, 94,* 133-139.

Tyler, R. S., Moore, B. C. J., & Kuk, F. K. (1989). Performance of some of the better cochlear implant patients. *Journal of Speech and Hearing Research, 32,* 887-911.

Verrillo, R. T., & Gescheider, G. A. (1992). Perception via the sense of touch. In I. Summers (Ed.), *Tactile aids for the hearing impaired* (pp. 1-36). San Diego: Singular.

Weinstein, S. (1968). Intensive and extensive aspects of tactile sensitivity as a function of body part, sex, and laterality. In D. R. Kenshalo (Ed.), *The skin senses* (pp. 195-222). Springfield: Thomas.

Weisenberger, J. M. (1986). Sensitivity to amplitude-modulated vibrotactile signals. *Journal of the Acoustical Society of America, 80,* 1707-1715.

Weisenberger, J. M. (1991). Issues in evaluating wearable multichannel tactile aids. *Journal of the Acoustical Society of America, 89,* 1958.

Weisenberger, J. M. (1992). Communication of the acoustic environment via tactile stimuli. In I. Summers (Ed.), *Tactile aids for the hearing impaired* (pp. 83-109). San Diego: Singular.

Weisenberger, J. M., Broadstone, S. M., & Kozma-Spytek, L. (1991). Relative performance of single-channel and multichannel tactile aids for the hearing-impaired. *Journal of Rehabilitation Research and Development, 28,* 45-56.

Weisenberger, J. M. Broadstone, S. M., & Saunders, F. A. (1989). Evaluation of two multichannel tactile aids for the hearing-impaired. *Journal of the Acoustical Society of America, 89,* 1764-1775.

Weisenberger, J. M., Heidbreder, A. F., & Miller, J. D. (1987). Development and preliminary evaluation of an earmold sound-to-tactile aid for the hearing-impaired. *Journal of Rehabilitation Research and Development, 24,* 51-66.

Weisenberger, J. M., & Russell, A. F. (1989). Comparison of two single-channel tactile aids for the hearing-impaired. *Journal of Speech and Hearing Research, 32,* 83-92.

Wilson, B. S. (1993). Signal processing. In R. S. Tyler (Ed.), *Cochlear implants: Audiological foundations* (pp. 35-85). San Diego: Singular.

SUGGESTED READING

Cooper, H. (Ed.). (1991). *Cochlear implants: A practical guide.* San Diego: Singular.

Summers, I. (Ed.). (1992). *Tactile aids for the hearing impaired.* San Diego: Singular.

10 |⌐

Speech and Language Characteristics of Children and Adults with Hearing Impairments

Lynne A. Davis

THE LINK BETWEEN HEARING AND SPEECH
Interpreting Audiograms and Applying Speech Acoustics

Before beginning treatment with any client with a hearing impairment it is crucial to obtain and analyze the client's audiogram, including both unaided and aided thresholds. If the information is not available or not current, the client should be referred for audiologic evaluation to obtain the audiometric information needed to develop an appropriate treatment plan.

The first step in analysis of the audiogram is to compare the intensities at which the person can hear each frequency with information regarding the acoustics of English phonemes. This identifies which phonemes should be audible to the child with aided and unaided hearing. It also helps predict what features of speech and language the child should be able to acquire through audition and which may require additional modalities such as vision and taction. For example, in Figure 10.1, the audiogram indicates that when using a hearing aid, the child can hear conversational speech through 2500 Hz. That means that suprasegmental information about pitch, intensity, and duration and the first and second formants of English vowels and the most intense regions of the consonants /b/, /m/, /w/, /ɹ/, /n/, /ł/, /g/, and /ŋ/ are available under good listening conditions. The child would be expected to develop these aspects of speech through audition. However, the consonants /f/, /v/, /p/, /t/, /d/, /l/, /s/, /z/, /ʃ/, /ʒ/, /θ/, /ð/, /t͡ʃ/, /d͡ʒ/, /j/, /k/, /h/, cues that allow discrimination of nasal consonants, and cues that allow discrimination of fricatives from affricates are not available to the child. This child would not be expected to acquire those aspects of speech spontaneously and, indeed, may require

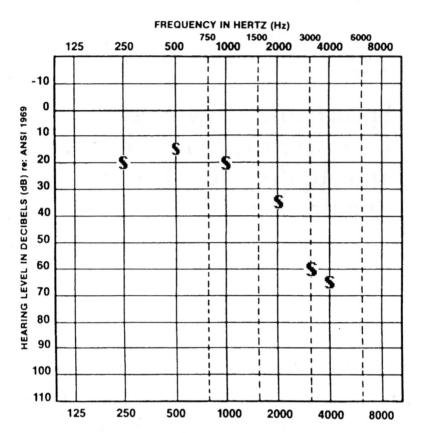

FIGURE 10.1 Audiogram. S indicates binaurally aided soundfield thresholds at 250, 500, 1000, 2000, 3000, and 4000 Hz.

additional modalities to acquire them. Careful analysis of each client's audiometric information makes it possible to predict aspects of speech that should be developing and to design treatment approaches to facilitate the development of those not available through audition.

The Role of Auditory Skills

Why is it important to start by evaluating auditory skills? The ability to hear and discriminate sounds is the basis for establishing the effective auditory feedback system necessary for development of natural-sounding speech (Ling, 1976). Although vision and proprioception allow for some acquisition and monitoring of speech production, they are inefficient substitutes for auditory feedback (Davis & Hardick, 1981). Therefore, acquiring speech sounds means also acquiring the ability to identify and imitate those sounds. An effective treatment program begins with evaluation of auditory skills in combination with speech production (Ling, 1976).

Although the specific aspects of speech available to a person with a hearing loss must be analyzed individually, it is possible to make some general statements about typical patterns of acquisition and errors for people with various degrees of hearing impairment. People with hearing losses labeled as mild or moderate, no more than a 55 dB to 60 dB hearing loss unaided, usually develop natural-sounding speech. Depending on audiogram configuration and use of appropriate amplification, these people may have some articulation errors on sibilants and /ɹ/ (Hudgins & Numbers, 1942; West & Weber, 1973). As hearing loss becomes more severe, it is typical to see problems involving place and manner of articulation, for example, /d/ for /g/ and /m/ for /b/. In addition, as the second formants of vowels become inaudible, vowel confusions and difficulty with acquisition of such contrasts as /i/ versus /u/ appear along with difficulty perceiving and producing sounds with a place of articulation in the middle of the mouth. In English many phonemes are produced with alveolar place of articulation, which means that fine distinctions and accurate articulator placements and uses of air are necessary for correct production. This causes problems for people with severe or profound hearing losses (Smith, 1975).

People who have access only to acoustic information below 1000 Hz essentially receive only suprasegmental information about speech; they hear only patterns of intensity and duration. These are the people for whom acquisition of natural-sounding speech through use of audition is extremely difficult, if not impossible. Such people have problems with all aspects of speech production, including control of respiration for speech (Forner & Hixon, 1977), control of the glottis for phonation (Monsen, 1979), control of velopharyngeal opening and closing, and timing and movement of the tongue, lips, and jaw (McGarr & Harris, 1983). As a result of these problems, it is typical to see problems with control of voicing, pitch, and air expenditure. These problems lead to speech that is slow and labored, often with only a few syllables per breath, either monotone or with wildly varying pitch, and with little differentiation of phonemes (Calvert, 1962; Levitt, 1971). Tye-Murray (1991) found that speakers who are deaf show a less flexible tongue body and tend to use the same tongue movements for all vowels. Because so much can be in error and individual patterns differ greatly, thorough evaluation of audition and a wide range of speech skills is necessary for adequate treatment approaches.

The Link Between Hearing and Language

Developmental Effects

Children who are born with a hearing loss or who acquire a hearing loss before 3 years of age are at high risk for language problems. Depending on the severity of the hearing loss, language difficulties may range from mild delays in language development to complete failure to develop a coherent body of language rules (Kretschmer & Kretschmer, 1978a). Such language problems appear to be a result of lack of exposure to concepts and rules.

There are two important contributors to the language problems. First, although the age at which hearing losses are identified is decreasing in the United States as neonatal registries and screenings become more common, many children are still not identified as having a hearing impairment until 16 to 22 months of age for moderate to profound hearing losses and 3 years for mild losses (Matkin, 1988). In addition, the lag between identification and fitting with amplification and beginning early communication programming is still more than 6 months. A child who is 18 months to 2 years of age has already missed many crucial language milestones and has considerable delays in language development (Davis & Hardick, 1981). Second, even after the hearing loss is identified and the child is fit with amplification and enrolled in treatment for developing communication skills, two additional factors work against remediation of the delays. First, because 90 percent of children with hearing losses are born to parents with normal hearing, these children often are not exposed to consistently appropriate language in a modality they can easily acquire and use. If the parents choose an auditory-oral approach to communication, the children must use damaged input systems and faulty speech production to communicate. They miss concepts and functions of language and are not easily understood when they speak.

On the other hand, if parents choose a total communication approach for communication development, parents rarely develop their sign communication skills to the point at which they can provide accurate, complete representations of English (Moeller & Luetke-Stahlman, 1990). Instead, the parents sign three- or four-word phrases and omit many of the function words. The children also often receive a limited number of content words because of the parents' limited sign vocabularies. In addition, much of children's language skill develops through peripheral, environmental exposure to the communication around them throughout the day. Children with hearing impairments do not acquire language without being focused on its presence and importance. Children with normal hearing hear a word many times before completely integrating it into their language systems. Children with hearing impairments are exposed to fewer words in an inconsistent manner, and they must attend directly to the words for adequate exposure to occur. They are, therefore, likely to develop language at a slower rate and with more deficits than children with normal hearing.

Over the years there has been an ongoing discussion about whether the language problems of children with hearing losses represent language delays that can be remedied with language treatment that involves increased exposure or whether these children have language deficits that require targeted remediation approaches (Kretschmer & Kretschmer, 1978a; Osberger, 1986). In all likelihood both approaches may be correct. Lack of consistent, appropriate exposure to language results in delays in its development. In addition, however, there are patterns of language difficulty that persist into adulthood for people with prelingual hearing losses. McAfee et al (1990) found problems with language functions in college students with hearing impairments, particularly in written language. Such patterns point to areas of language development that may be in need of specific targeting in communication treatment programs.

Effects of Hearing Loss in Language Comprehension and Production

As with speech skills in people with hearing losses, it is crucial to evaluate and treat each client as a person with individual strengths and weaknesses. However, with individual variations clearly in mind, some generalizations are possible. Again, as in speech development, the more severe the hearing loss, the greater the delays and deficits tend to be. For people with mild or moderate hearing losses, the problems include poor vocabulary, resulting from lack of exposure to different ways of expressing similar concepts; delays in the development of morphologic markers using high-frequency phonemes, such as plurals, third-person present tense, and regular past tense in English, because these sounds are among the more difficult to hear; and delays in the development of function words such as prepositions and articles (Davis & Hardick, 1981).

Function words are a problem area because they are quieter than content words and have poorer visual referents. Articles may prove especially difficult because they have the "hidden" use in English of coding new as opposed to old information. Prepositions are also a problem because they are so often used in idiomatic expressions as well as to represent actual locations.

Not surprisingly, as hearing losses become more severe, the patterns of deficits in language development increase. Along with the problems described earlier, people with severe or profound hearing losses often have difficulty with verbs and verb tenses, especially those that take auxiliaries (Davis & Hardick, 1981). These people also may have problems with word order, because they tend to understand and express content words to the exclusion of function words, and their representation of English syntax is extremely incomplete (Easterbrooks, 1987). Often the language skills of those with severe hearing losses resemble those of people with language or learning disabilities.

ASSESSING COMMUNICATION SKILLS OF CHILDREN WITH HEARING IMPAIRMENTS

Tests Designed for Children with Hearing Impairments

Speech

The following tests were specifically designed for evaluating the speech skills of people with hearing losses.

The Functional Speech Sound Test (FSST) (Levitt et al, 1990) is designed to assess pitch control, prosody, and articulation of vowels and consonants. The norm was based on degree of hearing loss (moderate to profound) in people 6 through

21 years of age. Stimuli include syllable repetition, counting, single words, sentences, and short stories for conversational samples.

The Phonetic Level Speech Evaluation (Ling, 1976) is designed to assess duration, intensity, pitch, and articulation of vowels and consonants. Subtests for assessing word-initial and word-final clusters are also available. The test may be used for people from preschool age through adulthood with any degree of hearing loss. There is no norm, but Ling's book provides a description to be used in analyzing results. Stimuli include consonant-vowel nonsense syllables in single productions, repeated productions, in alternation with other consonant-vowel syllables and produced over a five-tone pitch range. Ling's book also describes the use of phonologic level assessment.

Language

The Grammatical Analysis of Elicited Language (GAEL) (Moog & Geers, 1979) is designed to assess language skills in children 3 through 12 years of age with moderate through profound hearing impairments. The test is available in pre-sentence, simple sentence, and complex sentence versions. The pre-sentence version assesses comprehension and expression, and the other two assess expression only. The GAEL utilizes language elicited through play with toy figures both immediately after the tester's model and after a delay.

The Ski*Hi Language test (Watson & Clark, 1985) is designed to assess receptive and expressive language skills in children from birth through 4 years of age with hearing impairments. The test is designed for either oral or total communication and includes items that assess comprehension and use of concepts and syntax.

The Kretschmer Spontaneous Language Analysis Procedure (Kretschmer & Kretschmer, 1978b) is designed specifically for analysis of the semantics and pragmatics in language samples obtained from children with hearing impairments.

The Reynell Developmental Language Scales (Reynell, 1977) are designed to assess receptive and expressive language skills. It has norms for 3 through 8 years of age, both with normal hearing and with hearing impairments. The test was developed in England, and initial norm data were gathered there. American norms are now available. The test includes subtests for comprehension of single words through complex sentences and production from the single-word level through stories elicited with toys and sequenced pictures.

The Rhode Island Test of Language Structures (Engen & Engen, 1983) can be used to assess comprehension of syntactic structures. The norm was derived from people 3 through 20 years of age with hearing impairments. The test consists of 20 sentence types, which range from simple through complex, and uses a point-to-the-picture format.

The Teacher Assessment of Grammatical Structure Test (Moog & Kozak, 1983) was developed at the Central Institute for the Deaf. It consists of rating forms for evaluation of children's understanding and use of grammatical structures of English on the pre-sentence, simple sentence, and complex sentence levels. It is designed for children up to 8 years of age with hearing impairments. The results suggest a sequence for teaching skills not demonstrated.

The Test of Syntactic Abilities (TSA) (Quigley et al, 1978) is designed for the assessment of language skills of people 8 through 18 years of age with severe to profound hearing impairments. Stimuli are presented in written form with a multiple-choice format. Subtests available include a screening test, which is to be used to identify which specific-area subtests should be administered. Areas assessed include negation, complementation, relativization, question formation, conjunction, pronominalization, verb processes, and nominalization. A version of the test with automatic scoring is available on disk for use on Apple II computers (Apple, Cupertino, Calif.).

The Written Language Syntax Test (Berry, 1981) was developed at Gallaudet University for use in the assessment of 69 instructional objectives in children with hearing impairments who have at least basic language skills. The test results can be used to design language programming.

Auditory Skills

The Test of Auditory Comprehension (TAC) (Trammell et al, 1976) is designed to assess auditory skills in children 4 through 12 years of age with moderate to profound hearing losses. The norm is based on such a sample. The test includes ten subtests that cover identification of speech versus noise, discriminating speech and environmental sounds, understanding stereotypical messages, single-word vocabulary, two-element phrases, four-element phrases, recalling three elements in a story, recalling five elements in a story, discriminating and recalling three elements in noise, and discriminating and recalling five elements in a story. Stimuli are black and white drawings, and the child points to the picture as a response. The TAC is part of the Auditory Skills Instructional Planning System, which also includes The Auditory Skills Curriculum, a program for developing auditory skills.

The Ski*Hi program (Watson & Clark, 1985) includes materials and activities for the assessment of auditory skills in young children with hearing impairments and for a program of auditory skill development. It does not have a norm.

Using Tests Not Designed for Children with Hearing Impairments

Overall Philosophy

Although the number of tests designed for children with hearing losses and with a norm based on findings for such a group of children is increasing, it is still limited and does not include all skills that need to be assessed. Unfortunately, few tests not specifically designed for children with hearing impairments include norms for such children. A clinician who plans to perform a thorough assessment, including formal and informal measurements, of communication skills of a child with a hearing impairment needs to use some tests not designed for such children. There are two possible approaches to testing and analyzing test results in such circumstances. One is to present the tests according to the directions and score them as usual; age-equivalent scores or standard scores are calculated as if the hearing impairment were not present. Such an approach unfortunately has several problems. First, it may not be an accurate representation of the child's communication abilities, because the test instructions may have been too long for the child's auditory memory or may have included unfamiliar words. In those cases how do professionals know if the results represent communication skill or skill in understanding the test directions? They do not. Although it is possible to calculate age-equivalents or standard scores for the results, these scores say nothing about the pattern of errors seen. Some aspects of the communication skills of people with hearing impairments resemble those of normal acquisition, but others clearly do not. Therefore, achieving a certain numerical score equivalent to some age norm is not the same as performing as a child of that age. The patterns of strength and weakness can be very different.

Test Adaptations

How then can professionals use tests not designed for children with hearing losses in a valid way for communication assessment? The most reasonable approach seems to be to use the tests to develop descriptions of the children's skills and deficits. To accomplish this, testers must make some modifications. They must be sure the children understand what they are to do in the test. That may require repeating or modifying the instructions or even giving some practice examples to show how to respond. Testers may need to present test items more than once, although that can cause problems while solving others. For example, the repetition of an item helps ensure comprehension and testing of skill rather than hearing. However, children with hearing losses tend to believe they have responded incorrectly, and they often change their answers when items are repeated. The best way to avoid having to repeat items is to make sure to have the children's visual and auditory attention before presenting the items in the first place. Testers should not present items while children are looking away from them. If the test requires scanning several response options, a good approach is to allow time for the children to scan first, then look at the tester for the item, then return to the page to select the response.

Tests must be given in the modality or language in which the children communicate. Under ideal circumstances, should a total communication approach be needed, the tester should be able to sign well enough to communicate, give the test items, and interpret responses. Use of an interpreter is less desirable, because the tester loses control of exactly how items are presented and also may not receive the children's verbatim responses. To be valid, interpretation must be exact for both stimuli and responses. Anything less does not produce a valid result for these children. The test environment should be carpeted, as quiet as possible, and have good lighting. If the room has a window, the children should be placed with their backs to the window, so direct lighting without glare falls on the testers' faces.

Children who use auditory training systems, as is often true in schools, should use the device during the evaluation to improve the signal-to-noise ratio (S/N).

Precautions

After using appropriate methods to test children with hearing impairments, it is equally important to analyze the results properly. Rather than calculating age or standard scores with the information obtained through modified testing, it is necessary to analyze the items successfully completed and those missed. The tester should look at the particular skills involved in those items and derive patterns of strengths and weaknesses over several tests. It is important to look at whether the children performed better on structured items than on open-ended items; whether length of stimulus utterance affected performance; whether certain question forms interfered with or assisted performance; and whether the children know particular words or rules of grammar.

Although children with hearing impairments display a wide range of behavior while being tested, just as do children with normal hearing, testers must be aware of some general patterns of behavior when testing children with hearing impairments. Such children tend to be more impulsive when responding (Davis & Hardick, 1981). They may have difficulty scanning visual response choices or attending to auditory response choices without prompting from the tester. Impulsivity can have the effect of substantially lowering apparent level of skill. Therefore, in the modifications necessary for testing of skill it may be necessary to prompt the children repeatedly to identify the response options, then to attend to the item, and then to respond.

Children with hearing impairments tend to be very visually aware, and they often look at the tester for cues about the correct response (Davis & Hardick, 1981). Good ways to counter this behavior are (1) to watch the children's faces while presenting the items and follow the children to a response, rather than watching the test booklet, which could lead the tester to look at the correct response, and (2) to be sure to record all responses out of the children's visual ranges or to record something of relatively equal length after each response. Recording check marks for correct responses but writing children's entire responses for incorrect items can provide unintentional cues about test performance and lead some children to give up. Of course, the usual test procedures regarding giving positive feedback randomly not only after correct responses apply.

Informal Evaluation

As with communication skill evaluations for any children, a great deal can be learned by observing children with hearing losses in their typical environments and with people with whom they usually interact. Evaluating children informally after giving formal assessment measurements can allow the tester to focus on how areas of strength and weakness are expressed in everyday situations and to evaluate how the language they receive from those around them affects performance. A thorough description of communication skills includes both formal and informal measurements.

TREATING COMMUNICATION PROBLEMS IN CHILDREN WITH HEARING IMPAIRMENTS

Overall Philosophy

In the past, most treatment of children with hearing losses involved treatment sessions in which the children were removed from the home or school and the sessions are divided into parts. Portions of the sessions were devoted to developing speech skills, other portions to auditory skills, and still others to language skills. It has become increasingly clear that such an approach to development of communication is not ideal (Moeller et al, 1987), because communication skills are inextricably linked and dependent on one another. Children without good language skills have little ability or motivation to develop and use good speech skills, and the ability to discriminate speech sounds is crucial for the self-monitoring necessary for development and maintenance of intelligible speech. As a result, programs are increasingly changing to focus on integrated development of all areas of communication skill, including speech, audition, and language, both spoken or signed and, when appropriate, written. Such an integrated approach links content and production in a natural way, because skills in one area support the development of others. Treatment is no longer limited to the therapy room—more sessions are taking place in the home or classroom, where functional communication is truly important for the children. The more children see communication skills as helpful in daily life, the greater are their motivation and ability to generalize the skills.

Developing Speech and Auditory Skills

Although there have been many approaches to the development of speech skills in children with hearing losses, most of them do not incorporate auditory development. Two that do are the Functional Auditory Speech Treatment (FAST) program (Osberger, 1983) and the Ski*Hi program (Watson & Clark, 1985). The FAST program is based on Ling's (1976) system for the development of speech skills in children with hearing impairments. The program includes Ling's emphasis on the development of automaticity of movements for natural speech production in all vowel and consonant combinations with control of pitch and intensity. The FAST program also incorporates a systematic approach to the development of auditory skills with the goal of encouraging development of the auditory feedback loop. Each speech production goal requires discrimination of the professional's production from another word, sound, or sound pattern; imitation of the professional's production; and then independent production of the target. The program is applicable to people with any degree of hearing loss from preschool age through adulthood who require work on the development of auditory and speech skills. An excellent description of the program is available in Hochberg et al (1983).

The Ski∗Hi program (Watson & Clark, 1985) contains sections on speech, audition, and language skills, so they can be incorporated into an integrated approach to communication development. This program is aimed at young children with hearing losses and is designed for use by parents assisted by a professional. The Auditory Skills Curriculum (Stein et al, 1976) and its Preschool Extension (Head et al, 1986) can be used in conjunction with a speech development program but do not include such a component themselves.

The Development of Language Skills

Structured Approaches

Most programs for the development of language in children with hearing impairments have been highly structured, particularly in terms of syntax. Examples of such programs include the Fitzgerald key (Fitzgerald, 1949) and the Apple Tree curriculum (Anderson et al, 1980). Structured approaches select specific language targets to be introduced and developed based on the results of standardized tests that show particular weaknesses. Targets may be lists of vocabulary words, particular syntactic structures, or specific morphologic markers.

Several problems have been identified with structured approaches, however. First, they often do not take into account developmental patterns of acquisition in both children with normal hearing and those with hearing losses. This results in selection of targets that may be inappropriate for the developmental level of the children involved. Second, normal language acquisition does not involve exposure and drill on specific targets. Such approaches lack connection to concepts that have already been learned and exposure to language as it is normally used for daily communication in various settings. Structured approaches tend to lead to incomplete representations of English and overapplication of simple rote structures. Eccarius (unpublished manuscript, 1977) stated that in such approaches "the disorganization is deliberate," and that may be worse than random selection of goals.

Naturalistic Approaches

One solution to the problems apparent in the structured approaches to language development is the use of a naturalistic-conversational approach (Horstmeier & MacDonald, 1978). In a naturalistic approach children are exposed to language skills by family members, professionals, and others in the course of daily routines and play interactions. Such an approach tends to make use of informal and environmental assessments (MacDonald, 1978) and to focus on adult speaking style as the basis for the development of communication. Although the adult may have general targets in mind, or even specific goals, activities are based on following the children's leads and commenting on objects and actions in their immediate environment then waiting for the children to respond before providing more natural communication. Concepts and structures are introduced as they present themselves in the children's environment.

Cognitive Language Programming

Moeller et al (1987) developed an approach to language remediation for children with hearing impairments based on the work of Taba (1970) and the preschool curricula of Grammatico and Miller (1974), Weikart et al (1971), and Hohmann et al (1979) for children with normal hearing. This approach is, to some degree, an extension of the naturalistic approach in that it emphasizes giving children experiences and providing the language to help them organize those experiences. The cognitive approach goes beyond the naturalistic approach in using developmental cognitive skills as the basis for providing verbal labels and links for concepts the children have developed or are developing nonverbally. This approach utilizes both formal and informal assessments to evaluate children's areas of strength and weakness, focusing on identifying nonverbal and verbal skills the children apply to problem solving. Moeller et al (1987) provide excellent descriptions and examples of applications of the cognitive approach for various ages of children.

Communication Modalities: Myths and Realities

Selection of a communication mode for children with hearing impairments has been, and continues to be, one of the most important decisions facing parents and professionals who work with children with hearing impairments. Traditionally, the choices have been whether to use an auditory-oral or a total communication approach, but an increasing number of other options are available, including cued speech (Cornett, 1967), the unisensory approach (Pollack, 1970), and the use of American Sign Language initially with the introduction of English as a second language in a total communication approach in school (Johnson et al, 1989). Aspects often considered in making decisions about communication mode are age at identification, degree and configuration of hearing loss, age at which treatment began, and wishes of the parents. What is most needed for making good decisions about communication mode are controlled studies of levels of communication skills in people who have been exposed to the different methods.

Unfortunately, controlled studies are not in adequate supply, and those that do exist cannot be considered definitive for various reasons. Because of the impossibility of controlling for all of the factors on which children's cases might differ and coming up with two or more groups of precisely equivalent children, results may be interpreted as supporting a method but not as guaranteeing its superiority. Among the studies that have attempted to investigate the issue, several (Stevenson, 1964; Meadow, 1968; Brasel & Quigley, 1977) have found superior language skills in children using the total communication approach. Others

(Quigley & Frisina, 1961) have found oral skills to be superior in children who use the auditory-oral approach, although still others (Denton, 1966; Jensema & Trybus, 1978) have found few if any important differences between children who use the auditory-oral approach and those who use total communication. Controlled studies involving children who use the other communication methods are nearly nonexistent, although articles can be found to support any of them. Two facts are clear from the research on language acquisition and hearing impairment: (1) children who receive early, consistent, and clear language input, whatever the modality, later perform better on tests of language skill than those who do not, and (2) it is impossible given the status of current knowledge to determine which of the available communication modalities is best for any particular child.

Two Approaches to Selecting Communication Modality

Auditory-Oral Treatment Program

The first approach to selecting a communication modality for children appears to have developed because most professionals who have worked with children with hearing impairments have wanted to help the children communicate through hearing and speech. In this approach all children with hearing losses, except those with multiple handicaps or whose parents use a manual or total communication method, are placed first in an auditory-oral treatment program. The rationale for this approach stems from the belief that exposure to other communication modalities interferes with the acquisition of hearing and speech skills (Davis & Hardick, 1981). Visual representations of language are seen as easier for children with hearing losses to acquire and use than are auditory and oral skills. The use of manual representations of language is thought to discourage the development of auditory and oral skills.

In the auditory-oral–first approach, children who do not acquire and use intelligible speech and who do not understand the oral communication of others by a specified age are transferred to programs that use other communication modalities, usually sign language (Moores et al, 1978). An advantage of this approach is that parents with normal hearing do not need to spend time and effort learning a new system of communication at a time when they are most likely overwhelmed by the thought of coping with a child with a hearing loss.

There appear to be three disadvantages to the auditory-oral–first approach to selecting a communication modality. The first is that there simply are no data to support the idea that the use of additional communication modalities interferes with development of auditory and oral skills in most children with hearing impairments. In fact, studies have indicated the opposite; early acquisition of language with total communication encourages the development and use of auditory and speech skills (Moores et al, 1978). Second, by waiting until the children are substantially delayed in language development to change communication modality, the critical period for language development, 0 to 5 years (Chapman,

1978) is lost. Those delays are never made up, and the children are at a disadvantage the rest of their lives regardless of the communication modality chosen after they are removed from the auditory-oral program. Third, because parental involvement in the development of children's communication skills is emphasized in almost all early programming, parents may develop feelings of guilt if their children do not acquire good auditory and oral skills. They may feel that the reason their children did not succeed in the auditory-oral program was that they as parents did not do their part or did not do it well.

Total Communication Treatment Program

The other approach to selecting a communication modality is, in a sense, to allow the children to do the selecting. In such a total communication–first approach, children are given access to all modes of communication from the start of their treatment. People who communicate with the children use whatever way of presenting language is necessary for communication, including speech, signs, gestures, speech-reading, writing, and finger-spelling. The children respond using whatever means of communication they can. As the children develop communication skills, it likely they and the people who communicate with them will be able to drop some of the communication modalities. With the total communication–first approach, some children communicate orally, although others need one or more of the other modalities to communicate successfully.

The most important advantage of this approach is that all children have been guaranteed access to a complete system of communication. Another advantage is that the children are exposed to language as fully as possible as early as possible, which is known to provide the best chance for development of good language skills. Yet another advantage is that such an approach avoids any sense of failure or guilt on the part of the children or their parents. A substantial disadvantage of this approach is that it does require parents to learn additional methods of communicating with their children. A study by Moeller and Luetke-Stahlman (1990) found that most parents using an English-based sign language system with their children in a total communication approach do not develop adequate signing skills to represent English fully, leaving incomplete the input to their children. The level of proficiency the parents develop with any of the non-oral communication methods is a limiting factor in the success of a total communication approach.

Whose Decision Is It?

Although it may be tempting to professionals to believe they know which communication modality should be used with which children, the ultimate decision regarding selection of a communication modality rests with the children's parents. Public Law 94-142 (1977) provides that parents have the legal right to approve or reject any and all aspects of their children's treatment program, including communication modality. Unfortunately, that can lead professionals to withdraw entirely from the decision-making process under the guise of leaving the decision to the parents. Professionals have a responsibility in such situations. They must provide the parents access to the facts that bear on the decision, whether or not the parents ask for the information. The information must be presented in a form parents can understand.

If the parents make their informed decision regarding a communication approach, and their choice is not that of the professional, the professional must face his or her own ethical decisions. The professional must decide if he or she can commit to providing enthusiastically the best treatment possible using the communication modality the parents have chosen or if the parents should be referred to another professional for treatment with the chosen communication modality. If a referral is necessary, professionals best serve themselves and parents by wishing the parents well while leaving the door open for future services.

SPEECH-LANGUAGE PATHOLOGISTS AS CASE MANAGERS IN THE SCHOOLS

Programs with an Audiologist on Staff

Some schools employ one or more audiologists on a full-time basis, whereas others contract for services on a part-time basis or receive audiologic services through a regional educational service agency. The roles of speech-language pathologists are different for the two arrangements. When audiologists are available on a full-time basis, they take the lead in such areas as monitoring amplification systems, re-evaluating the audiologic status of students with hearing impairments, and interpreting audiologic findings and recommendations for other educators. In these situations, speech-language pathologists serve as members of the educational team, providing information from formal and informal assessments of communication skills, interpreting that information for other educators, and making recommendations regarding placement and treatment.

Programs Without Audiologists on Staff

When audiologic services are available only on a contracted basis, speech-language pathologists may need to provide some services otherwise provided by full-time audiologists. In effect, speech-language pathologists become the case managers in the schools for children with hearing losses. They may be the best-trained professionals available on a regular basis to answer questions about monitoring results from the children's hearing aids and frequency modulation (FM) systems, to consult on classroom acoustics, and to be involved in decisions about services needed by specific children. If the children in a school are mainstreamed and a teacher of children with hearing impairments is not available full-time, speech-language pathologists may also be called upon to provide information about the effects of hearing loss on language and learning skills and to assist classroom teachers in modifying materials and lessons.

Speech-language pathologists without special background or education in such areas must recognize areas in which to either acquire the necessary information or refer the teachers to another source.

Treatment: Consultation and Coordination with Classroom Teachers

An increasing number of speech-language pathologists who work in schools have begun to use a consultative approach to expanding their services in classrooms. The consultative approach is highly appropriate for use with children who have hearing losses, because it well suited for use of the cognitive and naturalistic approaches to the development of communication skills. Speech-language pathologists can select communication goals that reflect cognitive language skills, consult with teachers about current and upcoming units presented in the classroom, use the topic areas being covered in classes for individual treatment sessions, and work with classroom teachers to encourage the students to apply skills to master classroom tasks.

COCHLEAR IMPLANTS

The Device, Selection, and Fitting

Some people with profound hearing losses receive little if any benefit from conventional hearing aids because current hearing aid technology does not amplify sound sufficiently to make speech and environmental sounds audible. Some of these people are candidates for receiving cochlear implants (Chapter 9). Cochlear implants are designed to make auditory information audible by converting sounds to electrical signals that stimulate the fibers of the acoustic nerve. Cochlear implants currently consist of the following components: a microphone, an external digital processor, an internal receiver that is surgically placed under the skin behind the ear, and a set of small electrodes implanted in the cochlea (Figure 10.2). The microphone picks up sounds and converts them to electrical signals, and a cord carries the electrical signals to the digital processor. The digital processor extracts selected information from the signals and converts that information into a series of pulses that are carried by another cord to the internal receiver and finally to the electrodes in the cochlea. Circuitry within the external processor reduces levels of background noise (Cochlear Corporation, 1990). In the United States one multichannel cochlear implant system has completed Food and Drug Administration (FDA) testing for safety and effectiveness. This device was approved by the FDA in 1985 for use in specific populations of adults with postlingual deafness and in 1990 for use in children with profound hearing impairments (Cochlear Corporation, 1990).

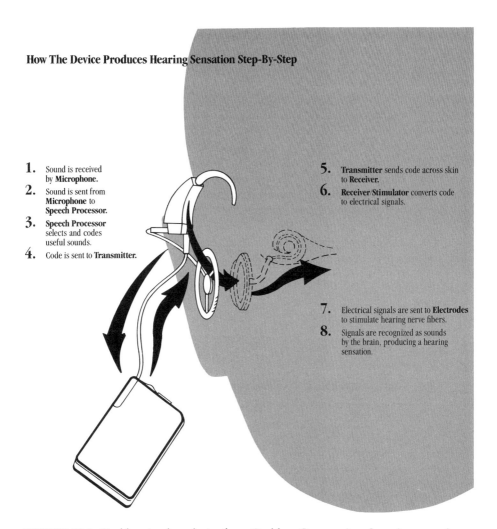

How The Device Produces Hearing Sensation Step-By-Step

1. Sound is received by **Microphone**.
2. Sound is sent from **Microphone** to **Speech Processor**.
3. **Speech Processor** selects and codes useful sounds.
4. Code is sent to **Transmitter**.

5. **Transmitter** sends code across skin to **Receiver**.
6. **Receiver/Stimulator** converts code to electrical signals.

7. Electrical signals are sent to **Electrodes** to stimulate hearing nerve fibers.
8. Signals are recognized as sounds by the brain, producing a hearing sensation.

FIGURE 10.2 Cochlear implant device from Cochlear Corporation. Steps in processing of sound signals and transmission to acoustic nerve.

(Reprinted with permission from Cochlear Corporation, Englewood, Colo.)

A cochlear implant team usually consists of an ear surgeon (an otologist or otolaryngologist), an audiologist, a psychologist, and a speech-language pathologist. If a pediatric candidate is involved, the team may also include teachers, rehabilitation specialists, and other school personnel. Several evaluations are conducted, including audiologic, medical, and psychological tests. The team works with people who are candidates for cochlear implants and with their families to establish realistic and appropriate expectations and to determine candidacy for implant use. Cochlear implants are considered an option for children with profound hearing impairments who meet the following criteria: age 2 to 17 years, profound sensorineural hearing loss in both ears, limited or no benefit from hearing aids or vibrotactile devices, no medical contraindications, enrollment in an educational program that emphasizes development of auditory skills, and high motivation and appropriate expectations on the part of the children and parents. Cochlear implants may be appropriate for adults who lost their hearing after developing speech and language skills and who meet the following criteria for candidacy: 18 years of age or older, profound bilateral sensorineural hearing loss, limited or no benefit from hearing aids or vibrotactile devices, no medical contraindications, and high motivation and appropriate expectations.

It generally requires 3 to 5 weeks after surgery for the incision to heal. After healing is complete, the implant recipient returns to the implant center to be fit with the external parts of the device. The audiologist programs the speech processor, setting the appropriate levels of stimulation for each electrode from soft to comfortably loud. Subsequent sessions are required to fine-tune the electrodes, changing the program as the client adjusts to the sounds.

Expected Benefits of the Use of Cochlear Implants

Most adult recipients of cochlear implants who have postlingual hearing losses receive substantial benefit from implant use. Improvement is seen in their ability to monitor their own speech in terms of vocal intensity and intelligibility. Almost all improve their communication ability when the device is used in conjunction with speechreading. The implant enables recipients to hear and recognize environmental sounds at comfortable loudness levels. Most implant users can detect speech at a conversational level, and more than half demonstrate some improvement in understanding speech without speechreading.

Like adults with postlingual deafness, children who become deaf after acquiring oral language seem to be able to connect the sounds from the implant with their memories of sound. They learn to identify meaningful sounds such as speech more quickly than children with prelingual deafness (deaf before language is developed) or perilingual deafness (deaf early in the period of language acquisition). However, even children with pre- and perilingual deafness children may use implants successfully if they are given proper support and training for a sufficient length of time (Cochlear Corporation, 1991a).

Cochlear implants do not provide normal hearing, and children with cochlear implants function as if they have a severe rather than a profound hearing loss. Studies of children with cochlear implants have shown the following benefits for more than half the children: the ability to detect conversational level environmental sounds, including speech, at comfortable loudness levels; the ability to differentiate speech patterns; and improvement in speech production and loudness control after training and experience with the implant. One-third to one-half of children with cochlear implants show the following skills: identification, from a closed set of alternatives, of everyday sounds such as car horns, doorbells, and birds singing; identification of speech in context; and improved speechreading. Less than one-third of children with cochlear implants can recognize speech without context.

The Role of the Speech-Language Pathologist

Speech-language pathologists are important in the cochlear implantation process. Although participation on the implant team is possible only at implant centers, speech-language pathologists in hospital, clinical, educational, and private settings may encounter questions regarding cochlear implants. They need to be aware of eligibility criteria, implantation sites, and the treatment process to provide accurate information in response to inquiries and to make appropriate referrals if clients appear to be candidates for implants.

In areas where a clinical audiologist is not available, speech-language pathologists may become the primary provider of postimplantation treatment. The kind, quantity, and frequency of training are based on the needs of the individual implant user. Important factors to consider when providing such treatment include age at onset of hearing loss, length of time between the onset of deafness and implantation, dependence on spoken language, and the auditory and speech demands of the environment (Brackett, 1991).

For people with postlingual deafness, training focuses on matching the sounds received through the cochlear implant with memories of sounds. Implant users with congenital or prelingual deafness, however, must be taught to attach meaning to the auditory signal in much the same manner used with children who wear hearing aids. If the hearing loss is postlingual but of more than 4 years duration, the implant users may need to readjust to the intrusion of sound and learn skills useful for receiving and monitoring speech information.

Professionals at the implant center may provide assistance in determining appropriate models and materials for the development of auditory skills. Training sessions may be scheduled at the implant center during the months after surgery, and the implant team generally consults with the treatment provider. Because much of the responsibility for planning and implementing treatment falls on therapists after implantation, it is important to recognize that success with an implant is highly related to two factors—the amount of exposure to meaningful sounds and the amount of time each day that the device is used (Brackett, 1991).

Auditory training materials are commercially available to make goal-setting and activity planning easier. Some of the commonly used curricula are as follows:

- The Auditory Skills Curriculum (Stein et al, 1976) is divided into areas of discrimination, memory sequencing, auditory feedback, and figure-ground with activities for each objective. There is also a preschool supplement (Head et al, 1986).

- The Developmental Approach to Successful Listening (Stout & Windle, 1986) has activities for sound awareness, phonetic listening, and auditory comprehension with specific cochlear implant information.
- The Ski*Hi Model (Watson & Clark, 1985) is designed for children from birth to 6 years of age. Additional information about cochlear implants can be found in Tyler (1992).

ADULTS WITH ACQUIRED HEARING LOSSES

Services Provided by Speech-Language Pathologists

Speech-language pathologists may have clients with hearing losses acquired in adulthood who have been referred to them for treatment. The professionals who refer them may be looking for treatment in the areas of speech maintenance, speech-reading, or general communication skills. Serving the needs of this group is very different from serving children with hearing losses, because language skills are not a concern, and these adults generally were adequate communicators before acquiring their hearing losses. However, speech-language pathologists who keep an orientation toward solving communication problems in situations and settings typical for their clients find commonalities in approaches.

Speech

One possible area of concern with adults who have acquired hearing losses is the effect of the hearing loss on maintenance of intelligible and natural speech. As with congenital and prelingual hearing impairments, the potential effect of hearing loss on speech skills depends on the degree and configuration of the loss. Hearing losses characterized as mild or moderate have not been found to have any effect on the quality or intelligibility of speech (Davis & Hardick, 1981), although sometimes adults with hearing losses change their vocal intensity because of difficulty monitoring it (Oyer, 1966).

Severe acquired hearing losses may have an effect on speech. Studies by Goehl and Kaufman (1984) and Cowie and Douglas-Cowie (1983), however, showed little change in intelligibility in most cases. It appears that many adults with acquired hearing losses, even profound losses, adapt and use other means of self-monitoring to maintain good intelligibility. There are, however, some changes in voice quality and articulation. The changes have been found to involve increased pharyngeal resonance and distortion of sibilants not severe enough to affect intelligibility (Bergman, 1952). Thus, research findings do not support routine recommendations for speech maintenance for adults with acquired hearing losses. In some instances, however, such adults may wish to be seen for treatment, and that could be appropriate if changes in their speech would handicap them in employment or other activities. Some people who have had profound hearing losses for many years do demonstrate problems with intelligibility (Cowie & Douglas-Cowie, 1983). Decisions about speech maintenance, therefore, need to made on an individual basis.

Speechreading

Another widely recommended component of treatment programs for adults with acquired hearing loss is speechreading instruction to improve use of vision for understanding speech. Several programs have been developed over the years for speechreading instruction. Some emphasize an analytic approach, which involves breaking down lip movements into precise sequences and learning to follow those sequences (Nitchie, 1912). Others use a synthetic approach, which involves acquiring an overall picture of facial expression and general patterns of information that is available visually (Bruhn, 1927). Binnie (1977), van Rooij and Plomp (1992), and Gagné et al (1991), among others, have questioned the efficacy of speechreading instruction. Their findings indicate that there is a wide range of ability to use visual cues to understand speech and that instruction does not change poor speechreaders into good ones. Walden et al (1977) found some improvement in scores on standard measurements of speechreading skill for most participants in speechreading programs whether an analytic or a synthetic approach was used. Most improvements were not statistically significant, however, and the relative rankings of skill did not change.

Another finding about speechreading is that people with good language skills perform better in general on speechreading measurements than those with poor language skills (Davis & Hardick, 1981). Because adults with acquired hearing losses have normal language skills, their speechreading ability has been found to be generally good, although with great individual variation (Davis & Hardick, 1981). Yet another finding regarding speechreading is that because adults acquire hearing losses gradually, as is typical, they rely increasingly on visual cues for speech comprehension (Davis & Hardick, 1981), and they do so without instruction. This does not mean that as people acquire hearing losses they become better speechreaders. In fact, Lyxell and Rönnberg (1989) found no differences in speechreading ability between people with normal hearing and those with hearing impairments. They also stated that the individual differences seen are best predicted by cognitive skills related to the use of contextual cues.

Is speechreading instruction a valuable part of treatment programs for adults with acquired hearing losses? The answer appears to be a qualified yes. Binnie (1977) suggested that although relative levels of speechreading skill are unlikely to change with treatment, absolute levels may improve. That is, ways of helping adults use their speechreading skills optimally include instruction in recognizing visual aspects of speech; learning limitations to speechreading, so people do not feel they must recognize every sound of every word to be a good speechreader; learning ways of improving the environment for speechreading; and learning how to make good use of context to assist comprehension. People whose hearing losses are sudden do not have the opportunity to learn the use of visual cues gradually and independently. They are likely to benefit from more specific instruction in recognizing visual patterns, learning groups of sounds that cannot be differentiated with only visual cues, and combining visual and auditory cues with contextual cues (Hardick, 1977; Schow & Nerbonne, 1980; Alpiner, 1982; Giolas, 1982; Sanders, 1982).

Strategies for Solving Communication Problems

In the past few years another aspect of treatment for people with hearing losses has been given attention—using problem-solving strategies to repair breakdowns in communication. Erber (1988) developed a comprehensive program of treatment for adults that is based on a conversational approach. Clients are taught how to make comprehension easier and more likely and how to solve misunderstandings when they do occur. Communication repair strategies include asking for repetitions of whole or parts of utterances, asking for the first letter of a word that was missed, and asking for key words to the topic of conversation. A complete description of repair strategies is available in Erber's book (1988), as well as in publications by Davis and Hardick (1981), Alpiner (1982), and Giolas (1982).

Additional Considerations in Treating Adults with Hearing Losses

Two additional comments need to be made about treatment programs for adults with hearing impairments. First, for most people the first step in an aural rehabilitation program is fitting and training with appropriate amplification, that is, hearing aids. In most cases speech-language pathologists should be certain that evaluation, fitting, and training have been completed before they institute other treatment. It then is simpler to identify remaining communication problems and select appropriate goals for treatment. Second, effective programs for adults with hearing impairments often include approaches to help them accept responsibility for their losses and for managing their surroundings for success. Many adults who acquire hearing losses adopt passive approaches, such as not acknowledging the hearing problem or trying to hide it, pretending to understand, and withdrawing from difficult listening situations (Bess et al, 1989). For these people, treatment to assist them in identifying passive, assertive, and aggressive techniques for solving communication problems can be highly appropriate. Treatment needs to involve people and situations important to the adults with hearing losses and needs to focus on improving function in daily life.

PSYCHOSOCIAL ASPECTS OF DEAFNESS

Hearing loss is now the most prevalent chronic health problem in the United States and in most scientifically advanced countries. It affects more people than heart disease and multiple sclerosis combined (Vernon & Andrews, 1990). Yet, in general, society demonstrates little understanding or tolerance of deafness. In many instances, as information is confused or misunderstood, people with hearing impairments become the target of anger, frustration, or rude jokes. As a result, deaf people may simply smile and nod to suggest understanding rather than risk a negative interaction.

Few professionals who have normal hearing and work with deaf clients have much knowledge of the deaf community or sign language. According to a survey reported by Levine (1974), 83 percent of psychologists in the United States who were working with children with hearing impairments had no special training for the assignment, and 90 percent of them were unable to communicate in sign language. For those in the field of speech and language remediation, it is important to gain some insights into deaf culture to provide appropriate services for people who have hearing impairments.

The Deaf Community

Audiologists and sociologists may define *a deaf person* very differently. Audiologists may quantify deafness in terms of decibel levels measured across specific frequencies, although sociologists may use attitudes, customs, and belief systems to determine membership in a specific cultural group. To understand how deaf people qualify as a cultural group, one must consider the idea that to be social, one must have language. Deaf people, however, cannot hear the sounds of speech. Therefore, they may need to develop language in a way that is not based on a sound system (Rutherford, 1988). The use of American Sign Language is the chief identifying characteristic of membership in the deaf community. The degree of hearing loss in the audiologic sense is not as important as the acceptance of deaf values. Some people with profound deafness and unintelligible speech are not socially deaf, whereas some people with less severe hearing losses and intelligible speech choose to become members of the deaf community. Hearing children of deaf parents may also consider themselves members of the deaf community (Vernon & Andrews, 1990). The literature generally uses the term *deaf* (with a lowercase *d*) to refer to people who have a clinically significant degree of hearing loss but who choose to interact primarily with the hearing majority. *Deaf* (with a capital *D*) includes people who subscribe to the social, behavioral, and cultural norms of American Deaf Society (Sachs, 1990).

Ninety percent of children with hearing impairments are born to hearing families. As a result these children are potential members of a different cultural group from their parents (Rutherford, 1988). It is a unique characteristic of this group that many of its members acquire their primary language from their peers and teachers rather than from their parents. In contrast, children of deaf parents acquire American Sign Language much as hearing children acquire their language, only through visual modes rather than auditory. Five-year-old native signers can express themselves as well as their hearing peers, who possess a vocabulary of approximately 5000 words (Sachs, 1990).

The Deaf community organized the National Association for the Deaf (NAD) to serve as an advocate for educational, employment, legal, and social concerns.

This organization, with more than 18,000 members and 50 state associations in the United States, is controlled exclusively by deaf people. The NAD also has a youth division, called the Junior NAD, which has chapters in most state residential schools and aims to promote leadership among deaf youth (Vernon & Andrews, 1990). At an international level, NAD belongs to the World Federation of the Deaf, although numerous regional and local clubs also exist.

Although deafness is stigmatized by the hearing majority, it has a very positive value within the Deaf community. Deaf people with a positive Deaf Identity see themselves not as handicapped or abnormal, but as intact, healthy Deaf people who belong to a larger cultural entity.

The Diagnosis of Deafness: Its Impact on a Family

Leading causes of childhood deafness include heredity (40 to 60 percent), Rh factor, prematurity, maternal rubella, meningitis, and ototoxic drugs, among others. However, determining the cause of deafness in children is sometimes difficult, particularly because there is often a time lag between the onset of the hearing loss and its diagnosis. It often surprises people that deafness can go undiagnosed until children are between 1 and 3 years of age. The time until diagnosis varies in direct relation to the degree of deafness, the alertness of the physician, the presence of a genetic history of deafness, the occurrence of prenatal disease known to cause deafness, and the familiarity of the parents with normal child development (Vernon & Andrews, 1990). Deaf parents, on the other hand, are well aware of the behaviors that indicate deafness and often desire deaf children. They frequently make the diagnosis when their child is as young as 2 to 3 months.

Reactions of hearing parents to the diagnosis of deafness parallel the reactions of parents who face any serious disease or other life tragedy. The initial blow is of such intensity that little of what is said immediately afterward is remembered. There is shock and disbelief, followed by denial. With deafness, the less intimate is the relationship to the deaf child, the greater is the tendency to deny. Thus, extended family members tend to deny more than parents, and fathers are frequently more denying than mothers.

Grief and depression frequently follow denial, often accompanied by anger, guilt, feelings of impotence, and blame directed toward the other parent or professionals involved in the diagnosis. This period of mourning eventually should lead to an acceptance of the situation and an ability to deal with reality.

The problem with deafness is that many parents never progress through these stages. Other parents do so at a time so late in their child's life that permanent social, psychological, and educational damage is done (Vernon & Andrews, 1990). Constructive and effective coping with permanent disability begins only after the patient and family are fully aware of the full range of its effects (Mindel & Vernon, 1971; Vash, 1981).

Adults with Acquired Hearing Loss

There is agreement that in general when the deafness occurs later in life, the sense of loss is much more intense (Pochapin, 1965; Vernon, 1980). A child born deaf has never known hearing and does not suffer trauma over its loss. When the deafness occurs in the preschool or elementary school years, or even as late as the college years, there is an intense shock and a period of grief, but people generally develop new social and educational ties. For middle-aged people, already married and established in a career, adapting can be more difficult. Hearing loss may threaten their financial stability, because it often appears during the years of maximal earning power. Compounding the problem is that many of these hearing losses are progressive, but providing an accurate prognosis is difficult. Thus, people who may have just enough hearing to get by professionally do not know how long they will be able to communicate adequately on the job (Vernon & Andrews, 1990).

An additional factor in late-onset hearing loss is its effect on marriage and social life. For a couple who has enjoyed an active social life, restaurants and parties may become places full of misunderstandings and tension. One-on-one communication, which is crucial for healthy relationships, may require more energy and empathy than either person has to give. Friends may limit interactions both in person and on the telephone, because they become frustrated by the effort required to communicate.

People with late-onset hearing losses may experience not only psychological pressures but also physical effects. The additional stress may cause problems such as hypertension, insomnia, and excessive smoking or eating. Few professionals are trained to help with these problems. Speech-language pathologists who are prepared to work with people who experience stress related to communication disorders can be a valuable resource for people with late-onset hearing loss.

Assessment of Psychological and Psychosocial Skills

Difficulty in understanding and expressing language has influenced the assessment of various psychosocial skills in people with hearing impairments. This is particularly true for measurements of intelligence and personality, although tools for evaluating social acceptance and self-concept also are affected (Davis & Hardick, 1981).

Psychological tests or interviewing procedures that depend on the use of verbal language to measure intelligence, personality, or other attributes almost inevitably measure the language difficulties of a person with a hearing impairment rather than that person's intelligence, psychodynamics, interests, or aptitudes (Vernon & Andrews, 1990). A valid measurement can be obtained only with a nonverbal performance type of measurement, and preferably one with norms for both children with normal hearing and those with hearing impairments. A sample of intelligence tests, adaptive and behavioral scales, personality tests, and educational achievement tests appropriate for use with people with hearing impairments is listed in this chapter's Appendix.

SOURCES OF FUNDING FOR TREATING AND SERVING PEOPLE WITH HEARING IMPAIRMENTS

Insurance

Private

Most personal and group insurance policies are not written to cover speech, language, and hearing services. Some states have passed laws stating that the option to purchase coverage for such services must be available from all insurance carriers that operate in those states, but most do not specify any need to offer such coverage. Some policies, however, do include coverage of speech-language services if provided by approved providers, that is those who are accredited and licensed, in states with licensure. Policies that cover speech-language services vary greatly in that coverage. Some specify a certain number of sessions, others a specific length of time, and still others have no predetermined limit. Policies also differ on whether or not physicians must certify a need for the service. Some policies allow for renewal or extension of covered services, either with or without physician certification, if the need for continuation is well documented. Because of the wide variety of coverage, professionals need to encourage those they serve to verify the terms of their policies with their insurance carriers.

Medicare

Medicare is the federally funded insurance program for older adults in the United States. It is divided into two parts, Part A and Part B. Neither part covers hearing aids or related services, but Part B may cover individual treatment under certain conditions. Physician certification of need for the services is necessary, and clients must meet other eligibility requirements in terms of hospitalization within the past 90 days and having no other insurance policies to cover the services. Medicare coverage and eligibility are periodically revised, and professionals who provide services are advised to obtain copies of the most recent regulations.

State Programs

Children with Medical Handicaps

States offer programs of coverage for services in speech, language, and hearing for children with sensory and developmental handicaps. Coverage varies from state to state, but eligibility is based on physician certification of the handicapping condition, income level of the family, and age of the child. Children are covered from age of certification until 16 or 18 years of age. States usually have lists of approved providers, and coverage applies only to those providers. Programs often cover at least one hearing aid and related services, including aural rehabilitation treatment. Children are generally approved to be covered for a specified number of sessions, which can be extended as long as the need is verified and family income remains within the eligible range. As is typical of governmentally funded programs, reimbursement is below the usual professional charges of speech-language pathologists.

Vocational Rehabilitation

All states offer funding for vocational training of adults with handicapping conditions. Eligibility requirements vary from state to state, and some states cover both unemployed and underemployed people, although other states cover only the unemployed. Coverage usually includes at least one hearing aid and related services, which may include aural rehabilitation treatment, depending on what is necessary for the person to be employable. Vocational rehabilitation programs start covering clients at the age level at which they are no longer eligible for funding through children's programs, generally 16 or 18 years of age. Some fund services for older adults to allow them to remain in their own homes rather than requiring residential placement.

Medicaid

All states offer Medicaid insurance programs to fund medical services for people with limited financial resources, but coverage is extremely variable from state to state. Some states do not cover speech, language, and hearing services, whereas others provide diagnostic services and one or more hearing aids over a certain time period. Treatment, including that provided by some school districts, may be funded through Medicaid programs for people or agencies approved as providers. Typical of governmentally funded programs, reimbursement is below the usual professional charges.

Service Organizations

Because private insurance and government programs do not cover many people in need of speech, language, and hearing services who do not have the resources to pay for such services themselves, several service organizations have developed funding programs. Service organizations available to assist with funding services for people with hearing impairments vary from area to area, but at least three are national in scope. One is the Easter Seal Society which provides prostheses and rehabilitation services for children with various handicapping conditions, including hearing losses. Another is the Lions Club International, which is well known for its vision program to supply eyeglasses to those in need. It also funds speech, language, and hearing services in some areas. A third program, somewhat less widely known, is Sertoma, which has speech and hearing as its primary philanthropic area and which may provide funding for speech, language, and hearing services either through community agencies or directly to professionals. In addition, some areas have other, local charitable organizations that may fund services. Professionals should make sure they are familiar with potential sources of funding in their areas.*

REFERENCES

Alpiner, J. (1982). *Handbook of adult rehabilitative audiology.* Baltimore: Williams & Wilkins.

Anderson, M., Boren, N., Caniglia, J., Howard, W., & Krohn, E. (1980). *Apple tree.* Beaverton: Dormac.

Bergman, M. (1952). Special methods of audiological training of adults. *Acta Otolaryngology, 40,* 336-345.

Berry, S. (1981). *Written language syntax test.* Washington, DC: Gallaudet University Press.

Bess, F., Lichtenstein, M., Logan, S., Burger, M., & Nelson, E. (1989). Hearing impairment as a determinant of function in the elderly. *Journal of the American Geriatric Society, 37,* 123-128.

Binnie, C. (1977). Attitude changes following speechreading training. *Scandinavian Audiology, 6,* 13-19.

Brackett, D. (1991). Rehabilitation strategies for children with cochlear implants. *Cochlear Corporation Clinical Bulletin, November.*

Brasel, K., & Quigley, S. (1977). The influence of certain language and communication environments in early childhood on the development of language in deaf individuals. *Journal of Speech and Hearing Research, 20,* 95-107.

Bruhn, M. (1927). *Elementary lessons in lipreading: The Mueller-Walle method.* Lynn, Mass.: Nichols Press.

Calvert, D. (1962). Speech sound duration and the surd-sonant error. *Volta Review, 64,* 401-402.

Chapman, R. (1978). Comprehensive strategies in children. In J. F. Kavanagh (Ed.), *Speech and language in the laboratory, school and clinic* (pp. 308-327). Cambridge: MIT Press.

Cochlear Corporation (1990). Issues and answers. *Cochlear Corporation Clinical Bulletin, August.,* Somerville, Mass.

Cochlear Corporation (1991a). Teacher guide to the Mini System 22 cochlear implant. *Cochlear Corporation Clinical Bulletin, March.*

*Acknowledgment: I wish to express my appreciation to Marcia Woodfill for her contributions to this chapter. She provided information that was the basis of the sections on cochlear implants and psychosocial aspects of hearing impairment, and for that I am most grateful.

Cornett, R. (1967). Cued speech. *American Annals of the Deaf, 112,* 3-13.

Cowie, R., & Douglas-Cowie, E. (1983). Speech production in profound postlingual deafness, In M. E. Lutman & M. P. Haggard (Eds.), *Hearing science and hearing disorders (*pp. 183-230*).* New York: Academic Press.

Davis, J., & Hardick, E. (1981). *Rehabilitative audiology for children and adults.* New York: Wiley.

Denton, D. (1966). A study in the educational achievement of deaf children. *Report of the proceedings of the 42nd meeting of the convention of American instructors of the deaf.* Washington, DC: US Government Printing Office, Rpt #4158, 428-433.

Easterbrooks, S. (1987). Speech/language assessment and intervention with school-age hearing impaired children. In J. Alpiner & P. McCarthy (Eds.), *Rehabilitative audiology: children and adults (*pp. 188-240*).* Baltimore: Williams & Wilkins.

Engen, E., & Engen, T. (1983). Rhode Island test of language structures. Baltimore: University Park Press.

Erber, N. (1988). *Communication therapy for hearing impaired adults.* Melbourne: Clovis.

Fitzgerald, E. (1949). *Straight language for the deaf.* Washington, DC: A.G. Bell Association for the Deaf.

Forner, L., & Hixon, T. (1977). Respiratory kinematics in profoundly hearing-impaired speakers. *Journal of Speech and Hearing Research, 20,* 373-408.

Gagné, J-P., Dinon, D., & Parsons, J. (1991). An evaluation of CAST: A computer-aided speechreading training program. *Journal of Speech and Hearing Disorders, 34,* 213-221.

Giolas, T. (1982). *Hearing handicapped adults.* Englewood Cliffs: Prentice Hall.

Goehl, H., & Kaufman, D. (1984). Do the effects of adventitious deafness include disordered speech? *Journal of Speech and Hearing Disorders, 49,* 58-64.

Grammatico, L., & Miller, S. (1974). Curriculum for the preschool deaf child. *Volta Review, 79,* 19-26.

Hard, E. (1977). Aural rehabilitation programs for the aged can be successful. *Journal of the Academy of Rehabilitative Audiology, 10,* 51-67.

Head, J., Fedorak, L., Gibbons, D., et al (1986). Auditory skills curriculum preschool supplement. North Hollywood: Foreworks.

Hochberg, I., Levitt, H., & Osberger, M. J. (Eds.) (1983). *Speech of the hearing impaired: research, training, and personnel preparation.* Baltimore: University Park Press.

Hohmann, M., Banet, B., & Weikart, D. (1979). *Young children in action.* Ypsilanti, Mich.: High/Scope Press.

Horstmeier, D., & MacDonald, J. (1978). *The environmental language intervention program.* Columbus: Merrill.

Hudgins, C., & Numbers, F. (1942). An investigation of the intelligibility of the speech of the deaf. *Genetic Psychology Monograph, 26,* 293-392.

Jensema, C., & Trybus, R. (1978). Communication patterns and educational achievement of hearing impaired students, Series T, Number 2. Office of Demographic Studies, Washington, DC.

Johnson, R., Liddell, S., & Erting, C. (1989). Unlocking the curriculum: Principles for achieving access in deaf education. Gallaudet Research Institute Working Paper 89-3. Washington, DC: Gallaudet University Press.

Kretschmer, R., & Kretschmer, L. (1978a). *Language development and intervention with the hearing impaired.* Baltimore: University Park Press.

Kretschmer, R., & Kretschmer, L. (1978b). Language assessment. In R. Kretschmer & L. Kretschmer, *Language development and intervention with the hearing impaired* (pp. 184-210). Baltimore: University Park Press.

Levine, E. (1974). Psychological tests & practices with the deaf: A survey of the state of the art. *Volta Review, 76,* 298-319.

Levitt, H. (1971). Speech production for the deaf child. In L. Connor (Ed.), *Speech for the deaf child: Knowledge and use* (pp. 59-83). Washington, DC: A.G. Bell Association for the Deaf.

Levitt, H., Youdelman, K., & Head, J. (1990). *Fundamental speech skills test.* Englewood Cliffs: Resource Point.

Ling, D. (1976). *Speech and the hearing impaired child.* Washington, DC: A.G. Bell Association for the Deaf.

Lyxell, B., & Rönnberg, J. (1989). Information-processing skill and speechreading. *British Journal of Audiology, 23,* 339-347.

MacDonald, J. (1978). *Environmental language inventory.* Columbus: Merrill.

Matkin, N. (1988). Re-evaluating our approach to evaluation: Demographics are changing—are we? In F. Bess (Ed.), *Hearing impairment in children* (pp. 101-111). Parkton, MD: York Press.

McAfee, M., Kelley, J., & Samar, V. (1990). Spoken and written English errors of postsecondary students with severe hearing impairment. *Journal of Speech and Hearing Disorders, 55,* 628-634.

McGarr, N., & Harris, K. (1983). Articulatory control in a deaf speaker. In I. Hochberg, H. Levitt, & M. J. Osberger (Eds.), *Speech of the hearing impaired: Research, training, and personnel preparation* (pp. 75-95). Baltimore: University Park Press.

Meadow, K. (1968). Early manual communication in relation to the deaf child's intellectual, social, and communicative functioning. *American Annals of the Deaf, 123,* 925-936.

Mindel, E. D., & Vernon, M. (1971). *They grow in silence.* Silver Spring, MD: National Association for the Deaf Press.

Moeller, M. P., & Luetke-Stahlman, B. (1990). Parents' use of SEE-II: A descriptive analysis. *Journal of Speech and Hearing Disorders, 55,* 327-338.

Moeller, M. P., & McConkey, A. (1984). Language intervention with preschool deaf children: A cognitive/linguistic approach. In W. H. Perkins (Ed.), *Current therapy of communication disorders.* New York: Thieme-Stratton.

Moeller, M. P., Osberger, M. J., & Morford, J. (1987). Speech-language assessment and intervention with preschool hearing impaired children. In J. Alpiner & P. McCarthy (Eds.), *Rehabilitative audiology: Children and adults* (pp. 163-187). Baltimore: Williams & Wilkins.

Monsen, R. (1979). Acoustic qualities of phonation in young hearing-impaired children. *Journal of Speech and Hearing Research, 22,* 270-288.

Moog, J., & Geers, A. (1979). *Grammatical analysis of elicited language.* St. Louis: Central Institute for the Deaf Press.

Moog, J., & Kozak, V. (1983). *Teacher assessment of grammatical structure.* St. Louis: Central Institute for the Deaf Press.

Moores, D., Weiss, K., & Goodwin, M. (1978). Early education programs for hearing impaired children: Major findings. *American Annals of the Deaf, 123,* 925-936.

Nitchie, E. (1912). *Lipreading: Principles and practice.* New York: Stokes.

Osberger, M. J. (1983). Development and evaluation of some speech training procedures for hearing-impaired children. In I. Hochberg, H. Levitt, & M. J. Osberger (Eds.), *Speech of the hearing impaired: Research, training, and personnel preparation* (pp. 333-348). Baltimore: University Park Press.

Osberger, M. J. (1986). Language and learning skills of hearing impaired students. *Asha Monographs, 23.*

Oyer, H. (1966). *Auditory communication for the hard of hearing.* Englewood Cliffs: Prentice Hall.

Pochapin, S. W. (1965). Some emotional aspects of deafness. *Laryngoscope, 75,* 57-64.

Pollack, D. (1970). *Educational audiology for the limited hearing infant.* Springfield: Charles C Thomas.

Quigley, S., & Frisina, D. (1961). *Institutionalization and psycho-educational development of deaf children.* Washington, DC: CEC Research Monograph.

Quigley, S., Steinkamp, M., Power, D., & Jones, B. (1978). *Test of syntactic ability.* Beaverton: Dormac.

Reynell, J. (1977). *Reynell developmental language scale.* Windsor, Ontario, Canada: NFER.

Rutherford, S. D. (1988). *The culture of American deaf people.* Reprint by Linstock Press for Summer Sign Language Studies, Silver Spring, MD.

Sachs, O. (1990). *Seeing voices* (p. xii). New York: Harper Perennial.

Sanders, D. (1982). *Aural rehabilitation: A management model* (2nd ed.). Englewood Cliffs: Prentice Hall.

Schow, R., & Nerbonne, M. (1980). *Introduction to aural rehabilitation.* Baltimore: University Park Press.

Smith, C. (1975). Residual hearing and speech production in deaf children. *Journal of Speech and Hearing Research, 18,* 795-811.

Stein, D., Benner, G., Hoversten, G., McGinnis, M., & Thies, T. (1976). *Auditory skills curriculum.* North Hollywood: Foreworks.

Stevenson, E. (1964). A study of the educational achievement of deaf children of deaf parents. *California News, 80,* 143.

Stout, B., & Windle, J. (1986). *Developmental approach to successful learning.* Houston: DASL.

Taba, H. (1970). *Curriculum development: Theory and practice.* New York: Harcourt, Brace and World.

Trammell, J., Farrar, C., Francis, J., et al (1976). *Test of auditory comprehension.* North Hollywood: Foreworks.

Tye-Murray, N. (1991). The establishment of open articulatory postures by deaf and hearing talkers. *Journal of Speech and Hearing Disorders, 34,* 453-459.

Tyler, R. (Ed.) (1992). *Cochlear implants: Audiological considerations.* San Diego: Singular.

van Rooij, J., & Plomp, R. (1992). Auditive and cognitive factors in speech perception by elderly listeners. III. Additional data and final discussion. *Journal of the Acoustical Society of America, 91,* 1028-1033.

Vash, C. (1981). *The psychology of disability.* New York: Springer Publishing.

Vernon, M. (1980). Perspectives on deafness and mental health. *Journal of Rehabilitation of the Deaf, 13,* 9-14.

Vernon, M., & Andrews, J. (1990). *The psychology of deafness.* White Plains: Longman.

Walden, B., Prosek, R., Montgomery, A., Scherr, C., & Jones, C. (1977). Effects of training on the visual recognition of consonants. *Journal of Speech and Hearing Disorders, 20,* 130-145.

Watson, T., & Clark, S. (1985). *The Ski*Hi Model: Programming for hearing impaired infants through home intervention.* Logan: Ski*Hi Institute.

Weikart, D., Rogers, L., Adcock, C., & McClelland, D. (1971). *The cognitively oriented curriculum.* Urbana: University of Illinois Press.

J West, J., & Weber, J. (1973). A phonological analysis of the spontaneous language of a four-year-old hard-of-hearing child. *Journal of Speech and Hearing Disorders, 38,* 25-35.

SUGGESTED READING

Alpiner, J., & McCarthy, P. (Eds.) (1987). *Rehabilitative audiology: Children and adults.* Baltimore: Williams & Wilkins.

Clickener, P. (1989). How can I keep from singing? A story about a cochlear implant. *SHHH, July/August,* 3.

Cunningham, J. K. (1990). Parents' evaluations of the effects of the 3M/House cochlear implant on children. *Ear and Hearing, 11(5),* 375-381.

Defilippo, C., & Sims, D. (Eds.) (1988). New reflections on speech reading. *Volta Review, 90,* 1-313.

Eisenberg, L. (1985). Perceptual capabilities with the cochlear implant: Implications for aural rehabilitation. *Ear and Hearing, 6 (Suppl.),* 605-695.

Hellman, S. A., Chute, P. M., Kretschmer, R. E., & Nevins, M. E. (1991). The development of a children's implant profile. *American Annals of the Deaf, 136,* 77-81.

Kileny, P. R., Kemink, J. L., & Zimmerman-Philips, S. (1991). Cochlear implants in children. *American Journal of Otology, 12,* 144.

Moog, J. S., & Geers, A. E. (1991). Educational management of children with cochlear implants. *American Annals of the Deaf, 136,* 69.

Osberger, M. J. (1990). Audiological rehabilitation with cochlear implants and tactile aids. *Asha, 32(4),* 38-43.

Osberger, M. J., Miyamoto, R., McConkey-Robbins, A., et al. (1990). Performance of deaf children with cochlear implants and vibrotactile aids. *Journal of the American Academy of Audiology, 1,* 7-10.

Perkins, W. H. (Ed.) (1984). *Current therapy of communication disorders.* New York: Thieme-Stratton.

Quigley, S., & Paul, P. (1984). *Language and deafness.* San Diego: College Hill Press.

Simon, C. (1979). Communicative competence: A functional-pragmatic approach to language therapy. Tucson: Communication Skill Builders.

Staller, S. J., Beiterm, A. L., Brimacombe, J. A., & Mecklenburg, D. J. (1988). Clinical trials of a cochlear implant in children. *Hearing Instruments, 39(11),* 22-24, 86.

Subtelny, J. (1980). *Speech assessment and speech improvement for the hearing impaired.* Washington, DC: A. G. Bell Association for the Deaf.

APPENDIX

The following is a brief summary of evaluations that have proved useful in the measurement of the intelligence, behavior, and personality of people with hearing impairments. It is by no means complete. Many of these tools require fluent sign language on the part of the examiner and client or excellent oral communication skills by both parties.

Test	Age	Publisher
Intelligence Tests		
Arthur Adaptation of the Leiter Performanc Scale (1952)	4–12 y	Chicago: Stoelting International
Developmental Activities Screening Inventory (DASI) (DuBose & Langley, 1977)	6 mo–5 y	New York: *New York Times* Teaching Resources
Hiskey-Nebraska Test of Learning Aptitude (Hiskey, 1966)	3–17 y	Lincoln: Union College Press
Merrill-Palmer Scale of Mental Tests (Stutsman, 1931)	2–5 y	Chicago: Stoelting
Ravens Progressive Matrices (Raven, 1948)	5 y–adult	Los Angeles: Western Psychological Corporation
Smith-Johnson Nonverbal Performance Scale (Smith & Johnson, 1977)	2–4 y	Los Angeles: Western Psychological Corporation
Wechsler Performance Scale for Children–Revised (Wechsler, 1974)	6–16 y	New York: Psychological Corporation
Wechsler Performance Scale for Adults–Revised (Wechsler, 1981)	6–16 y	New York: Psychological Corporation
Adaptive and Behavioral Scales		
AAMD Adaptive Behavior Scale (Nihira et al, 1974)	3–69 y	Washington: American Association of Mental Deficiency
Alpern-Boll Developmental Profile (Alpern & Boll, 1972)	Birth–12 y	Indianapolis: Psychological Development Publication
Behavior Problem Checklist (Quay & Peterson, 1967)	6–18 y	Champaign: University of Illinois Press

Test	Age	Publisher
Adaptive and Behavioral Scales *Continued*		
Brunschwig Personality Inventory for Deaf Children (Brunschwig, 1936)	School age	New York: Teachers College Contribution to Education, No. 687
School Behavior Check List (Miller, 1974)	Grades 1–6	Louisville: University of Louisville Press
Vineland Social Maturity Scale (Doll, 1953)	1–25 y	Princeton: Educational Testing Service
Personality Tests		
Children's Apperception Test (CAT) (Bellak & Bellak, 1975)	6–12 y	New York: Psychological Corporation
Draw-A-Person (Machover, 1949)	Through adult	New York: Psychological Corporation
Education Apperception Test (Thompson & Jones, 1973)	6–12 y	Los Angeles: Western Psychological Services
House-Tree-Person (Buck, 1949)	Through adult	New York: Psychological Corporation
Make-A-Picture-Story (MAPS) (Schneidham, 1951)	6–12 y	New York: Teachers College Press
Thematic Apperception Test (TAT) (Bellak & Bellak, 1974)	Through adult	New York: Psychological Corporation

GLOSSARY

Auditory feedback loop   The process of listening to one's own speech sounds and using what one hears to monitor, and perhaps change, speech output.

Auditory-oral approach   A method of communicating for people with hearing impairments. It includes use of residual or aided hearing, speechreading, and speech production.

Cued speech   A method of communicating with people who have hearing impairments. It was developed by Cornett at Gallaudet University and involves the use of a small group of handshapes and positions to make the listener aware of differences among speech sounds that appear similar when speechreading.

Directional microphone   A microphone that partially cancels sounds coming from certain directions. Used in hearing aids and cochlear implants to decrease the signal level coming from behind the wearer.

Pharyngeal resonance   A voice quality produced by using predominantly the pharynx rather than the oral cavity. Speech with pharyngeal resonance usually sounds muffled or "swallowed."

Postlingual hearing loss   Hearing loss that occurs after normal basic speech and language skills are mastered, usually after 3 to 5 years of age.

Prelingual hearing loss   Hearing loss that occurs before normal basic speech and language skills are mastered. May be present at birth or acquired before 3 to 5 years of age.

Proprioception (for speech)   The process of feeling the positions and movements of one's own speech sounds and using what one feels to monitor, and perhaps change, speech output.

Segmental aspects of speech   The articulatory and acoustic characteristics of specific speech sounds.

Suprasegmental aspects of speech   The loudness, duration, and intonation of the pitch for speech.

Total communication   A method of communicating for people with hearing impairments or other disabilities. It involves using any or all of the following that results in successful communication: residual or aided hearing, speechreading, speech production, fingerspelling, sign language, writing, gestures, and pantomime.

Unisensory approach   A method of communicating for children with hearing impairments. It was developed by Pollack and includes the use of residual or aided hearing and speech production, with no use of speechreading by the children. It was designed to encourage maximum development and use of residual hearing.

Viseme group   Two or more speech sounds that cannot be differentiated from each other with speechreading alone. For example, /p/, /b/, and /m/ are a viseme group.

11 ⌐⌐

Intervention with the Elderly

Kevin M. Fire

Most audiologists, speech-language pathologists, health care professionals, and educators are aware of the basic demographic facts about the elderly in society. The elderly constitute the fastest growing segment of the population. This chapter provides an overview of some of the physiologic, sociologic, and psychological factors the speech-language pathologist should consider while working with the elderly. Given the prevalence of disorders of communication among the aged, and the special problems that may exist while providing rehabilitation services to this population, effective clinical interaction can be enhanced by an understanding of some of the special needs and challenges of this heterogeneous group.

Senescent (age-related) changes affect the entire body, including the auditory system. These age-related changes occur not only in peripheral auditory structures but also in central auditory structures. The following section describes the anatomic alterations that occur at various sites in the auditory system during the aging process.

PERIPHERAL PHYSIOLOGIC CHANGES OF THE AUDITORY SYSTEM

External Ear

Pinna

The pinna of an aged person may change in size, shape, and flexibility over time. In fact, the pinna may become longer and wider by several millimeters (Tsai et al, 1958). An increase in the growth of hair may be noted, especially on the tragus (Hull, 1978). Age-related changes in the pinna raise questions about concomitant changes in sound transmission.

The ridges of the pinna can affect the characteristics of incoming signals, most notably providing an acoustic gain in the high frequencies (Shaw & Teranishi, 1968). This enhancement of the high frequencies seems to aid speech discrimination (Maurer & Rupp, 1979). The pinna also plays a small role in the localization of sound, particularly in the vertical plane (Fisher & Freedman, 1968). It seems unlikely that typical changes in the structural characteristics of the pinna of an elderly person have an important impact on auditory function, although there may be a slight change in the frequency response of the auditory system (Maurer & Rupp, 1979; Corso, 1977).

External Auditory Meatus

Atrophy and structural changes of the supporting walls of the external auditory meatus have been reported in elderly people (Magladery, 1959). Loss of the elasticity of the external auditory meatus may partially or completely occlude the canal and increase the likelihood that the canal will collapse upon placement of headphones during audiometric testing. If this happens, an elderly person demonstrates a conductive hearing loss that is more severe in the high frequencies (Chandler, 1964).

Accumulations of excessive cerumen are often observed in the elderly population (Perry, 1957). This may be related to the narrowing of the external canal due to loss of elasticity of supporting structures. A complete occlusion of the external auditory meatus with cerumen causes a conductive hearing loss (Corso, 1977). The severity of this conductive component depends on the quantity of cerumen occluding the canal.

The skin of the external auditory meatus of an elderly person is often quite dry, which may lead to inflammation and itching (Anderson & Meyerhoff, 1982). The number of tumors in the external ear increases in with advancing age. However, these tumors also are seen in much younger patients and therefore cannot be considered exclusively a result of aging.

It seems unlikely that the changes in the external ear due to aging will have any clinically significant long-term effect on audition. A slight change in the frequency response of the system may be noted, but the extent of these slight changes is unclear. Any conductive loss in this population should receive prompt medical attention.

Middle Ear

A nondiseased middle ear undergoes several changes with aging, including osteosis of the ossicles (Hinchcliffe, 1962), stiffening of the ossicular chain (Etholm & Belal, 1974), thinning and loss of mobility of the tympanic membrane (Covell, 1952), atrophy of the middle ear muscles (Hull, 1978), and atrophy of the fibers of the middle ear ligament (Covell, 1952). Newman and Spitzer (1981) demonstrated a decrease in eustachian tube ventilating efficiency in a group of elderly people.

However, the most common cause of conductive hearing loss in the elderly is not due to age-related structural changes but to disease. Most often, these diseases have been present for many years. The most commonly encountered pathologic conditions of the middle ear in an elderly population are cholesteatomas, chronic suppurative otitis media, otosclerosis, tumors of the middle ear, and serous otitis media (Ruby, 1986).

A mixed hearing loss may occur in elderly people. An example is otitis media superimposed on the sensory manifestations of presbycusis. The symptoms of a sudden reduction in hearing sensitivity, tinnitus, and vertigo may lead to the incorrect diagnosis of a sudden severe cochlear lesion along with a poor prognosis for recovery. In fact, the person may have a conductive hearing loss that can be readily treated through medical or surgical means. Changes in a single area of the auditory system do not negate the possibility of associated lesions in other regions, which may or may not be directly due to aging (Zikk et al, 1985).

Inner Ear

Many changes occur throughout the entire auditory system with aging, including the cochlea. It has been suggested that four general classes of disorders result from these changes (Schuknecht 1974). These classifications include sensory, neural, metabolic, and inner ear conductive presbycusis. *Sensory presbycusis* is caused by atrophy of the organ of Corti and degeneration of cochlear hair cells. The loss of hair cells begins at the basal turn of the cochlea and progresses toward the apex. *Neural presbycusis* results from the loss of auditory neurons. *Metabolic presbycusis* is caused by atrophy of the stria vascularis. *Inner ear conductive presbycusis* is theoretic and is likely caused by an increase in the stiffness of the supporting cells of the cochlear duct, which results in a change in the vibration pattern of these structures.

Advancing age is also associated with hair cell and nerve cell degeneration, which usually begins in the basal turn of the cochlea. Hair cell degeneration precedes nerve cell degeneration. Changes in peripheral vestibular structures often coexist with cochlear changes (Johnsson & Hawkins, 1972).

People with presbycusis often exhibit bilateral, symmetric sensorineural hearing loss, but some evidence suggests there are general audiometric patterns associated with subtypes of presbycusis (Jerger & Jerger, 1981). Sensory presbycusis results in a sloping high-frequency loss. Neural presbycusis has an adverse effect on speech discrimination that is greater than would be predicted by pure-tone sensitivity. Metabolic presbycusis is characterized by a flat audiometric configuration. Mechanical presbycusis generally involves a hearing loss that is initially found in the high frequencies and then progresses to the low frequencies.

Some investigators report that there are two additional categories of presbycusis (Johnsson & Hawkins, 1972). These include vascular presbycusis, resulting from a loss of blood supply to the stria vascularis and tympanic lip, and central presbycusis, which is characterized by a loss of neurons in the cochlear nucleus and other central auditory nerve centers.

CENTRAL AUDITORY CHANGES

Degenerative changes due to aging occur in retrocochlear structures. This section examines the central auditory pathways and brain structures that are affected by aging.

Central Auditory Pathways

Postmortem microdissections of the central auditory pathways of elderly people show consistent changes in structures. These include a decreased number of ganglion cells in the ventral cochlear nucleus, cell shrinkage of the remaining cells in the ventral cochlear nucleus, degeneration of the inferior colliculus, degeneration of cell bodies in the dorsal cochlear nucleus, and degeneration of cells in the cochlear nerve (Kirikae et al, 1964; Johnsson & Hawkins, 1972; Hansen & Riske-Nielsen, 1965; Hinchcliffe, 1962; Schuknecht, 1964).

There is little question that the functional findings of presbycusis stem in part from lesions of the inner ear; however, changes in the nerve cells of central auditory pathways are also an important factor in the origin of presbycusis (Kirikae et al, 1964). The elevation of auditory threshold, poor speech discrimination, and poor binaural hearing are likely because of senile retrocochlear changes.

Auditory Centers in the Brain

Changes in the structures of the central auditory nervous system are often found among the elderly. Loss of neurons have been reported in the superior and inferior temporal gyrus (Bergman, 1980), precentral gyri, striate area (Brody, 1955), and some areas of the auditory cortex (Hinchcliffe, 1962; Welsh et al, 1985). Other changes that may occur include degeneration of the white matter of the brainstem and auditory centers in the cortex, ganglion cell loss, and an accumulation of degenerative products in the cytoplasm (Hansen & Riske-Nielsen, 1965).

It is reasonable to expect that the changes in the structures of the central and peripheral auditory system that occur with aging will have some detrimental effect on hearing ability. The following is a discussion of the changes in hearing that result from anatomic changes in the central auditory nervous system.

Auditory Performance

There is ample evidence in the scientific literature that physical changes in the auditory structures have deleterious effects on hearing. This section reviews literature concerning the changes in auditory performance found among the aged. Several problems may complicate the interpretation of data from early field studies that investigated age and hearing (1935-1936 National Health Survey, 1939 World's Fair, and 1948 San Diego County Fair Hearing Survey; Kopra, 1982). The data collection may not have been done by qualified technicians. Control of the testing environment was often less than rigid. Differences in procedures for establishing thresholds and differences in instrumentation were common among the investigations. Finally, subject selection procedures did not ensure a random sample of the population.

Even with the aforementioned methodologic problems, these early studies provided important insights into the changes in auditory sensitivity associated with aging. Several of these procedural difficulties were addressed during the Health Examination Survey of 1960-1962 (Glorig & Roberts, 1965). The hearing levels of nearly 7000 randomly selected people were tested at 500, 1000, 2000, 3000, 4000, and 6000 Hz by competent technicians with calibrated equipment. In addition, there was a controlled acoustic environment and a physician performed an otoscopic examination on all of the participants. The data indicated a progressive decrease in auditory sensitivity in older cohort groups with women demonstrating better auditory threshold sensitivity than men. Once again, the decrement in hearing sensitivity was greatest in the higher frequencies (above 1000 Hz). These findings agreed with those of earlier investigations.

Prevalence of Pure-Tone Sensitivity Loss

Whereas the aforementioned field studies indicate that thresholds for pure tones tend to increase in the elderly, not all elderly people demonstrate a loss of auditory sensitivity. Estimates of the prevalence of hearing loss among elderly people varies widely, depending on such factors as procedures used to establish hearing ability and the threshold level that the investigator chooses to define as a hearing loss. Interviews or clinical threshold procedures may be used to establish the existence of a loss of auditory sensitivity.

In a study in which the investigators conducted personal interviews, it was found that 20 to 25 percent of a population 65 years of age and older were in need of auditory rehabilitation (Shanas, 1962). A study conducted in Great Britain in 1965 concluded that approximately 33 percent of the elderly people in Great Britain demonstrated auditory difficulties (Townsend & Wedderburn, 1965).

Widely varying estimates of hearing loss based on audiometric thresholds are common, primarily because of the criteria used to define a clinically significant hearing loss. A relatively lax criterion may indicate a low prevalence of hearing difficulties. Conversely, a very strict criterion, such as that applied to the members of the Framingham Heart Survey, results in a high estimate of hearing loss (Moscicki et al, 1985). In this investigation, a single threshold over 20 dB in either ear at octave intervals from 1000 to 8000 Hz was sufficient evidence for a hearing loss. Using this very strict criterion, 83 percent of people older than 65 years exhibit a hearing loss. The United States Public Health Service in 1971 reported that 28 percent of the population 65 to 75 years of age and 48 percent of the population older than 75 years have some hearing difficulties. Regardless of the criteria used to establish the presence of a hearing loss, it is apparent that loss of auditory function in elderly people is a common occurrence.

Speech Discrimination Ability

A large number of researchers have demonstrated a decrease in the ability to understand speech messages among the elderly. Speech discrimination scores for monosyllabic words decline progressively with advancing age (Goetzinger et al, 1961). Decreased speech discrimination ability in aged listeners often is not associated with abnormal tone decay; thus it may be postulated that dysfunction of cranial nerve VIII is not the cause of the reduced speech discrimination (Harbert et al, 1965). It is possible that in many instances senescent changes in central auditory structures are responsible for the reduced speech understanding if the peripheral damage is too minimal to account for the findings.

Several researchers report very poor speech discrimination ability in aged listeners, even in the presence of only mild hearing losses (Pestalozza & Shore, 1955). In addition, there is often relatively poor agreement between pure-tone averages and spondee thresholds. Even with control for peripheral auditory sensitivity loss, the elderly consistently show a disproportionate loss of speech discrimination ability (Gaeth, 1948).

Performance-intensity (PI) functions of phonetically balanced (PB) words in elderly people reveal a systematic decrease in maximum PB score (PBmax) with increasing presentation level (Jerger, 1973). Rollover, which is poorer speech discrimination performance at high intensity levels than at low intensity levels, is also often found in elderly people. This finding is associated with eighth-nerve or brainstem dysfunction in younger listeners, thus providing functional evidence of a retrocochlear site of lesion in the elderly.

Degraded Speech Perception

Along with reduced sensitivity for pure tones and decreased discrimination ability for undistorted speech, elderly people often have reduced discrimination ability for time-altered or acoustically degraded speech (Corso, 1977). The inability of elderly people to understand speech under stressful listening conditions is often quite marked. These findings are consistent with the descriptions of elderly people; they have no trouble understanding speech in quiet listening situations, but they experience a great deal of difficulty when there is background noise (Kopra, 1982).

This marked change in the speech discrimination ability of older people in the presence of a competing message may be explained by structural changes in the central auditory nervous system. The normal auditory system has an overabundance of neuronal connections, which is termed *neural redundancy* or *intrinsic redundancy* (Bocca, 1967). Language is also inherently redundant. This is termed *external redundancy*. A speech signal may be quite distorted acoustically and yet be easily understood by a listener with an intact auditory system because the message has linguistic redundancy and is processed by a neurally redundant system (Kopra, 1982). When the number of neuronal connections is reduced, a corresponding loss of internal redundancy results. As long as external redundancy is high, speech processing may not be affected. However, if both internal and external redundancy are reduced, a considerable reduction in speech perception may result.

This is the rationale for using distorted speech tasks to evaluate central auditory function in the elderly. The status of the central auditory nervous system is assessed by stressing the system through a reduction in external redundancy. External redundancy may be reduced by acoustically changing the speech signal in any of several ways. When words are temporally overlapped or are interrupted at a rate of eight times per second, discrimination of the words is often reduced among the elderly (Bergman, 1971). This reduction in discrimination starts in the fourth decade of life and gradually worsens with advancing age. In fact, by the seventh decade, elderly people may have less than half of the discrimination ability of young listeners. There is also a decreased ability among elderly people to understand speech with a long reverberation time.

Elderly people consistently demonstrate poorer speech recognition abilities than younger listeners for other types of impoverished speech signals. Spectral alterations, such as passing speech through band-pass filters, cause a greater decrement in speech recognition performance in older than in younger listeners (Palva & Jokinen, 1970). Temporal alterations in the speech signal, such as time-compression of speech (Konkle et al, 1977; Sticht & Gray, 1969; Wingfield et al, 1985) or accelerated speech (Calearo & Lazzaroni, 1957), are associated with a greater reduction in speech recognition abilities among older listeners. Speech that is rapidly alternated between the ears (RASP) is also difficult for the elderly listener to discriminate (Welsh et al, 1985).

Several investigators (Jerger & Hayes, 1977; Otto & McCandless, 1982; Shirinian & Arnst, 1982) suggest that a comparison of the PI functions for synthetic sentences (SSI) and PB words is useful to differentiate between peripheral and central sites of auditory disorders. When the PBmax falls considerably above the maximum SSI score (SSImax) a central auditory dysfunction exists. A peripheral site of lesion is suggested when PBmax falls considerably below SSImax. This comparison of PBmax to SSImax is called the *central-peripheral ratio* (Jerger & Hayes, 1977).

In studies of elderly people, central-peripheral ratios consistent with a central auditory dysfunction often exist among older people independent of their hearing thresholds (Jerger & Hayes, 1977). A longitudinal study was conducted on an elderly patient with presbycusis over a 9-year interval using the central-peripheral ratio. Although there was little change in peripheral hearing sensitivity, central auditory function was found to decline substantially (Stach et al, 1985). Traditional air, bone, and speech testing often does not reveal central and neural changes in the senescent auditory system, whereas the central-peripheral ratio reveals consistent age effects (Otto & McCandless, 1982).

IMPACT OF AUDITORY DYSFUNCTION ON ELDERLY PEOPLE
Hearing Handicap

Audiometric data can provide important information, such as the degree of hearing impairment, the configuration of hearing loss, and the type of hearing impairment (Katz & White, 1984). This information is valuable for planning intervention strategies for a person with a hearing impairment. Because audiometric tests assess only sensory variables, however, they offer only indirect information regarding the actual communicative handicap of a person with a hearing impairment (Giolas, 1982b). Because nonsensory factors, such as general communication skills (Demorest & Walden, 1984), contribute to hearing handicap, it is apparent that procedures other than audiometric tests must be used to evaluate a person's hearing handicap.

Several variables influence the degree to which a particular hearing impairment handicaps a given person. These factors include age of onset, severity, site of lesion, and the presence of other nonauditory impairments (Davis & Hardick, 1981; Giolas, 1982b). These contributing factors help explain why two people with essentially equivalent hearing impairments may exhibit vastly different hearing handicaps (Weinstein & Ventry, 1983; Giolas, 1982b).

In an attempt to quantify the handicapping nature of hearing loss, a number of self-report instruments have been proposed (High et al, 1964; Noble & Atherly, 1970; Ewertsen & Birk-Nielson, 1973; Alpiner et al, 1978; Giolas et al, 1979). In general, these scales present a person with a hearing impairment with a series of questions concerning potentially handicapping conditions and require the person to rate their overall auditory function in these specific situations. Consequently, these hearing handicap scales provide valuable insights into a person's perception of the handicapping nature of the hearing impairment.

Historically, the use of handicap scales with the elderly has been limited because normative data for this population were not available (Ventry & Weinstein, 1982). In addition, except for the Denver Scale of Communication Function for Senior Citizens Living in Retirement Centers (Zarnoch, J., & Alpiner, J., unpublished study, 1976), these handicap scales are designed for use with the general population and do not take into account the unique situations and problems that affect older people. These problems were remedied in 1982 by the Hearing Handicap Inventory for the Elderly (HHIE) (Ventry & Weinstein, 1982). This scale assesses the effects of auditory impairment on the emotional and social adjustment of people 65 years of age and older. The HHIE was designed solely for use with elderly people, and all of the normative data for this scale were obtained from people 65 years of age and older. The screening version of the HHIE is included in Chapter 5.

Several investigations found that with an elderly population speech recognition abilities account for no more than 20 percent of the variance in handicap scores, and pure-tone sensitivity accounts for only 36 to 38 percent of handicap scores (Weinstein & Ventry, 1983). In addition, the greatest variability in self-rating of hearing handicap among elderly people was found in people with mild sensitivity losses. It is apparent that factors other than loss of pure-tone sensitivity and speech recognition abilities must contribute to hearing handicap. Measurements of hearing handicap allow a clinician to probe the impact of an auditory disorder on an elderly person and may reveal information not garnered from a clinical audiometric assessment.

Other Physiologic Concerns

Other changes in the physiologic status of an aging person may have an impact on the aural rehabilitation strategy used. These changes in systems other than the auditory system may have considerable impact on the handicapping nature of a hearing loss. Thus, factors other than changes in auditory performance must be taken into consideration to develop an effective intervention strategy for the elderly. This section describes some of the physical changes that may occur in the principal organ systems of the elderly.

Visual System

The aging visual system undergoes predictable changes in structure and function similar to those found in the auditory system. The development of lens opacities (cataracts) is a very common finding in the elderly eye (Abrahamson, 1984). Cortical cataracts are the most common type of lens opacity associated with aging. This cataract appears in the outer layers of the lens, is slow-growing, and may not initially interfere with vision. Because of the predominantly central location of the cataracts, visual reduction is likely to occur, especially in bright light with the associated pupillary constriction.

The development of cataracts seems to be associated with the structural design of the lens itself. The crystalline lens does not replace its cells or dispose of old ones (Sperduto & Seigel, 1980). This leads to regularly increasing annular layers of the lens cortex, with the associated progressive compression of the nuclear or central components of the lens (Said & Weale, 1959). The result is a reduction in the clarity of the lens.

Another common finding in the lenses of geriatric patients is presbyopia, in which the lens loses its ability to change diameter (accommodation) (Corso, 1977). Accommodation involves an adjustment of the ciliary muscle around the lens of the eye, which results in a shape change. This leads to an alteration in the focal length of the eye so that the light rays are brought to bear on the retina. In accommodation, the lens becomes thicker when an person looks at a near object and thinner when a person looks at a distant object. The difference between the closest point and the farthest point of focus is called the *range of accommodation*. As a person grow older, the near point of vision recedes so that the range of accommodation becomes much less. The cause of presbyopia is not completely clear, however, the condition is believed to be due to loss of the elastic properties of the lens or changes in the ciliary muscle itself (Weale, 1986).

With advanced age there is an increased danger of abnormally high fluid pressure in the eyes. Two processes affect the pressure of the fluids in the senile eye. These are the reduction of aqueous secretion and the decrease in aqueous outflow with advanced age. These processes compensate for each other with the net result that the intraocular pressure remains essentially unchanged in old age or demonstrates only a slight increase (Armaly, 1965). A disruption in this balance often leads to increased intraocular pressure (glaucoma). This condition is one of the most common causes of impaired vision or blindness in an elderly population; the reported prevalence is 2 to 5 percent (Graham, 1972).

The structural changes often found in the visual system of an elderly person may have many functional consequences on that person's vision. In a study of an aged population, researchers reported a significant decline in the function of visual acuity (Slataper, 1950), color vision (Kalmus, 1987), dark adaption (McFarland, 1960), visual field (Wolf, 1960), and contrast sensitivity (Sekular & Hutman, 1980). It should be noted that these changes in visual function are not likely to be found in isolation. An elderly person with dysfunction in the visual system may experience declining driving abilities; problems with face recognition; difficulty completing household tasks; problems reading, watching television, or other leisurely pursuits; and even a reduction in the ability to walk independently (Hakkinen, 1984). The extent of these consequences is quite variable among elderly people. It depends to a large extent not only on their functional visual changes but also on other personal variables,   such as concomitant physical disabilities. A professional working with elderly clients should be aware of the common conse- quences of visual deterioration in the elderly when planning intervention. In particular, attention should be given to lighting, contrast, and light reflection. The occurrence of visual dysfunction in an elderly person with other coexisting sensory deficits, such as hearing loss, may make intervention such as speech training impractical.

Pulmonary Function

Changes in the lung and associated tissues accompany advancing age. The aggregate of these changes is a reduction in the function of the respiratory system. The aged healthy person has function that is adequate for normal breathing at rest, but there is a loss of reserve, so large volumes or high rates of breathing are lost (Turner et al, 1965). This reduction in breath support may affect the sustained and dynamic speech production capabilities of an elderly person. Thus, if speech improvement is a goal in therapy, the professional must be cognizant of possible reduction in breath support.

Pharmacology and Aging

An elderly person often is exposed to a wide array of medical treatments. The action of these agents on an older person may have a drastic effect. The elderly tend to take considerably more medication for a longer period of time than younger people. This, combined with a reduction in the performance of the liver and kidneys (the former to metabolize and the latter to excrete the agents), may affect an elderly person in a way that is not the intended action of the medication (Bender, 1974). The speech-language pathologist and health care professional should be aware of the medications taken by a client and of the intended actions and possible side effects of the agents.

Absorption of the medication may be influenced by changes in the aging gastrointestinal tract. Slowed motility and lowered acidity affect the rate of absorption. Changes in the proportion of adipose and lean tissue can result in changes in distribution of water and fat-soluble medications. Lowered renal and hepatic function often leads to an increased time for excretion or metabolism of drugs.

Elderly people often demonstrate an enhanced response to drugs that sup-press the central nervous system. This includes drugs for seizures and sedatives. This enhanced response may lead to confusion, incoordination, or changes in the production of speech. Similar findings have been reported for some antidepressant medications.

The Aging Nervous System

Several marked changes occur throughout the aging nervous system. Brain mass decreases in advanced age. This reduction is primarily due to loss of neurons and their sensory and motor processes. This loss occurs rather slowly during the third decade of life but increases in rate beginning in the seventh decade. This change happens slowly so new connections between surviving cells are established, and often little functional loss is found in a healthy aged person (Vernadakis, 1985).

There is a reduction in the conduction speed of neuronal information by about 30 percent from early adulthood to the age of 80 years. This reduction in neural transmission speed is in addition to the reduced numbers of neuronal connections. This may lead to a reduction in sensory sensitivity, alterations in cognition, and changes in posture and gait.

Sociologic Issues and the Elderly

Advancing age may be associated with alterations in the social status and effectiveness of a person. Although it is not the purpose of this chapter to detail these sociologic issues, some of the common sociologic consequences of aging may have an impact on clinical intervention. A brief description of these considerations follows.

Demographic Factors

The growth of the segment of the population older than 65 years has been dramatic through the second half of the twentieth century, and this trend is accelerating. At the beginning of the twentieth century, people older than 65 years composed approximately 4 percent of the population, and by 1980 this proportion had increased to 11 percent. Current estimates (U.S. Bureau of the Census, 1990) indicate that by the year 2000, more than 36 million people in the United States will be older than 65 years. Not only are more people reaching the age of 65 years, but also elderly people are living much longer in general. People older than 85 years is a segment of society that is growing considerably faster than any other at this time (U.S. Bureau of the Census, 1990). This trend is expected to continue for at least the next 20 years. There is also a steady improvement in the general health of the elderly population.

This tremendous increase in the elderly population seems to be due to better health care, immigration, and the fact that a large number of people were born in the early part of this century. These increases in the number of people in the population with the greatest need for intervention in disorders of communication will have significant implications for providers of these services well into the next century.

Financial Considerations

Sparse financial resources are a fact of life for many older people. This may limit their transportation and even limit the purchase of many essential daily items. It is not surprising that the elderly have difficulty finding adequate resources to pay for direct clinical services. Often, the expenses not covered by third-party reimbursement agencies may not be payable by the older client. In addition, even though augmentive communication devices may be appropriate to enhance communication, the older person may not be able to afford them.

Professionals may need to be creative in finding sources to fund clinical activities for elderly patients. A large number of agencies other than private insurance companies or federal agencies such as Medicaid and Medicare provide funding. Several national foundations provide funding for clinical service if there is a justification based on financial need. Federal agencies that provide funds for research on aging (eg, the National Institute on Aging) also have funds available for clinical intervention. An elderly person may also be eligible for services provided by the Veterans Administration. State and local agencies should not be overlooked as potential funding resources.

Mobility

An important concern of elderly people in need of communicative intervention may be their inability to travel to the site where services are provided. These problems may be physical or fiscal in nature. Ambulatory restrictions may make travel outside of the home difficult for an elderly person. Financial limitations also may restrict travel, especially if the person has special transportation requirements. Thus, the professionals involved with remediation must be aware that clinical intervention with the elderly is often most efficient when performed in the patient's residence, whether it is a private home visitation program or an extended-care facility.

Psychologic Aspects of Aging

Advancing age is often associated with changes in a person's psychological characteristics. Personal, cognitive, and emotional changes are commonly found among senescent people and may have a direct bearing on the efficacy of clinical intervention.

Cognitive Considerations in the Elderly

While age-related changes in the function of the central and peripheral auditory mechanisms influence the perception of speech by elderly people, other nonsensory factors contribute to the ability to communicate. Changes in memory and use of linguistic cues may affect the auditory understanding of speech by an elderly person. Speech understanding depends not only on the signal received at the ear and passed through the auditory system (bottom-up processing) but also on the expectations (such as semantic memory and syntactic constraints) that the person has about the incoming signal (top-down processing) (Committee on Hearing, Bioacoustics, and Biomechanics [CHABA], 1988). A clinician must have some understanding of both bottom-up and top-down processing to understand age-related changes in the understanding of speech.

Memory Changes

Most cognitive theorists consider memory not to be a unidimensional phenomenon but to have several components. The most common model for describing memory processes differentiates sensory memory, primary memory, and secondary (or long-term) memory (Klatzky, 1980).

Sensory memory is the most short-term of the memory components. It retains a brief image of the sensory stimulus to facilitate higher level processing. Auditory sensory memory (called *echoic memory*) does not seem to be influenced by advancing age and is probably not responsible for declining verbal communication performance among the aged (Arenberg, 1976).

Short-term memory has a limited capacity and likely provides a workspace for the information on which the person is currently concentrating. While absolute short-term memory capacity has not been shown to decline considerably with advancing age, it has been demonstrated that the ability of an older person to accurately utilize short-term memory may be compromised when stimuli are presented rapidly (Coyne, 1985). This may have some relation to the impaired understanding of temporally altered speech signals that is often reported among older listeners. Decreases in short-term memory performance have been reported among elderly listeners when they are required to attend to several stimuli (Craik, 1973). This task requirement may be comparable to the processing of a speech message, in which part of the message must be held in memory while the remainder of the signal is analyzed for syntactic and semantic relations.

Long-term or secondary memory is often described as being composed of episodic memory, or the memory of time or place specific information, and semantic memory, or the recognition of concepts and the underlying rules of language. Large age-related differences favoring the young are often found in secondary episodic memory, (Perlmutter & Mitchell, 1982). This decline in secondary memory skills often seen in the elderly may in some way contribute to communication difficulties.

Understanding speech requires the use of semantic memory, that is, knowledge of word meanings, syntactic structure, and other rules of language. There is little research that examines the possible changes in semantic memory among the aged. There are many similarities in the organization of semantic memory between young and older adults. Both groups recognize words of frequent occurrence more rapidly than infrequent words (Bowles & Poon, 1981). No decline in vocabulary size as measured by intelligence tests with advancing age has been noted. Any differences in semantic memory demonstrated between young and old people are of small magnitude and not easily generalized. It is important to remember that little research exists on this topic area to date, thus the possible relation between changes in semantic memory and the perception of speech are unclear at this time. In addition, little research has investigated the relation between cognitive factors and the handicapping nature of a hearing loss. More research is needed to establish these relationships.

Consistent slowing in cognitive processing is associated with advancing age (Birren et al, 1980). Some researchers have postulated that this slowing causes many of the changes in sensory processing that occur in the elderly (Birren, 1974). This slowing may manifest itself in any area of cognitive function. It would not be surprising if many of the difficulties in speech understanding experienced by elderly people were related to this general cognitive slowing. There is evidence that older people take longer to retrieve a word from the lexicon than do younger people (Petros et al, 1983). In addition, elderly people seem to be slower at preparing and carrying out responses (Salthouse, 1980).

Use of Linguistic Information

Comparatively little research has addressed age-related differences in the use of syntactic or semantic cues to facilitate receptive communication. Several researchers investigated the effects of speed of auditory processing of older listeners for speech strings with varying degrees of semantic and syntactic information (Wingfield et al, 1985). Wingfield et al noted a large reduction in overall performance by older listeners compared with younger listeners as the speed of presentation was increased. This relative decline in performance was less apparent when syntactic and semantic cues were available. Thus, it may be postulated that there is a statistically significant cognitive slowing in the older listeners, but they are able to make use of syntactic and semantic cues to overcome most of these difficulties.

To assess processing of semantic predictability with age, clients are given the Speech Perception in Noise (SPIN) test (Kalikow et al, 1977). In this test, subjects must identify the final word of a sentence. In half of the sentences, the correct response is cued by the semantically related words preceding it. The other half of the sentences do not provide such cues. A comparison of the high- and low-predictability sentences gives some indication of the effect of semantic predictability on word recognition. There is an overall decrease in word recognition performance with increasing age. There is not a statistically significant difference between old and young listening groups in manipulating semantically predictable information. The overall poorer performance in the older group may be explained at least in part by the higher auditory thresholds found in these participants.

Use of Visual Information to Assist in Verbal Communication

There are no differences in the effect of speechreading on the speech reception thresholds of older listeners compared with younger listeners (Middlelweerd & Plomp, 1987). Young and elderly listeners are generally able to take advantage of syntactic-semantic structure in sentence strings to facilitate word recognition (Holtzman et al, 1986). Overall performance is higher among the younger listeners, however, the use of percentage-facilitation scores indicate that there is no significant difference between age groups in the effect of sentence structure on performance. In other words, the proportional increase in performance when linguistic cues are available is comparable in the two age groups. It seems likely that there is little difference between younger and older listeners in the amount of benefit associated with speech recognition that can be gained from syntactic or semantic structure.

Motivation of the Elderly

Many investigations have demonstrated poor performance among elderly people on many tests of cognitive function. This may be the result of several factors. First is an overall decrement in performance that may be associated with general cognitive slowing or decline. Another possible cause of reduction in communication on the part of elderly people may be due to a more conservative response criterion than is typically found in younger people (Marshall, 1981). It appears as if elderly listeners have a more conservative criterion for response and therefore may be less likely to respond to stimuli that are unclear.

Signal detection analysis may be used to quantify response criteria among listeners separate from their auditory sensitivity. However, one group of investigators was unable to establish differences in response willingness between young and old listeners (Yanz & Anderson, 1984). Other investigators (Blood & Blood, 1984) have reported that the elderly participants in their study tended to set a conservative response criterion, regardless of degree of auditory impairment. Still other investigators (Marshall & Jesteadt, 1986) demonstrated very small differences in response bias between young and old listeners; the older people had a slightly more conservative criterion. Differences in response bias between young and old listeners in an opposite direction to that reported in the foregoing study have been reported (Gordon-Salant, 1986). That is, the older participants in several investigations exhibited less strict response criteria than younger listeners. Clearly, more research is needed to investigate these relationships.

Psychiatric Function and Disorders

The most common psychiatric disturbances of advanced age are depression, dementia, and paranoia. Most estimates are that approximately 10 percent of people older than 65 years have dementia, and this proportion rises to approximately 20 percent among people older than 80 years. Clinical depression is found in 2 to 4 percent of elderly people, and paranoia and adjustment disorders have an impact on many elderly people (Moore, 1988).

Dementia

Dementia is one of the most common disorders of advanced age (Moore, 1988). Most people who experience dementia have dementia from Alzheimer disease, but it is important to remember that several other diseases may produce dementia. Metabolic disturbances and nutritional deficiencies also may produce symptoms of dementia. It is therefore important that a complete physical evaluation be conducted for any client who shows symptoms of dementia.

Adjustment Disorders

An adjustment disorder may be defined as an abnormal reaction to a psychosocial stress. The most frequent adjustment disorders of later life are depressed mood, anxious mood, or mixed emotional features. The loss of a spouse is the most common precipitating factor, with bereavement leading to an adjustment disorder (Moore, 1988).

Affective Disorders

The most common affective disorder of senescence is depression; bipolar disorder the second most common disorder. Bipolar disorder consists of an alteration in mood from a manic state to a depressive state. The manic episode is characterized by talkativeness, expansive mood, flight of ideas, grandiose self-image, distractibility, and overactivity. Manic episodes must be interspersed with clinically significant depression to be classified as a bipolar disorder (Gillis & Zabrow, 1982).

Clinically significant depression is manifested as a change in appetite, a blue mood, change in sleep patterns, loss of interest in usual activities, poor concentration, and suicidal thoughts. These symptoms must be present for at least 2 weeks. These people may also be described as psychotic or melancholic (Blazer & Williams, 1980).

Although speech-language pathologists do not have the training to provide intervention for psychiatric disorders, awareness of the symptoms is critical. Modifications in clinical intervention are necessary for elderly clients with these common psychological problems. The speech-language pathologist or health care professional should try to ensure that the elderly person who manifests the symptoms of the common psychological problems receives appropriate medical, psychological, sociological, and rehabilitative intervention.

CLINICAL INTERVENTION WITH ELDERLY PEOPLE

Minimizing the Impact of an Auditory Disorder

Auditory dysfunction is one of the most common handicapping conditions among the elderly. There are several ways to minimize the impact of these disorders. These include modifications in the environment to make communication easier and the use of auditory communication aids such as personal amplification devices. In addition, speaking in a normal conversational manner, the speech-language pathologist or health care professional should take the following steps to enhance communication:

1. Increase the volume of your voice slightly *if necessary* but do so sparingly.
2. Speak at a normal rate. Rate reduction strategy should be used conservatively.
3. Do not obstruct your mouth while speaking.
4. Do not speak with anything in your mouth.
5. Move the lips normally, without exaggerated movements.
6. Reduce environmental noise.
7. Reduce the distance between the listener and the speaker.
8. Communicate in an environment with little sound reverberation. Reverberation is a problem in an environment with hard, flat surfaces. Absorbent material (such as carpeting and drapes) improve a reverberant environment.

Attention to the following details in the visual environment may enhance verbal communication:

1. Use of facial expressions and gestures.
2. Position yourself so that your face is well lit. Do not stand with your back to a window or bright light.
3. Not hiding or covering the mouth while talking.
4. Facing the person with the hearing impairment.
5. Communicating from a position close to the client.
6. Not speaking with anything in the mouth, which distorts the visual cues the listener may be using to aid understanding.

It is helpful to pay attention to the following aspects of the linguistic environment:

1. If the hard-of-hearing listener appears to have lost the subject of the conversation, take a moment to inform him or her of the topic.
2. Repetition may be necessary. If such repetition is necessary, changing the wording of the message may help communication. Sentences should not be too long or complex.

The following general recommendations help enhance communication:

1. *Touch.* Gently placing a hand on the listener may help him or her to focus attention on the speaker.
2. *Honesty in communication.* Do not indicate you understand if that is not the case. A paper and pencil may be used if all else fails.
3. *Composure.* Do not appear upset or uncomfortable if the client has difficulty understanding. Negative reactions encourage listeners to act as if they understand, even when they do not.
4. *Awareness of physical condition.* A person with a hearing disability may understand less well when tired or ill. Listening in the presence of a hearing loss is hard work and requires great effort.
5. *Compassion and patience.* Both factors help bridge the communication gap.

Other Aids to Communication

Hearing Aids

With the prevalence of auditory dysfunction among the aged, it would seem that the use of amplification would be widespread among this population. However, many people who could benefit from amplification do not use hearing aids. There are several reasons for this phenomenon.

First, the cost of hearing aids may place the devices out of the reach of many older people. The small controls may be difficult for a person with reduced tactile sensitivity to manipulate. Poor vision may lead to difficulty in management of small amplification devices. Many studies have found that cosmetic concerns convince many older people not to try amplification.

Even if an older person wears amplification, he or she does not receive as much benefit as a younger person with a similar hearing loss. Several researchers have postulated that this occurs because of central auditory dysfunction that often accompanies advanced age. It has been found that elderly people who have a severe central auditory aging effect do not receive as much benefit from amplification as elderly people with similar sensitivity losses but with no central component. The hearing aid rejection rate among people who exhibit neural lesions is higher than for those with cochlear abnormalities alone. A longitudinal investigation (Stach et al, 1985) demonstrated that diminished success as a hearing aid user seemed to parallel a decline in central auditory function. Thus, it is possible that a central auditory dysfunction may limit the benefit of amplification and indeed any aural rehabilitation of an elderly person.

Some clinicians advocate the evaluation of central auditory function in both ears of elderly listeners with a hearing impairment. In some patients one ear might exhibit a central auditory dysfunction while the other ear does not. This difference in central auditory function between ears may be found even when no difference is detected with routine audiometric tests. Therefore, the evaluation of central auditory function may provide useful information about the appropriate ear to fit with a hearing aid. It is apparent that the evaluation of speech perception both in a quiet environment and in the presence of background noise may reveal important information to aid in the effective planning and implementation of a successful aural rehabilitation program.

Assistive Listening Devices

Along with hearing aids, many devices are available to aid a person in certain listening situations. These devices are described in Chapter 8. Many older people who could benefit from these devices do not have amplification. A professional working with elderly people should consider providing a portable desktop assistive listening device to aid in communication with an elderly person with a hearing impairment. Many churches, theaters, and auditoriums have installed frequency modulation (FM), infrared, or hardwired assistive listening devices to aid the patrons with hearing impairments.

An Aural Rehabilitation Program for the Elderly

The purpose of any aural rehabilitation program is to minimize the impact of a hearing loss on a person's function. A typical aural rehabilitation program for the elderly may consist of the following components:

1. A thorough evaluation of the degree of hearing impairment. This should include auditory sensitivity assessment (pure-tone audiometry) sufficient to establish the type and degree of hearing loss. This should include an assessment to determine if the elderly person has a clinically significant central auditory disturbance. Some research has shown that as the auditory dysfunction moves from a more peripheral to a more central locus, the impact of the disorder increases (Otto & McCandless, 1982). In addition, the understanding of speech at threshold and under optimal and degraded listening environments should be evaluated.

2. An assessment of the handicapping nature of an auditory impairment. The most commonly used instrument to assess the impact of an auditory dysfunction on an elderly person is the HHIE (Ventry & Weinstein, 1982).

3. Selection of the most appropriate amplification system. This selection should be based on lifestyle, hearing loss, communication environment, and perception of the auditory difficulties (Ross, 1994).

4. A hearing aid orientation and follow-up program.

5. Possible formalized speechreading training. This should include not only visual information from the articulators of the speaker but also additional environmental and interpersonal visual information, such as communicative context, facial expression, and gestures.

6. Possible formalized auditory training. Garstecki (1981) described a method that manipulates the redundancy in the message, the competing noise in the environment, and the type and amount of auditory and visual cues. In this way, the listener can be exposed to messages that can vary a great deal in auditory content and linguistic complexity. This is a very formalized procedure to train a listener to make use of auditory messages in less than ideal communicative environments. An important consideration of this technique is that it requires the use of audiometric equipment and a sound-treated booth.

7. Education about hearing loss, assistive listening devices, effective communication strategies, the psychosocial impact of hearing loss, and coping strategies when a communication breakdown occurs.

8. Information about environmental modifications to enhance auditory understanding.

Much information can be provided as part of group activities. Interactions among the participants with hearing impairments and their spouses, partners, or family members may be beneficial (Giolas, 1982a). Individual counseling sessions may be appropriate and may be preferable for some elderly people with a hearing impairment.

Modifications in Assessment and Intervention

Environment

The assessment of communicative function should be conducted in an environment that enhances the evaluation. There should be accommodations for a wheelchair if necessary. The acoustic environment should be quiet and free of excessive reverberation. There should be strong lighting, and provisions should be made to reduce glare. Because there may be a reduction in visual contrast sensitivity, particularly with blue-green discrimination, the testing table should be covered with red, orange, or yellow. A person with cataracts may benefit from rather dim, indirect lighting during the evaluation.

Procedures

Adequate response time by an elderly person needs to be considered. Because of generalized cognitive slowing, an elderly person may need as much as twice as much time as a younger person to respond accurately. The clinician should ensure adequate time to provide instructions and allow time between the instructions and the initiation of the task. The instructions may need to be rephrased and given slowly at an adequate distance and volume so the client can take advantage of auditory and visual cues.

Fatigue

An older person may tire easily. This may have adverse effects on the behaviors measured and the efficacy of clinical intervention. When possible, sessions should be broken into short periods to avoid overtiring an elderly person. Fatigue may be avoided by choosing clinical activities that are stimulating or interesting, not overly difficult, and not overly time-consuming. Sleep disturbances and side effects of medication also may cause fatigue in a client.

SUMMARY

The elderly will make up an increasing proportion of the caseload of speech-language pathologists and health care professionals in coming years. Physiologic and psychological changes within this population can present a number of challenges to successful clinical assessment and intervention. Changes in vision, hearing, and other physiologic systems must be considered when planning for effective and appropriate clinical activities. Psychological changes, including changes in intellectual function, cognitive processing, and affective state all have an impact on the success or failure of clinical intervention. Reduced financial resources may limit the types of services that an older person can utilize. These changes cause the elderly to be a more heterogeneous population than other age groups. Each professional must be creative and adaptable to modify clinical strategies to best meet an older person's needs. The challenges and rewards of meeting the special needs of the aging population can provide a great deal of satisfaction to the professional motivated enough to provide them services.

REFERENCES

Abrahamson, I. (1984). Eye changes after forty. *American Family Physician, 29,* 171-181.

Alpiner, J., Chevrette, W., Glascoe, G., Metz, M., & Olsen, B. (1978). The Denver Scale of Communication Function. In J. Alpiner (Ed.), *Handbook of adult rehabilitative audiology* (lst ed.) (pp. 53-56). Baltimore: Williams & Wilkins.

Anderson, R., & Meyerhoff, W. (1982). Otologic manifestations of aging. *Otolaryngology Clinics of North America, 15,* 353-370.

Arenberg, D. (1976). The effects of input condition on free recall in young and old adults. *Journal of Gerontology, 31,* 551-555.

Armaly, M. (1965). On the distribution of applanation pressure. I. Statistical features and the effect of age, sex, and family history of glaucoma. *Archives of Ophthalmology, 62,* 11-18.

Bender, A. (1974). Pharmacodynamic principles of drug therapy in the aged. *Journal of the American Geriatric Society, 13,* 192-198.

Bergman, M. (1971). Hearing and aging. *Audiology, 10,* 164-171.

Bergman, M. (1980). *Aging and the perception of speech.* Baltimore: University Park Press.

Birren, J. (1974). Translations in gerontology—from lab to life: Psychophysiology and speed of response. *American Psychologist, 29,* 808-815.

Birren, J., Woods, A., & Williams, M. (1980). Behavioral slowing with age: Causes, organization, and consequences. In W. Poon (Ed.), *Aging in the 1980's.* Washington, DC: American Psychological Association.

Blazer, D., & Williams, C. (1980). Epidemiology of dysphoria and depression in an elderly population. *American Journal of Psychiatry, 137,* 439-444.

Blood, I., & Blood, G. (1984). Cautiousness and hearing acuity in elderly women: A signal detection approach. *Journal of Communication Disorders, 17,* 255-230.

Bocca, E. (1967). Distorted speech tests. In Graham, A. (Ed.), *Sensorineural hearing processes and disorders* (pp. 359-370). Boston: Little, Brown.

Bowles, N., & Poon, L. (1981). The effect of age on the speed of lexical access. *Experimental Aging Research, 7,* 417-425.

Brody, H. (1955). Organization of the cerebral cortex: A study of aging in the human cerebral cortex. *Journal of Comparative Neurology, 102,* 511-556.

Calearo, C., & Lazzaroni, M. (1957). Speech intelligibility in relation to the speed of the message. *Laryngoscope, 67,* 410-419.

Chandler, J. (1964). Partial occlusion of the external auditory meatus: Its effect upon air and bone conduction hearing acuity. *Laryngoscope, 74,* 22-54.

Committee on Hearing, Bioacoustics, and Biomechanics (CHABA) (1988). Speech understanding and aging. *Journal of the Acoustical Society of America, 83,* 859-893.

Corso, J. (1977). Auditory perception and communication. In J. Birren & K. Schaie (Eds.) *Handbook of the psychology of aging* (pp. 535-551). New York: Van Nostrand Reinhold.

Covell, W. (1952). Histologic changes in the aging cochlea. *Journal of Gerontology, 7,* 173-177.

Coyne, A. (1985). Adult age, presentation time, and memory performance. *Experimental Aging Research, 11,* 147-149.

Craik, F. (1973, August). Signal detection analysis of age differences in divided attention. Presented at the Annual Meeting of the American Psychological Association, Montreal, Canada.

Davis, J., & Hardick, E. (1981). *Rehabilitative audiology for children and adults.* New York: Van Nostrand Reinhold.

Demorest, M. E., & Walden, B. E. (1984). Psychometric principles in the selection, interpretation, and evaluation of communication self-assessment inventories. *Journal of Speech and Hearing Disorders, 49,* 226-240.

Etholm, B., & Belal, A. (1974). Senile changes in the middle ear joints. *Annals of Otology, Rhinology, and Laryngology, 23,* 49-54.

Ewertson, H., & Birk-Nielson, H. (1973). Social hearing handicap index: Social handicap in relation to hearing impairment. *Audiology, 12,* 180-187.

Fisher, H., & Freedman, S. (1968). The role of the pinna in auditory localization. *Journal of Auditory Research, 8,* 15-26.

Gaeth, J. (1948). A study of phonemic regression in relation to hearing loss. Chicago: Northwestern University. Dissertation.

Garstecki, D. (1981) Audiovisual training paradigm for hearing-impaired adults. *Journal of the Academy of Rehabilitative Audiology, 14,* 223-228.

Gillis, L., & Zabrow, A. (1982). Dysphoria in the elderly. *South African Medical Journal, 62,* 410-413.

Giolas, T. G. (1982a). A sample eight-week aural rehabilitation program. In T. G. Giolas. *Hearing handicapped adults.* Englewood Cliffs: Prentice Hall.

Giolas, T. G. (1982b). *Hearing handicapped adults.* Englewood Cliffs: Prentice Hall.

Giolas, T., Owens, E., Lamb, S., & Schubert, E. (1979). Hearing performance inventory. *Journal of Speech and Hearing Disorders, 44,* 169-195.

Glorig, A., & Roberts, A. (1965). Hearing levels of adults by age and sex (United States 1960-1962). National Center for Hearing Statistics Series, II, No. 11. Washington, DC: United States Department of Health, Education, and Welfare.

Goetzinger, C., Proud, G., Dirks, D., & Emberg, J. (1961). A study of hearing in advanced age. *Archives of Otolaryngology, 73,* 662-674.

Gordon-Salant, S. (1986). Effects of aging on response criteria in speech-recognition tasks. *Journal of Speech and Hearing Research, 29,* 155-162.

Graham, P. (1972). Epidemiology of simple glaucoma and ocular hypertension. *British Journal of Ophthalmology, 56,* 223-229.

Hakkinen, L. (1984). Vision in the elderly and its use in the social environment. *Scandinavian Journal of Social Medicine, 35* (Suppl.), 5-60.

Hansen, C., & Riske-Nielsen, E. (1965). Pathological studies in presbycusis. *Archives of Otolaryngology, 82,* 115-133.

Harbert, F., Young, I., & Menduke, H. (1965). Audiologic findings in presbycusis. *The Journal of Auditory Research, 6,* 297-312.

High, W., Fairbanks, C., & Glorig, A. (1964). Scale of self-assessment of hearing handicap. *Journal of Speech and Hearing Disorders, 29,* 215-230.

Hinchcliffe, R. (1962). The anatomical locus of presbycusis. *Journal of Speech and Hearing Disorders, 27,* 301-310.

Holtzman, R., Familitant, M., Deptula, P., & Hoyer, W. (1986). Aging and the use of sentential structure to facilitate word recognition. *Experimental Aging Research, 12,* 85-88.

Hull, R. (1978). Hearing evaluation of the elderly. In J. Katz (Ed.), *Handbook of clinical audiology* (pp. 426-441). Baltimore: Williams & Wilkins.

Jerger, J. (1973). Diagnostic audiometry. In J. Jerger (Ed.), *Modern developments in audiology* (2nd ed.) (pp. 75-116). New York: Academic Press.

Jerger, J., & Hayes, D. (1977). Diagnostic speech audiometry. *Archives of Otolaryngology, 103,* 216-222.

Jerger, S., & Jerger, J. (1981). *Auditory disorders.* Boston: Little, Brown.

Johnsson, L., & Hawkins, J. (1972). Sensory and neural degeneration with aging, as seen in microdissections of the human inner ear. *Annals of Otology, Rhinology, and Laryngology, 81,* 179-194.

Kalikow, D. N., Stevens, K. N., & Elliot, L. L. (1977). Development of a test of speech intelligibility in noise using sentence materials with controlled word predictability. *Journal of the Acoustical Society of America, 61,* 1337-1351.

Kalmus, H. (1987). Decline of contrast perception and colour sensitivity with age. In G. Verriest (Ed.), *Color vision deficiencies VIII.* Boston: Nijhoff/Junk.

Katz, J., & White, T. (1984). Introduction to the handicap of hearing impairment: Hearing impairment versus hearing handicap. In R. Hull (Ed.), *Rehabilitative Audiology* (pp. 1326). New York: Grune & Stratton.

Kirikae, I., Sato, T., & Shitara, T. (1964). Study of hearing in advanced age. *Laryngoscope, 74,* 205-221.

Klatzky, R. L. (1980). *Human memory: Structures and processes* (2nd ed.). San Francisco: Freeman.

Konkle, D., Beasley, D., & Bess, F. (1977). Intelligibility of time-altered speech in relation to chronological aging. *Journal of Speech and Hearing Research, 20,* 108-115.

Kopra, L. (1982). The auditory-communicative manifestations of presbycusis. In R. Hull (Ed.), *Rehabilitative audiology* (pp. 243-270). New York: Grune & Stratton.

Magladery, J. (1959). Neurophysiology of aging. In J. Birren (Ed.), *Handbook of aging and the individual* (pp. 117-148). Chicago: University of Chicago Press.

Marshall, L. (1981). Auditory processing in aging listeners. *Journal of Speech and Hearing Disorders, 46,* 226-240.

Marshall, L., & Jesteadt, W. (1986). Comparison of pure-tone audibility thresholds obtained with audiological and two-interval forced-choice procedures. *Journal of Speech and Hearing Research, 29,* 82-91.

Maurer, J., & Rupp, R. (1979). *Hearing & Aging.* New York: Grune & Stratton.

McFarland, R. (1960). Dark adaption as a function of age. I. A statistical analysis. *Journal of Gerontology, 15,* 149-154.

Middelweerd, M., & Plomp, R. (1987). The effect of speechreading on the speech-reception threshold of sentences in noise. *Journal of the Acoustical Society of America, 82,* 2145-2147.

Moore, J. (1988). Common psychiatric problems in the elderly. In B. Shadden (Ed.), *Communication behavior and aging: A source book for clinicians.* Baltimore: Williams & Wilkins.

Moscicki, E., Elkins, E., Baum, H., & McNamara, P. (1985). Hearing loss in the elderly: An epidemiologic study of the Framingham Heart Study cohort. *Ear and Hearing, 6,* 184-190.

Newman, C., & Spitzer, J. (1981). Eustachian tube efficiency of geriatric subjects. *Ear and Hearing, 2,* 103-107.

Noble, W., & Atherly, G. (1970). The hearing measurement scale: A questionnaire for the assessment of auditory disability. *Journal of Auditory Research, 10,* 229-250.

Otto, W., & McCandless, G. (1982). Aging and auditory site of lesion. *Ear and Hearing, 3,* 110-117.

Palva, A., & Jokinen, K. (1970). Presbycusis: Filtered speech tests. *Acta Otolaryngologica, 70,* 232-241.

Perlmutter, M., & Mitchell, D. (1982). The appearance and disappearance of age differences in adult memory. In F. Craik & S. Trehub (Eds.), *Aging and cognition processes.* New York: Plenum.

Perry, E. (1957). *The human ear canal.* Springfield: Charles C Thomas.

Pestalozza, G., & Shore, I. (1955). Clinical evaluation of presbycusis on the basis of different tests of auditory function. *Laryngoscope, 65,* 1136-1163.

Petros, T., Zehr, H., & Chabot, R. (1983). Adult age differences in assessing and retrieving information from long-term memory. *Journal of Gerontology, 38,* 589-592.

Ross, M. (1994) Overview of aural rehabilitation. In J. Katz (Ed.), *Handbook of clinical audiology.* Baltimore: Williams & Wilkins.

Ruby, R. (1986). Conductive hearing loss in the elderly. *Journal of Otolaryngology, 14,* 245-247.

Said, F., & Wall, R. (1959). The variation with age of the spectral transmissibility of the living human crystalline lens. *Gerontologia, 3,* 213-231.

Salthouse, T. (1980). Age and memory: Strategies for localizing the loss. In W. Poon (Ed.), *New directions in memory and aging.* Hillsdale: Erlbaum.

Schuknecht, H. (1964). Further observations on the pathology of presbycusis. *Archives of Otolaryngology, 80,* 369-382.

Schuknecht, H. (1974). *Pathology of the ear.* Cambridge: Harvard University Press.

Sekular, R., & Hutman, L. (1980). Spatial vision aging. I. Contrast sensitivity. *Journal of Gerontology, 25,* 692-699.

Shanas, E. (1962). *The health of older people: A social survey.* Cambridge: Harvard University Press.

Shaw, E., & Teranishi, R. (1968). Sound pressure generated in an external ear replica and real human ears by a nearby point source. *Journal of the Acoustical Society of America, 44,* 240-249.

Shirinian, M., & Arnst, D. (1982). Patterns in the performance-intensity functions for phonetically balanced word lists and synthetic sentences in aged listeners. *Archives of Otolaryngology, 108,* 15-20.

Slataper, F. (1950). Age norms of refraction and vision. *Archives of Ophthalmology, 43,* 466-481.

Sperduto, R., & Seigel, D. (1980). Senile lens and senile macular changes in a population-based sample. *American Journal of Ophthalmology, 90,* 86-91.

Stach, B., Jerger, J., & Fleming, K. (1985). Central presbycusis: A longitudinal case study. *Ear and Hearing, 6,* 304-306.

Sticht, T., & Gray, B. (1969). The intelligibility of time-compressed words as a function of age and hearing loss. *Journal of Speech and Hearing Research, 12,* 443-448.

Townsend, P. & Wedderburn, D. 1965. *The aged in the welfare state.* London: C. Bell.

Tsai, H., Fong-Shyong, C., & Tsa-Jung, C. (1958). On changes in ear size with age, as found among Taiwanese-Formosans of Fulienese extraction. *Journal of the Formosa Medical Society, 57,* 105-111.

Turner, J., Mead, J., & Wohl, M. (1965). Elasticity of human lungs in relation to age. *Journal of Applied Physiology, 25,* 664-671.

U.S. Bureau of the Census (1990): Number of persons age 65 and older under 18, per 100 persons aged 18-64, 1930-1990 and projections to 2050. Washington, DC: US Government Printing Office.

Ventry, I., & Weinstein, B. (1982). The hearing handicap inventory for the elderly: A new tool. *Ear and Hearing, 3,* 128-134

Vernadakis, A. (1985) The aging brain. *Clinical Geriatric Medicine, 1,* 61-94.

Wall, R. (1986). Aging and vision. *Vision Research, 26,* 1507-1512.

Weinstein, B., & Ventry, I. (1983). Audiometric correlates of the hearing handicap inventory for the elderly. *Journal of Speech and Hearing Disorders, 48,* 379-384.

Welsh, L., Welsh, J., & Healy, M. (1985). Central presbycusis. *Laryngoscope, 95,* 128-136.

Wingfield, A., Poon, L., Lombardi, L., & Lowe, D. (1985). Speed of processing in normal aging: Effects of speech rate, linguistic structure, and processing time. *Journal of Gerontology, 40,* 579-585.

Wolf, E. (1960). Glare and age. *Archives of Ophthalmology, 64,* 502-514.

Yanz, J. L., & Anderson, S. M. (1984). Comparison of speech perception skills in young and old listeners. *Ear and Hearing, 5,* 134-137.

Zikk, D., Himelfarb, M., & Shannon, E. (1985). Sudden hearing loss in the elderly. *Clinical Otolaryngology, 10,* 191-194.

SUGGESTED READING

Alpiner, J., & McCarthy, P. (Eds.) (1993). *Rehabilitative audiology: Children and adults* (2nd ed.) Baltimore: Williams & Wilkins.

Beasley, D., & Davis, G. A. (1981). *Aging communication processes and disorders.* New York: Grune & Stratton.

Lubinski, R. (Ed.) (1991). *Dementia and communication.* Philadelphia: Dekker.

Mueller, H. G., & Geoffrey, V. (Eds.) (1987). *Communication disorders in aging: Assessment and management.* Washington, DC: Gallaudet University Press.

Perlmutter, M., & Hall, E. (1985). *Adult development and aging.* New York: Wiley.

Ripich, D. (Ed.) (1991). *Handbook of adult communication disorders.* Austin: Pro-Ed.

Sanders, D. (1993). *Management of hearing handicap: Infants to elderly* (3rd ed.). Englewood Cliffs: Prentice Hall.

Schow, R., Christiansen, J., Hutchinson, J., & Nerbonne, M. (1978). *Communication disorders of the aged: A guide for health professionals.* Baltimore: University Park Press.

Schow, R. R., & Nerbonne, M. (1989). *Introduction to aural rehabilitation.* Austin: Pro-Ed.

Shadden, B. (1988). *Communication behavior and aging: A sourcebook for clinicians.* Baltimore: Williams & Wilkins.

Williams, T. F. (1984). *Rehabilitation in the aging.* New York: Raven.

Willott, J. (1991). *Aging and the auditory system: Anatomy, physiology, and psychophysics.* San Diego: Singular.

GlOSSARY

Accommodation   The adjustment of the eye to focus for various distances.

Atrophy   A wasting or decrease in size.

Central auditory system   The structures and pathways of the auditory system from the brainstem to the auditory cortex.

Cerumen   A waxy secretion found in the external auditory meatus.

Cholesteatoma   A pocket filled with keratin debris that may occur in the middle ear.

Conductive hearing loss   A hearing loss due to a dysfunction in the outer or middle ear.

Eustachian tube   A tube leading from the middle ear to the pharynx.

External auditory meatus   The ear canal leading from the pinna to the tympanic membrane.

Glaucoma   A disorder of the eye associated with abnormally high fluid pressure.

Hearing handicap   The impact of a hearing loss on the daily psychological state of a person.

Hearing impairment   The degree of hearing loss as measured by clinical tests.

Osteosis   Bony growths.

Otosclerosis   A growth of bone in the middle ear, most involving the footplate of the stapes.

Otitis media   An inflammation of the middle ear. Serous otitis media is associated with a watery fluid in the middle ear. Suppurative otitis media is associated with an active infection in the middle ear.

Performance-intensity function   A test performed with speech stimuli to investigate speech understanding at various presentation levels.

Peripheral auditory system   The auditory system from the pinna to the eighth cranial nerve.

Phonemic balance   The situation in which the proportion of sounds in a set of speech stimuli is representative of the occurrence of sounds in a language.

Pinna   The outermost structure of the ear. The visible portion of the external ear.

Presbycusis   A hearing loss associated with advanced age. May be classified as sensory, neural, metabolic, inner ear conductive, central, or vascular.

Presbyopia   Loss of ability of the aged eye to change focal status.

Retrocochlear   Dealing with structures in the auditory system beyond the cochlea.

Senescence   Related to aging.

Synthetic sentences   Series of words used in auditory testing that are sentence-like but do not make sense. Each word in the sentence only semantically and syntactically agrees with the two previous words.

Tragus   Cartilaginous projection in front of the external auditory meatus.

12

Noise and Hearing Loss

William Melnick

Excessive noise exposure from nonoccupational as well as occupational noise sources has been identified as one of the main causes, if not the main cause, of sensorineural hearing loss. In most instances this hearing loss can be prevented. Prevention depends on educating the public regarding the effects of noise on hearing. The speech-language pathologist, school health nurse, and educator are all in the position to serve as a prime educational resource. Speech-language pathologists are recognized experts for understanding and managing communicative disorders. They frequently represent the first professional contact for people seeking information and assistance with these problems. In some circumstances, however, this educational opportunity may fall to the school nurse or classroom teacher. All of these professionals can provide information to students, teachers, and parents about the importance of prevention of hearing loss due to noise.

Hearing conservation programs have been required by federal legislation and regulation. Two major components of these programs are hearing testing and the education of both employers and employees. A speech-language pathologist, health care professional, or educator knowledgeable about the development of hearing loss from noise and about the technique of basic audiometric screening can play an active role in these conservation programs. The purpose of this chapter is to provide information on the acoustic properties of noise important in the production of hearing loss and on the principal elements of programs designed to conserve hearing in a hazardous occupational noise environment.

In our society, hearing loss resulting from exposure to intense sound is widespread. In January of 1990, it was estimated that approximately 28 million people in the United States exhibited hearing loss and that 10 million of these impairments could be at least partially attributed to damage from exposure to loud sound (National Institutes of Health [NIH], 1990). More than 20 million people are exposed to hazardous noise levels on a regular basis. The most common overexposure occurs in the occupational environment. Hearing loss from noise has been documented in construction and factory workers, military personnel, truck drivers, police officers, firemen, musicians, and farmers.

Exposure to hazardous levels of noise does not occur only in a person's occupational setting. A number of nonoccupational noise sources exist in our fast-paced society, including live or recorded high-intensity music, recreational vehicles such as snowmobiles, airplanes, lawn-care equipment, woodworking tools, chain saws, some household appliances, and guns used in hunting or target shooting. The pervasiveness of this noxious ototoxic agent makes it one of the principal causes of sensorineural hearing loss among the adult population.

Hearing loss from noise is preventable in all cases except for instances of accidental exposure. Laws and regulations have been enacted on the federal, state, and local level for the protection of workers from hazardous noise levels in the workplace and for the protection of consumers from hazardous noise in leisure activities. Hearing loss resulting from overexposure to sound, particularly in the occupational environment, is compensable in most states and, therefore, represents a serious economic issue for management in business and industry.

Although this chapter emphasizes concern with the effects of noise on hearing, the concern should be with exposure to all forms of acoustic energy, regardless of whether it is considered noise by the person experiencing the exposure. The ear damage and the hearing loss that follow exposure to noise depend on accumulation of exposure of the ear to sound from all sources. Nevertheless, hearing loss that results from overexposure to acoustic energy has become known as a hearing loss from noise. For convenience, *noise* is used herein to refer to all types of hazardous sound exposure.

Environmental noise has several effects on human listeners besides producing hearing loss. These effects include interference with speech communication, annoyance, and stress on body systems. These effects are important and have motivated regulations, national and local, on noise control in the community. The responsibility for coordinating these efforts was delegated to the Environmental Protection Agency (EPA) by the Noise Control Act of 1972. Although these effects are important, this chapter focuses on hearing loss resulting from noise.

Sounds of sufficient intensity and duration can damage structures in the ear and result in either temporary or permanent hearing loss. The range of the hearing loss can be from a mild impairment to total deafness. Tinnitus (head noise) frequently accompanies this hearing loss and is often a more distressing condition than the actual loss of hearing. Hearing loss from repeated overstimulation by sound is cumulative over a lifetime and, when permanent, has no known medical or surgical treatment. Although a hearing loss from noise is preventable in most cases, the increasingly noisy environment of today's society increases the number of people at risk for this impairment and the resulting adverse effects on the quality of life.

The effect of noise that has received the most attention is the loss of hearing sensitivity. This hearing loss may be temporary, in which hearing sensitivity returns to pre-exposure sensitivity after a period of recovery, or it can be permanent. The principal indication of the effect of noise on hearing sensitivity is a change in threshold hearing levels. These changes are described as threshold shifts and are estimated by the comparison of threshold hearing levels measured before and after exposure to noise. Shifts that are temporary have been designated as temporary threshold shifts (TTS), and those that are permanent are called permanent threshold shifts (PTS).

Acoustic exposures hazardous enough to produce permanent loss usually produce some additional temporary change in hearing sensitivity. The determination of permanent hearing loss from noise without contamination from the temporary component requires a suitable recovery interval before this assessment is made. The recovery interval depends on the exposure and the purpose of assessment. Federal regulations for hearing conservation programs (U.S. Department of Labor, 1983) require periods of 14 hours between exposure to hazardous noise and the measurement of a person's hearing to reduce the influence of temporary loss. When hearing loss is being assessed for compensation purposes, many states require at least a month of recovery between exposure to intense noise and the final hearing measurement.

ANATOMIC AND PHYSIOLOGIC PATHOLOGY

At least two types of injury from noise have been reported—that which results from acoustic trauma and that which results from chronic noise exposure resulting in what has been called noise-induced hearing loss. Acoustic trauma is the result of exposure to short-duration sounds of high intensity, for example, a gunshot or an explosion. Acoustic trauma may result in immediate, permanent hearing loss of varying degrees. Almost all of the structures of the ear can be damaged by this exposure. In these traumatic events, the fragile structures of the inner ear, particularly the delicate sensory cells (hair cells), may be torn and disintegrate. The traumatic sound energy may also damage the middle ear, perforating the eardrum and fracturing or dislocating the ossicular bony chain. Similar traumatic effects on the auditory structures can result from blows to the head.

Traumatic hearing losses are usually the result of accidents and, therefore, are not usually preventable. Fortunately, most cases of hearing loss from noise result from a cumulative experience over a period of many years. This noise-induced hearing loss can be prevented. Exposure to moderate levels of noise may initially cause temporary hearing loss or TTS. The anatomic changes associated with TTS include subtle intracellular changes in the hair cells, vascular changes, and changes in the stiffness of the cilia of the hair cells.

Repeated exposure to sounds that cause temporary hearing loss may gradually result in permanent loss of hearing sensitivity. At this stage cochlear blood flow may be impaired, and there may be scattered hair cell damage with each exposure. As the noise experience continues, the number of damaged hair cells increases. Once a sufficient number of hair cells is lost, the nerve fibers to that region also degenerate. Degeneration of cochlear nerve fibers (eighth cranial nerve) may result in corresponding neural degeneration within the central nervous system.

Chronic exposure to moderate sounds restricted to high frequencies confines the damage in the cochlea to a relatively narrow region involved in the processing of high-frequency information. When there is a comparable exposure to low-frequency noise, the hair-cell damage is confined not only to the low-frequency region but also may spread to include the areas of the cochlea responsible for processing high-frequency information.

Noise with energy distributed over a broad frequency range, typically encountered in industrial situations, tends to produce the greatest damage in the basal region of the inner ear. This pattern of damage seems to be the consequence of the characteristics of the external and middle ear. Although the noise may be relatively flat and broad in the working environment, by the time it reaches the structures in the inner ear, it is affected by the frequency response of the external and middle ear. These structures transmit sound energies best in the frequency range between 1000 and 4000 Hz. Usually then the pattern of hearing loss clinically observed as a consequence of working in noisy industrial environments is one of high frequency, particularly in the 3000 to 6000 Hz region. When the hazardous properties of noise are measured with a sound-level meter, the sound is filtered through a network that approximates the filtering effect of the external and middle ear on the sounds that reach the inner ear. This filter is called the A scale and the units of measure for this network are called dBA.

RELATIONSHIP BETWEEN NOISE AND HEARING LOSS

Four acoustic factors have been identified as contributing to the hazards of noise in relation to hearing: the distribution of sound energy over frequency (spectrum), the overall intensity, the total duration, and the temporal pattern of exposure. Each of these factors interacts with the other three. The interaction of two of these factors, intensity and duration, is particularly important, and the effects of one of these two factors should not be considered without specifying the other. The integration of noise intensity with noise duration is the basis of the concept of noise exposure. Noise exposure is not equivalent to noise level. Exposure is defined as a noise level (decibels) for a specified duration (seconds, minutes, hours, or days).

The most widely used measurement of sound magnitude or strength is sound level, which is measured in decibels with a sound-level meter. Sound levels less than 75 dBA are considered safe regardless of the duration of the exposure. Sounds that exceed this level can be hazardous and depend on the relationship of the four acoustic properties of noise listed earlier.

The noise conditions encountered by most people vary in temporal pattern. Noise levels usually are fluctuating or intermittent. In general, the hazard posed by time-varying noise exposure is less than would be observed if the noise were continuous.

The precise relationship between the temporal pattern of exposure and hearing loss is complicated; noise spectrum and a great variety of temporal patterns must be considered. The following simplifying principle has been applied for describing the hazards of the varying noise patterns. Time-varying noises are described in terms of being equivalent in energy to steady-state noises of constant intensity of a specified duration, usually 8 hours. For example, exposure to a fluctuating noise might be identified as equivalent in energy to that experienced in an 8-hour exposure to 95 dBA.

Noises that have high peak levels for a short duration are impulsive (gunshot) or impact (hammering) noises. Important characteristics that influence impulsive and impact noises are peak level, peak duration, number of impulses experienced, and time interval between impulses. If all other properties remain the same, impulsive noise becomes more hazardous as the peak level increases. Again, if other factors are constant, the hazard from impulse and impact noises increases in proportion to the number of the impulses experienced over a period of time. When the peak levels for these transient noises are 140 dB or less, the underlying mechanism for damaging auditory structures is the same as for chronic noise exposure. When the levels of the impulse and impact noises exceed 140 dB, the damaging mechanism is that seen in acoustic trauma.

Although the potential of sounds for a hazardous effect on hearing is usually defined in terms of sound level, duration, and frequency bandwidths, several simple observations indicate a potentially hazardous sound exposure. Noise may be suspected as hazardous if the listener experiences difficulty communicating while in the noise, ringing in the ears after noise exposure, or muffled speech or a change in the quality of other sounds following the noise exposure. In the identification of sounds that can produce damage to hearing, the acoustic energy of the sound and not its source is important. When it reaches a certain level, the acoustic energy experienced by the inner ear can produce damage, regardless of whether the noise source was experienced at work, at school, in a person's home, or in a recreational facility.

AUDIOLOGIC CHARACTERISTICS

Although the pattern of hearing loss from noise exposure depends on the spectrum of the noxious noise, most people with this type of hearing loss have been affected by chronic exposure in an industrial or occupational environment. Despite the fact that there is considerable short-term variation in these environments, the long-term spectrum of the noise background is generally broad and flat. Exposure to this type of noise produces systematic audiometric progression and a recognizable pattern of hearing loss. Progression in the audiometric configuration of noise-induced hearing loss as a consequence of an increase in the number of years of exposure is illustrated in Figure 12.1. These hearing losses resulted from occupational exposure to broadband noise of approximately 100 dBA (Taylor et al, 1965).

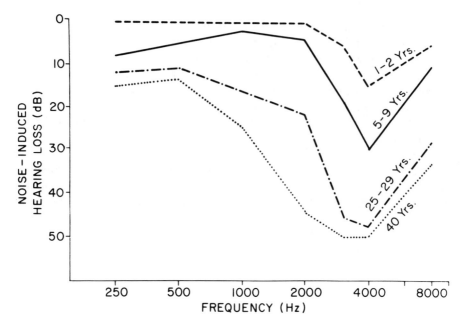

FIGURE 12.1 Audiometric pattern of hearing loss from exposure to broadband noise at sound pressure levels ranging from 95 to 100 dB as a function of the number of years worked in the noise.

(Data reprinted from Taylor et al, 1965.)

The earliest change is a slight decrease in sensitivity in the frequency range 3000 to 6000 Hz, 4000 Hz being the most affected. As the exposure continues, the hearing loss at 4000 Hz increases, but the loss is still contained in the relatively constricted range of 3000 to 6000 Hz. As the years of exposure continue to increase, the rate of change at 4000 Hz decreases, but the effects of the noise exposure spread to frequencies above 6000 and below 3000 Hz. With the spread of hearing loss, the frequencies important for speech sounds are affected and problems arise in receiving and understanding speech. It is usually at this stage that hearing difficulties first become noticeable to the person experiencing noise exposure.

Because the principal location in the auditory system of damage due to noise is the cochlea, the resulting hearing loss is sensorineural and the pattern of audiologic response is cochlear. Audiometric measurements of hearing sensitivity by bone conduction are virtually identical to those by air conduction. A person with noise-induced hearing loss shows signs of loudness recruitment, mild tone decay, and latency patterns in the auditory brainstem response consistent with the cochlear abnormality.

A hearing loss that results from chronic exposure to noise is usually binaural. Mild degrees of asymmetry are not unusual, however, particularly when there are lateralized noise sources (such as rifles) or when a worker habitually orients one ear toward the noise source (such as a truck driver, who has one ear closer than the other to the exhaust system of the engine).

Another common auditory effect of noise exposure is the development of subjective tinnitus. Subjective tinnitus is the perception of auditory sensations not audible to anyone except the person experiencing them. Tinnitus is not in and of itself a disease but is a symptom of an underlying auditory pathologic condition. A number of underlying mechanisms for the development of tinnitus secondary to noise-induced hearing loss have been proposed. Unfortunately, no completely acceptable explanation exists. Subjective tinnitus is not unique to noise exposure; it can result from a number of causes, including physical trauma, infectious diseases, and ototoxic drugs.

The sensorineural hearing loss that results from noise exposure is not progressive. When a person who experiences this hearing loss is removed from the noise environment or when the person is prevented from additional hazardous noise exposure from other sources, no additional hearing loss due to noise should occur. When additional hearing loss has been reported after removal from noise, the additional loss is usually related to another etiologic factor, such as aging.

SUSCEPTIBILITY

There can be large differences in the amount of noise-induced hearing loss measured in people with similar noise histories. Even though apparently exposed to the same noise conditions, some people can experience extreme losses in hearing whereas others retain their normal hearing sensitivity. At this point in time, it is not possible to predict a person's susceptibility to hearing loss due to noise. There does not seem to be one group of people who is susceptible and another group who is resistant to the hazards of noise. Susceptibility to noise-induced hearing loss seems to be normally distributed.

Individual variation in measured noise-induced hearing loss is due to physiologic differences both among people and within a given person at any given time. Other contributions to this variability may be inherent in audiologic measurement itself or in the methods used to measure the magnitude of noise exposure. Assessment of the noise environment is represented by a simplified average of sound energy over space and time. Individual workers in a given industrial environment or in similar occupations could very possibly experience considerably different amounts and types of noise exposure.

Several factors have been explored in an effort to explain differences in noise-induced hearing loss among individuals. These factors include the person's age, gender, skin color, drug history, and the presence of hearing loss from other causes.

Age

Two opposing notions have been proposed concerning the effects of aging and susceptibility to noise. One hypothesis is that young ears are more tender than older ears and therefore more vulnerable to the effects of noise. An opposing hypothesis is that young ears are more resilient than older ears and are, as a result, better able to withstand noise than are older ears. Although some studies have shown that there are critical stages of development during which laboratory animals are more susceptible to noise than in other stages, there is no conclusive evidence from studies of humans to show that age has an effect on susceptibility. There is also no experimental support for the frequently stated notion that working in noise toughens the ear. From the available evidence, age in and of itself does not seem to be a factor that directly influences the amount of hearing loss produced by a particular noise exposure.

Gender

In industrial situations where men and women work, audiometric surveys indicate that women, on the average, have better hearing than the men. This observation could lead one to believe that women are somehow less susceptible to the hazards of noise than men. The evidence for this condition is equivocal at best. Laboratory investigations of temporary hearing loss have not shown this gender difference. Field studies that reported men to be more vulnerable to noise than women were not controlled for other important differences in the social and occupational experience of men and women.

Women have been much less likely than men to have noisy hobbies such as hunting, automobile racing, and snowmobiling. Women in industry have been given more rest periods during the workday, resulting in interruptions of noise exposure, thereby rendering the noise environment less hazardous. Women have shown a higher absentee rate and experience less cultural and social pressures if they choose to leave a job that is uncomfortably noisy. Although it is possible that an inherent factor in the physiologic nature of the auditory system of women is responsible for less noise-induced hearing losses than among men, social factors could account for these reported measurements.

Skin Color

Reports, particularly a survey that compared the hearing of white and black workers in the southeastern United States (Royster et al, 1980), have indicated that blacks have slightly better hearing than their white counterparts. The implication is that pigmentation of the skin is also accompanied by similar pigmentation in the cochlea, which renders a person less susceptible to damage from noise. As in the case of gender differences, it is not clear whether the observed difference in hearing sensitivity is due to sociologic factors or is indeed the result of an inherent resistance related to pigmentation.

Drugs

Laboratory studies of animals have shown an apparent synergistic effect between some drugs and noise. More organic damage was observed with combined administration of drugs and noise than was observed when either of these two ototoxic agents was used alone. Investigated drugs have included aspirin, quinine, kanamycin, streptomycin, and neomycin. No definitive data have been reported demonstrating similar interactive drug and noise effects for humans. From the standpoint of hearing conservation, it is reasonable to assume a similar effect on people as on laboratory animals until there is evidence to the contrary. There have been reports of increasing susceptibility to temporary hearing loss in humans who have ingested aspirin (McFadden & Plattsmier, 1983).

Other Hearing Losses

Investigations of temporary hearing loss indicate that people with pre-existing hearing losses show less of a change in threshold hearing level from a given noise exposure than people with normal hearing. This condition also has been assumed to be true for noise-induced, permanent hearing loss even though there is an absence of investigative evidence. Because the amount of damage done by noise is related to the acoustic energy that reaches the inner ear, conductive hearing loss produced by an external or middle ear disorder renders a person less susceptible to the hazardous effects of noise. The conductive hearing loss simply serves as a hearing protector.

People with cochlear hearing losses also show less shift in hearing level than people with normal hearing exposed to similar noise levels. For a person with a cochlear abnormality, the sound that reaches the cochlea is the same as for listeners with normal hearing. However, because sensory cells are missing or nonfunctioning, not as many cells are available to become damaged resulting in additional hearing loss. There is no conclusive evidence to suggest that a person with a sensorineural hearing loss is more or less susceptible to damage from additional noise exposure.

LEGISLATION AND REGULATION

The Congress of the United States in 1970 passed the Occupational Safety and Health Act, which mandated compliance with safety regulations issued by the

Table 12.1 Permissible Noise Exposures

Duration per day (h)	Sound level (dBA slow response)
8	90
6	92
4	95
3	97
2	100
1½	102
1	105
½	110
¼ or less	115

From the Noise Standards of the Occupational Safety and Health Administration (OSHA) of the U.S. Department of Labor (1983).

Department of Labor (Public Law 91-596). This law extended regulatory activity to all industries participating in interstate commerce. From the standpoint of noise-induced hearing loss, regulations issued by the Department of Labor specified limits of noise level and duration that constitute permissible noise exposure in the occupational environment (U.S. Department of Labor, 1969). These limits are contained in Table 12.1. These noise regulations required the implementation and continuation of an effective hearing conservation program in instances in which the noise environment exceeded the specified limits. In 1983, the U.S. Department of Labor established the elements and procedures it considered to be an acceptable hearing conservation program, including noise exposure monitoring, audiometric testing, record keeping, and employee education.

Additional motivation for the establishment of industrial hearing conservation programs were statutes that provided for compensation for occupationally caused hearing loss. Worker compensation programs are principally the jurisdiction of the individual states. A survey of worker compensation statutes in 1986 (Fodor & Oleinick, 1986) indicated that all 50 states considered occupational hearing loss to be compensable. However, there is wide variation among these statutes both in the definition of compensable hearing loss and in the amount of compensation awarded. Federal regulations apply to most of the noisy industries in this country. Hearing loss prevention would be advanced if these regulations were to apply to all industry and if the regulations were adequately and evenly enforced.

HEARING CONSERVATION

The American Academy of Otolaryngology–Head and Neck Surgery lists as the important elements of an occupational hearing conservation program the following: sound surveys to assess the magnitude of hazardous noise exposure, engineering and administrative noise controls to reduce exposure, education of employers and employees about the hazards of noise and the prevention of hearing loss, hearing protection devices designed to reduce the sound energy reaching the inner ear, and audiometric evaluations for early detection of hearing loss (Osguthorpe, 1988). These are essentially the same elements described by Department of Labor regulations as the components of an effective hearing conservation program (U.S. Department of Labor, 1983).

As mentioned earlier, exposure to hazardous noise occurs in both occupational and nonoccupational settings. Hearing conservation should begin with providing information about noise-induced hearing loss. People should be aware that this hearing loss increases gradually, and once it becomes permanent is untreatable medically or surgically. Eventually the hearing loss can affect a person's ability to communicate and substantially affect that person's quality of life. Although hearing aids may assist auditory function, these aids do not restore normal hearing. People should be made aware of situations where they may be exposed to loud noise and either avoid these situations or protect themselves by using hearing protection devices.

Many potentially hazardous noise sources exist outside the occupational environment, including guns, power tools, chain saws, airplanes, farm implements, cordless telephones, toys, and household appliances. All may produce hazardous noise. A person may encounter hazardous noise levels at events such as rock-and-roll concerts, automobile races, and athletic events, which attract large and noisy crowds. Personal listening devices, such as stereo headphones and loudspeakers, also represent hazardous noise sources. Both adults and children must be aware of the risk from these exposures and how they can be managed safely.

Hearing loss due to nonoccupational noise is common, but the public generally is not aware of this hazard. Educational programs should be designed and directed toward children, parents, social groups, and professionals in influential positions, such as teachers, architects, engineers, legislators, and health care professionals, including physicians, audiologists, and speech-language pathologists. Consumers can be aided with product noise labeling. The public should have access to affordable, effective hearing protectors that are simple to use. Basic audiometric evaluations should be widely available. People who have had serious noise exposures should have access to appropriate counseling. The main objective of programs and actions designed to conserve hearing from the hazards of noise is the early detection of noise-induced damage and the interruption of its progression before it becomes an impediment to communication.

REFERENCES

Berge, E. H., Ward, W. D., Morrill, J. C., Royster, L. H. (Eds.) (1986). *Noise and Hearing Conservation Manual* (4th ed.) Akron: American Industrial Hygiene Association.

Feldman, A. S., & Grimes, C. T. (Eds.) (1985). *Hearing Conservation Industry*. Baltimore: Williams & Wilkins.

Fodor, W. J., & Oleinick, A. (1986). Workers' compensation for occupational noise-induced hearing loss: A review of science and the law, and proposed reforms. *Saint Louis University Law Journal, 30,* 703-804.

McFadden, D., & Plattsmier, H. S. (1983). Aspirin can potentiate the temporary hearing loss induced by intense sounds. *Hearing Research, 9,* 295-316.

Melnick, W. (Ed.) (1988). Noise and hearing. *Seminars in Hearing, 9,* 255-349.

National Institutes of Health (1990). Consensus Development Statement, Noise and Hearing Loss. Washington, DC: National Institutes of Health.

Noise Control Act (1972). Public Law 92-596.

Occupational Safety and Health Act (1970). Public Law 91-596.

Osguthorpe, J. D. (Ed.) (1988). Subcommittee on the Medical Aspects of Noise, Committee on Hearing and Equilibrium. Guide for conservation of hearing in noise (revised edition). Washington, DC: American Academy of Otolaryngology—Head and Neck Surgery.

Royster, L. H., Royster, J. D., & Thomas, W. G. (1980). Representative hearing levels by race and sex in North Carolina industry. *Journal of the Acoustical Society of America, 68,* 551-556.

Taylor, W., Pearson, J., Mair, A., & Burns, W. (1965). Study of noise and hearing in jute weaving. *Journal of the Acoustical Society of America, 38,* 113-120.

U.S. Department of Labor, Bureau of Labor Standards (1969). Occupational noise exposure. *Federal Register, 34,* 7946.

U.S. Department of Labor, Occupational Safety and Health Administration (1983). Occupational noise exposure: Hearing conservation amendment; final rule. *Federal Register, 48,* 9738.

SUGGESTED READINGS

Axelsson A., Dengerink H., Hellstrom P. A., & Mossberg A. M. (1993). The sound world of the child: The relationship between daily activities and hearing acuity. *Scandinavian Audiology, 22,* 117-124.

Brookhouser P. E., Worthington D. W., Kelly W. J., & Pillsbury H. C. (1992). Noise-induced hearing-loss in children. *Laryngoscope, 102,* 645-655.

Broste, S. K., Hansen, D. A., Strand, R. L., & Stueland, D. T. (1989). Hearing loss among high school farm students. *American Journal of Public Health, 79,* 619-622.

Catalano P. J., & Levin S. M. (1985). Noise-induced hearing loss and portable radios with headphones. *International Journal of Pediatric Otorhinolaryngology, 9,* 59-67.

Committee on Children, Youth, and Families (1991). Turn it down: Effects of noise on hearing loss in children and youth. Hearing Before the Select Committee on Children, Youth, and Families, House of Representatives, 102nd Congress, 1st Session. July 22, 1991, Washington.

Finitzo T. (1988). Classroom acoustics. In: F. J. Roeser & M. P. Downs (Eds.), *Auditory disorders in school children* (2nd ed.) (pp. 221-233). New York: Thieme.

Lankford J. E., & West D. M. (1993). A study of noise exposure and hearing sensitivity in a high school woodworking class. *Language, Speech and Hearing Services in Schools, 24,* 167-173.

13

Central Auditory Processing Disorders in Children and Adults

Jane A. Baran and Frank E. Musiek

Central auditory processing disorder (CAPD) is a term that has become well known not only in the field of audiology, but also in the fields of speech-language pathology, education, psychology, and in some medical specialties. Many children with learning disabilities and many adults with neurologic involvement of the auditory system are believed to have CAPDs. The area of central auditory function and dysfunction has a relatively large and rapidly growing research base in both the clinical and basic sciences. Procedures and professionals are available that can make valuable contributions to the proper identification and management of CAPDs. CAPDs are recognized as one of the many types of communication disorders of which specialists in a variety of professions should have an understanding. All people with hearing losses regardless of site of lesion (peripheral or central) can be considered at risk for CAPD.

DEFINITIONS AND SYMPTOMS

To paraphrase Efron (1985), *central auditory processing* is a popular term of postcomputer vintage. As are most new areas of study, the concept is seen differently by different professionals, making the term difficult to define. Many definitions exist; here are but a few that should provide the reader with a sense of the topic.

> Auditory processing involves attention, detection, and the identification of the signal
> . . . and the decoding of the neural message (Katz et al, 1992, p. 5).
>
> [Central auditory processing] refers to the functional role of those parts of the auditory
> system which lie within the brain itself as distinct from the cochlea and its neural
> output through the eighth cranial nerve (Efron, 1985, p. 43).

> [Central auditory processing refers to] the manipulation and utilization of sound
> signals by the central nervous system—what we do with what we hear (Lasky &
> Katz, 1983, p. 4).

More encompassing or exclusionary definitions are difficult to come by
because of the complex nature and multiple and varied facets of behavior and
neural functions that play a role in CAPD. It is important not to spend too much
time and effort searching for the perfect definition because it may never evolve,
and many other issues are more deserving of attention and work.

Although definitions of CAPD have their limitations, the symptoms associated with CAPD are sometimes quite revealing (Willeford, 1985; Musiek, 1985).
Adults and children with CAPD often have problems following complex auditory
directions and hearing in noise or poor acoustic environments. Symptoms less
frequently noted are lack of music appreciation, not hearing well on the telephone,
difficulty localizing sounds, presence of tinnitus localized in the head, inordinate
difficulty learning a foreign language, missing subtle acoustic signals, and trouble
participating in long, quickly spoken conversations.

Children in school often have difficulty with verbally based subjects such as
reading and spelling but may do well in less verbally based subjects such as
mathematics. Children with CAPD may also be easily distracted, shy, and unwilling
to ask questions in class. Some children with CAPD have documented speech and
language problems, and others do not. Moreover, some children with CAPD may
have attention deficit disorders with or without hyperactivity and vice versa. In
some children, the more prominent problem is the attention deficit, in others it is
the CAPD. Finally, learning disabilities often occur with CAPD, but not all children
with learning disabilities have auditory processing deficits. Although the focus of
the comments in this section has been on children, it should be noted that similar
problems can be (and are) experienced by adults, although the incidence appears
to be not as high.

THE BASES OF CENTRAL AUDITORY
PROCESSING DISORDERS

Neurologic insult to the central auditory nervous system is clearly one of the
bases for CAPD (Reeves, 1985). Degenerative disorders such as multiple sclerosis,
vascular problems such as strokes, mass lesions such as tumors, seizure disorders,
and normal aging all can cause CAPD in adults if the auditory tracts are affected.
Vascular problems, mass lesions, seizure disorders, and various neurologic syndromes can occur in children as well and can be the reason for CAPD. Fortunately,
these types of disorders are relatively rare in children; however, they do occur and
should not be overlooked as possible causes of CAPD. Detailed information
regarding the neurologic bases for CAPD is contained in Musiek et al (1994).

Children with learning disabilities may have two additional, more common
bases for their difficulties processing acoustic stimuli. Postmortem studies of the

brains of people with learning disabilities have revealed interesting findings that implicate the auditory system from an anatomic standpoint (Galaburda & Kemper, 1979; Galaburda et al, 1985). These studies indicated that there is a high incidence of heterotopias (nests of cells in improper locations) in the brains of people with learning disabilities. More specifically, these morphologic abnormalities are located primarily in the left hemisphere in Heschl gyrus and the planum temporale. These are known to be key auditory and language areas.

Magnetic resonance imaging (MRI) studies of children with learning disabilities have shown other areas of the brain to be smaller than in controls without learning disabilities. These include the auditory region of the corpus callosum, the insula, and a unusual symmetry of the planum temporale for the left and right sides (Hynd et al, 1990; 1991a; 1991b). If anatomic regions that involve auditory areas are different in children with learning disabilities than in normally developing children, it is reasonable to expect auditory function to be different, and it is.

Another basis for central auditory dysfunction in children with learning disabilities is the maturational lag of the central auditory system. It has been shown that myelination of the interhemispheric and intrahemispheric auditory areas continues into adolescence and beyond (Yakovlev & LeCours, 1967). It also has been shown that there are vastly different individual rates of brain maturation (Staudt et al, 1993). Hence, if one child's rate of neuromaturation is slower than that of another child, delays in the development of certain central functions such as auditory processing may be expected. This may be why, for example, some children who are 9 years of age perform more like 7-year-olds on tests of central auditory function. These differences in the maturational development of the central nervous system are likely to be the basis for the improvements over time noted in some children on tests of central auditory function.

It is likely that the bases of some of these deficits carry over into adulthood. Recently, many adults with auditory problems but with apparently normal audiograms have begun to seek additional assessment. In the past, many of these people were dismissed as overly anxious because their hearing was determined to be normal on the basis of routine peripheral auditory assessment. Fortunately, many audiologists now recognize the potential for CAPD in this population and have begun to test for it. For several years we have been assessing young adults who present with auditory problems in the presence of normal otologic and neurologic histories. Some of these individuals have been previously diagnosed as learning disabled and some have not. It is interesting to note that a number of these people do show auditory deficits when assessed with a central test battery.

Similar observations have been reported by Saunders and Haggard (1989), who coined the term *obscure auditory dysfunction* to describe the problems of a group of healthy people with auditory problems but normal audiograms. Given our clinical experience and intuitions, we believe that there are a number of people who in fact experience "real" auditory deficits despite the fact that their audiograms are normal. In some of these people, the basis of the problem may be emotional or psychological. In another small segment, the basis may be some type of subclinical compromise of the peripheral hearing mechanism. However, in a large number of these people the deficits may be centrally mediated.

A final factor to consider in discussing the bases for CAPD is peripheral hearing loss. A number of studies have demonstrated an alteration of the central auditory nervous system subsequent to peripheral hearing loss. Auditory deprivation secondary to peripheral hearing loss has been shown to result in transynaptic degeneration of the brainstem auditory neurons and changes in the tonotopicality of the auditory cortex (Morest & Bohne, 1983; Schwaber et al, 1993). Given these findings, it is reasonable to expect that central auditory compromise may accompany clinically significant peripheral hearing loss. The assessment of central auditory function and dysfunction in the presence of peripheral hearing loss presents a challenge, and interpretations of test findings must be made with extreme caution; however, professionals must be aware of the clinical implications of such data for the assessment and management of a client with a hearing loss.

ASSESSMENT OF THE CLIENT WITH A CENTRAL AUDITORY PROCESSING DISORDER

Assessment of central auditory processing represents a relatively new clinical arena for audiologists. The impetus was provided by a landmark investigation conducted in Italy in the early to mid-1950s. Bocca et al (1954) used a low-pass filtered speech test to assess central auditory function and dysfunction in a group of patients with lesions of the temporal lobe. Their research was motivated by a desire to document auditory difficulties in patients who presented with auditory problems that were not supported by routine peripheral auditory assessments. Convinced that auditory deficits were present, these researchers set their sights on developing a test that would document these difficulties. To do so they administered their low-pass filtered speech test to a number of patients with confirmed temporal lobe lesions and found that word recognition scores tended to be depressed in the ear contralateral to the lesion. Since that investigation, a number of developments have occurred that have led to more sophisticated and sensitive tests.

We will not be able to review all of the tests that are used in CAPD assessments. Many tests are available, and often one test is modified in a variety of ways depending on the intuitions and clinical experience of the audiologist. The tests, however, can be classified into five categories. What follows is a brief discussion of the underlying rationale for each category and a description of a representative test (or in some cases two or more tests) so that the reader may develop an appreciation of each test category and its potential application. A list of some of the commonly used tests of central auditory function along with a brief description of test parameters and a reference for each is provided in Table 13.1. Comprehensive coverage of the topic is contained in Baran and Musiek (1991).

Low Redundancy Speech Tests

Low redundancy speech tests use distorted speech materials as the stimuli. The speech stimuli can be nonsense syllables, monosyllabic words, multisyllabic words, or sentences that have been subjected to frequency, temporal, or spectral distortion. An example is the compressed speech test (Beasley et al, 1972a; 1972b). In the original version of this test, the word lists from the Northwestern University Auditory Test Number 6 (Tillman & Carhart, 1966) were compressed by means of a method of electromechanical time compression introduced by Fairbanks et al (1954). The words were compressed according to a number of compression ratios ranging from 0 to 70 percent in 10 percent intervals. Clinically, the most commonly used compression ratio appears to be 60 percent. The rationale for use of this particular compression ratio is that normal performance tends to decline gradually as the compression ratio increases from 0 to 60 percent but then drops off dramatically at 70 percent compression to the point where performance by a normally hearing listener is quite compromised. The compression of the signal results in both temporal and spectral distortion of the original words.

The stimuli are presented at a 40 dB sensation level (SL) in relation to the speech recognition threshold (SRT), and the client is asked to repeat each word presented. Clients are encouraged to guess when unsure of a response. A total of 50 items are presented to each ear and percentage-correct identification scores are derived for each ear. Scores below 82 percent correct for either ear are considered abnormal by our clinic's norms for adults.

A number of investigators have evaluated the sensitivity of low redundancy speech tests to compromise of the central auditory nervous system. A comprehensive listing of these investigations is beyond the scope of this chapter, but such information can be found in Baran and Musiek (1991). The collective results of numerous investigations have shown that monaural low redundancy speech tests are moderately sensitive to lesions of the central auditory nervous system and are more likely to be affected by lesions that involve the auditory areas of the cortex as opposed to lesions lower in the auditory system or in the interhemispheric fibers.

Dichotic Speech Tests

Dichotic speech tests use speech materials that are presented to both ears in a dichotic manner. The speech stimuli presented to the two ears differ in terms of their acoustic properties, and attempts are made to carefully align the onsets of the two stimuli. A popular dichotic speech test is the dichotic digits test (Musiek, 1983). In this test the numbers from 1 to 10 (excluding 7) are presented dichotically to the clients. Both single-digit and double-digit versions of the test are available, but the double-digit version tends to be used more frequently, especially with adult clients. In this version of the test, four digits (two to each ear) are presented in a dichotic manner to the two ears of a client and he or she is asked to repeat all

Table 13.1 Behavioral Tests Used in the Assessment of Central Auditory Processing Disorders*

Test	Stimulus	Mode	Onset	Result	Reference
Compressed speech	Monosyllabic words	Monaural	Not applicable	Percent correct	Beasley et al (1972a, b)
Low-pass filtered speech	Monosyllabic words[†]	Monaural	Not applicable	Percent correct	Willeford (1976)
Synthetic sentence index with ipsilateral competition	Third-order sentence approximations with a story as competition	Monaural	Not applicable	Percent correct	Jerger & Jerger (1974)
Dichotic digits	Digits (1 to 10, not 7)	Dichotic	Simultaneous	Percent correct	Musiek (1983)
Staggered spondaic words	Spondees	Dichotic	Staggered, overlapping	Percent correct	Katz (1962)
Dichotic CVs	Consonant–vowel combinations	Dichotic	Simultaneous or delayed	Percent correct	Berlin et al (1972)
Dichotic sentences	Third-order sentence approximations	Dichotic	Simultaneous	Percent correct	Fifer et al (1983)
Synthetic sentence index with contralateral competition	Third-order sentence approximations with a story as competition	Dichotic	Not applicable	Percent correct	Jerger & Jerger (1974)
Competing sentences	Sentences	Dichotic	Simultaneous	Percent correct	Willeford (1976)
Frequency pattern sequences	Sequences of three tonal stimuli	Monaural	Not applicable	Percent correct	Pinheiro & Ptacek (1971)
Auditory duration patterns	Sequences of three tonal stimuli[‡]	Monaural	Not applicable	Percent correct	Musiek et al (1990)

Table 13.1 *Continued*

Test	Stimulus	Mode	Onset	Result	Reference
Rapidly alternating speech perception	Sentences	Binaural	Alternating segments (300 msec)	Percent correct	Willeford (1976)
Binaural fusion	Spondees**	Binaural	Simultaneous	Percent correct	Willeford (1976)
Masking level difference	Pulsed pure tone in noise	Binaural/diotic	Simultaneous	dB difference	Olsen et al (1976)

*The descriptions presented represent the test parameters that appear to be most common in clinical use. There are a number of variations for many of these tests. Whenever attempting to interpret test results, it would be prudent to determine the parameters used by the tester because different parameters may affect normative data.

†The stimuli are passed through low bandpass filter with a 500-Hz cutoff frequency and an 18 dB per octave rejection rate.

‡The stimuli consist of long (500 msec) and short (250 msec) pure tones of a constant frequency (1000 Hz) in the following six sequences (LLS, LSS, LSL, SSL, SLL, and SLS).

**The stimuli are passed through a low bandpass filter (500–700 Hz) and a high bandpass filter (1900–2100 Hz). The low bandpass filtered information is presented to one ear and the high bandpass filtered information to the other ear. The order of presentation may then be reversed.

numbers heard. The test stimuli are presented to the client at 50 dB SL in relation to SRT, and percentage-correct scores are derived for each ear. For adults, the lower cutoff for normal performance is 90 percent correct for each ear.

In an earlier investigation of dichotic speech perception, Kimura (1961a, 1961b) documented depressed scores in the ear contralateral to the hemisphere that was compromised by a confirmed central nervous system abnormality. This lesion effect was found unless the left hemisphere was compromised; in that case, either contralateral or bilateral ear deficits were noted. These findings led to the development of a theory about the processing of speech under dichotic conditions that has done much to advance our knowledge of normal auditory function and increase our ability to detect the presence of central auditory dysfunction. It is well known that the auditory system has both ipsilateral and contralateral pathways that connect the cochleae to the auditory reception areas of each hemisphere. There is also evidence to suggest that the fibers in the contralateral pathways are more numerous and stronger than those of the ipsilateral pathways and that under conditions of dichotic stimulation the ipsilateral pathways are suppressed. Therefore, if deficits are noted in one ear, then either a lesion in the auditory areas of the contralateral hemisphere is indicated or a compromise of the interhemispheric pathways may exist. Such deficits have been documented extensively in the literature for a number of different dichotic tests (Baran & Musiek, 1991).

Dichotic speech tests have proved to be useful in the assessment of the development of the auditory nervous system. Myelination of the auditory system is not complete until adolescence. Given dichotic stimulation and the fact that the interhemispheric fibers are the last to develop, it is not uncommon to note depressed left ear scores relative to right ear scores for linguistically loaded stimuli in young children (Musiek et al, 1994).

As a child matures, left ear scores tend to improve noticeably, whereas minimal (or no) changes are noted in right ear scores because these scores tend to be similar to those of adults even at relatively young ages. Comparison of test scores with age-appropriate norms can provide insights into the extent of maturational delay a child is experiencing. Moreover, periodic re-evaluation over time may help to identify maturational lags in development as opposed to more static deficits.

Temporal Patterning Tasks

Tests that involve temporal patterning tasks involve the presentation of sequences of nonspeech stimuli to one ear at a time. The stimuli vary along some parameter such as frequency (pitch), and when the stimuli are presented, the client is asked to describe each sequence heard. Because the stimuli are nonspeech in nature, the assumption is that the acoustic envelope of the stimulus sequence is initially processed in the right hemisphere and that communication between the two hemispheres occurs via the interhemispheric pathways since a verbal response is required of the client and necessitates involvement of the left hemisphere. Because processing occurs in both hemispheres, a lesion in either hemisphere or of the interhemispheric fibers is likely to cause bilaterally depressed scores. For this reason, an audiologist may elect to conduct testing in the soundfield or diotically with headphones.

A representative test that involves temporal patterning tasks is the frequency patterns test (Pinheiro & Ptacek, 1971). The test was originally developed by Pinheiro and Ptacek and subsequently modified to consist of a total of 60 test items plus a number of practice items. Each test sequence contains three tone bursts composed of high (1122 Hz) and low (880 Hz) frequencies. The sequences were constructed so that one of the tone bursts in each sequence differs in frequency from that of the other two tone bursts. This allows the generation of a total of six different tone sequences (HHL, HLL, HLH, LLH, LHH, and LHL). Each of the tones has a 10 msec rise-and-fall time and a duration of 150 msec. The interval between the tones in each sequence is held constant at 200 msec.

Thirty items are presented to each ear at 50 dB SL in relation to SRT and the client is asked to describe each pattern verbally. If the client is unable to describe the patterns, an alternative method of responding may be attempted (humming, gesturing). Use of an alternative method, however, affects the test results and their potential interpretation because nonverbal responses do not require the verbal processing activities of the left hemisphere. A number of practice items are administered and a percentage-correct score is obtained for each ear (unless a soundfield or binaural presentation is used). Normal adult performance is 75 percent correct or better in the identification of the sequences if a verbal response is required.

Research with pattern tests has shown that people with lesions in either hemisphere or of the interhemispheric pathways have difficulty verbally describing the patterns. For the most part, bilateral deficits are noted on this test because some processing of the stimuli occurs in both hemispheres, and the interhemispheric pathways must be intact to allow for communication between the two hemispheres if a verbal report is required. Temporal patterning tasks are highly sensitive to cerebral lesions and to compromise of the interhemispheric auditory pathways; however, they are considerably less sensitive to brainstem compromise (Baran and Musiek, 1991).

Binaural Interaction Tests

The tests discussed thus far are most sensitive to compromise of the higher auditory pathways, but they can be affected by brainstem lesions. The reverse is true of binaural interaction tests. Although it is true that deficits may be noted if compromise of the higher auditory centers is present, the nature of the tasks in binaural interaction tests is such that deficits are typically not seen unless extensive and strategically positioned compromise is present. The tests that fall into this group are not nearly as homogeneous as those that have been discussed thus far.

Test stimuli can consist of either speech or nonspeech stimuli and can be presented in a dichotic or alternating ear type of test paradigm. For example, one version of a rapidly alternating speech perception test (Willeford, 1976) alternates 300 msec segments of sentences between the two ears. The integrity of the segments presented to either ear alone is so degraded that a person with normal hearing is unlikely to be able to identify much more than 10 to 20 percent of the sentences. However, when the alternating information is presented to both ears, recognition improves and the client is largely unaware that pieces of information are missing from the stimuli presented to each ear. It is at the level of the brainstem that information from the two ears is combined or fused as it is at this level that the major crossover of auditory fibers from one side of the head to the other side occurs. If this crossover is compromised, deficits on this test are expected.

A second binaural interaction test is the masking level difference (MLD) test. For this test, a signal (either a pulsed low frequency pure tone or a spondee) is presented diotically to the two ears in the presence of a noise source (either white noise or speech noise). Two thresholds are then established—one in which both the stimulus and the noise are in phase between the two ears (S_oN_o) and one in which either the stimulus ($S_{\pi}N_o$) or the noise (S_oN_{π}) is presented 180° out of phase between the two ears. In people with normal central auditory systems the threshold established in either of the latter two conditions is usually lower (ie, more sensitive) than the threshold in the first condition, demonstrating a phenomenon known as release from masking. The second threshold is subtracted from the first to establish a difference score (in dB) which is compared with normative values. Clinically, we use a 500 Hz pulsed tone with an on-and-off rate of 200 msec/200 msec. The pulsed tone is presented in the presence of a broad-band noise presented at a constant level of 60 dB hearing level (HL). The pulsed tone is varied in 2 dB increments and a threshold is established in both the S_oN_o and the $S_{\pi}N_o$ conditions. Differences of greater than 6 dB are considered abnormal for our test parameters.

As discussed earlier, these tests are more sensitive to compromise at the level of the brainstem than to cerebral lesions; however, they can be affected by cortical involvement in some patients. Compromise of the interhemispheric pathways is not likely to affect performance on these tests (Baran & Musiek, 1991).

Electrophysiologic Tests

Electrophysiologic tests have become increasingly more popular since the early 1970s. These tests are often referred to as auditory evoked potentials. The underlying premise of these tests is that electrical potentials generated within the brain in response to an auditory stimulus can be recorded, separated from the ongoing electrical activity of the brain, and measured. An acoustic signal is delivered to one or both ears, and electrical potentials are measured from electrodes placed at various positions on the client's scalp. The number and locations of the electrodes vary according to the response being elicited and the preferences of the tester. In addition, a number of other test parameters are varied according to the potential being elicited and the preferences of the tester. These parameters include the number of responses averaged, the filter settings used to exclude unwanted random brain activity, the polarity of the acoustic signal, and so forth.

Table 13.2 lists these stimulus and acquisition parameters and some commonly used specifications. A brief description of three of the more popular responses follows. There are, however, a number of additional potentials that have been used clinically or are currently being investigated that are not discussed herein. Some of these potentials (eg, mismatch negativity) may hold considerable clinical promise, but as of now, they are used much more frequently as research procedures than routine clinical assessment procedures. Additional information on electrophysiologic testing is contained in Hall (1992).

Auditory Brainstem Response

The auditory brainstem response (ABR) is a robust potential that typically occurs within the first 10 msec after a stimulus (click or tone pip) is presented. Because these potentials are small and often embedded in the random electrical activity of the brain, a number of trials or sweeps is required to detect the presence of the response. As can be seen in Figure 13.1, a number of positive peaks in the waveform suggest electrical activity in response to the auditory stimuli. A number of measurements are taken and compared with norms to determine if the waveform recorded represents a normal response to the eliciting stimuli or is an abnormality that suggests dysfunction within the auditory nervous system. As indicated in Figure 13.1, these measurements include the absolute latencies of waves I, III, and V; the interwave latency differences for waves I through III, III through V, and I through V; and the amplitude ratio between waves V and I. Not shown in this figure, but also derived, is the interear difference between the absolute latency of wave V of one ear compared with the other.

The ABR has been shown to be highly sensitive to compromise of the acoustic nerve. Abnormalities also have been documented for a variety of disorders that have compromised the auditory areas of the lower brainstem (eg, tumors, vascular disorders, demyelinating disease) (Hall, 1992; Musiek et al, 1994).

Middle Latency Response

The middle latency response (MLR) can be evoked with a click stimulus or a tonal stimulus. The response in a person with a normal auditory system should occur within a time window of 10 to 70 msec after presentation of the stimulus (Figure 13.2 on page 428). The response is presumed to be generated by activity high in the auditory system (subcortex and cortex). The MLR is somewhat more variable than the ABR, which makes interpretation more difficult. Because of the

Table 13.2 Stimulus and Acquisition Parameters Commonly Used in the Derivation of the Auditory Brainstem Response (ABR), the Middle Latency Response (MLR), the Auditory Late Response (ALR), and the Auditory Cognitive Potential (P3)*

Parameter	ABR	MLR	ALR	P3
Stimulus	Click	Click	Tone burst	Tone burst
Duration	100 μsec	100 μsec	40 msec	40 msec
Rise-and-fall time	Not applicable	Not applicable	10 msec	10 msec
Plateau	Not applicable	Not applicable	20 msec	20 msec
Frequency	Broadband	Broadband	1000 Hz	2000 Hz (rare)/1000 Hz (frequent)
Rate	<20/second	<10/second	<1/second	<1/second
Polarity	Rarefaction	Condensation	Rarefaction	Rarefaction
Intensity	70–90 dB nHL[†]	70–80 dB nHL	70–80 nHL	70–80 nHL
Presentation	Monaural	Monaural	Monaural	Monaural
Transducer	Phone/insert receiver	Phone/insert receiver	Phone/insert receiver	Phone/insert receiver
Analysis time	10 msec	100 msec	500 msec	800 msec
Amplification	×100,000	×75,000	×50,000	×50,000
Sensitivity	25 μV	50 μV	100 μV	100 μV
Filters	15–3000 Hz	20–3000 Hz	1–30 Hz	1–30 Hz
Electrodes-active	Fz-A1[‡]	C3-A1, C4-A2	C3-A1, C4-A2	Cz-A1, Cz-A2
Electrode-ground	Ac[‡]	Fpz	Fpz	Fpz
Sweeps (no. of responses averaged)	2000	1000	300	300**

*The specifications listed are those used for neurodiagnostic purposes and are intended to provide a representation of some commonly used parameters. Virtually all of these parameters can be and often are modified. It is important that one determine the parameters used because different parameters have different effects on the response and its interpretation (Hall, 1992).

[†]nHL, normal hearing level

[‡]A1 is used to refer to the mastoid or earlobe ipsilateral to the ear receiving the stimulus (ie, A1 if the left ear is stimulated and A2 if the right ear is stimulated). Ac refers to an earlobe or mastoid placement on the side contralateral to the ear receiving the stimulus. The other abbreviations (eg, Fz) refer to standard electrode placements specified in the 10–20 electrode system of the international federation (Jasper, 1958).

**Typically, 80 to 85% of averaged responses are elicited by the frequent tone, whereas 20 to 15% of the averages are for presentations of the rare tone.

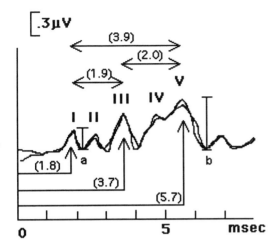

FIGURE 13.1
A normal ABR tracing and its replication showing the presence of waves I through V. Latency measurements for waves I, III, and V are indicated below the tracings; interwave latencies for waves I to III, III to V, and I to V are indicated by arrows and the associated values above the tracings. The line markers above *a* and *b* indicate peak to trough measurements used to derive the amplitudes of waves I and V. Actual amplitude measurements are not specified.

variability of the response, intrasubject comparisons are often advocated. Two negative potentials (Na and Nb) and two positive potentials (Pa and Pb) are often observed. Clinically significant findings include the absence of Pa, an extended latency for Pa, an amplitude difference for Na-Pa of greater than 50 percent for waveforms derived from the right ear and the left ear (ear effect), and an amplitude difference of greater than 50 percent for Na-Pa as measured over two corresponding hemispheric electrode sites (eg, C3 versus C4) with the stimulus presented to the same ear (electrode effect). Abnormalities have been demonstrated in patients with a variety of pathologic conditions that have compromised subcortical as well as cortical structures (Hall, 1992; Musiek et al, 1994).

Late Auditory Evoked Response

The late auditory evoked response can be elicited by a variety of auditory stimuli; the most common is a pure tone. The generators of the late potentials are presumed to be cortical sites, and a negative potential (N1) and a positive potential (P2) are noted. In addition to these potentials, which require no active participation from the client, an additional potential can be derived if the client is asked to attend to a stimulus that differs in some noticeable way from a second stimulus. Usually the stimuli are presented in what is referred to as an oddball paradigm in which one stimulus is presented frequently (eg, a 1000 Hz tone) and a second stimulus is presented infrequently (eg, a 2000 Hz tone). The client is asked to ignore the frequent stimulus and to count the number of occurrences of the infrequent, or rare, stimulus. The responses to the two different stimuli (frequent and rare) are then averaged in two different memory stores. The frequent tracing is the same as that discussed above.

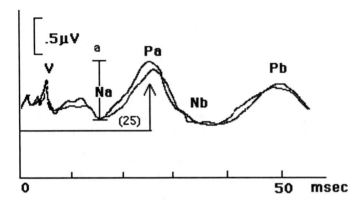

FIGURE 13.2 A normal MLR and its replication showing the presence of two negative potentials (Na and Nb) and two positive potentials (Pa and Pb). Also shown is wave V from the ABR. The latency of Pa is indicated below the tracings; the line marker below *a* indicates the peak to trough measurement that would be used to derive the Pa-Na amplitude. The actual amplitude is not specified.

In the rare tracing, however, an additional positive potential (P3) and two negative potentials (N2 and N3) are noted (Figure 13.3). The P3 has been shown to be abnormal in a number of patients with pathologic conditions, including patients with frank neurologic impairment involving the auditory areas of the cortex and a variety of psychological disorders such as schizophrenia and dementia of the Alzheimer type (Hall, 1992; Musiek et al, 1994). The P3 is also often abnormal in elderly people. The morphology of the waveforms is so variable, however, that questions have been raised regarding its reliability. Therefore, the test results must be interpreted by an experienced clinician, and care must be taken not to overinterpret test results. As with the MLR, intrasubject differences are often more diagnostically significant than intersubject differences.

Use of a Test Battery

A number of tests can be used to assess central auditory function. The audiologist selects from among the available tests those tests that will provide the most information regarding a given client's dysfunction. For example, if a cortical lesion is suspected, the administration of the ABR test is not indicated unless it is needed to document peripheral auditory sensitivity. Tests such as dichotic digits and possibly the MLR or late potentials should provide more valuable information. If, on the other hand, a brainstem lesion is suspected, use of the ABR, MLD, and other tests sensitive to dysfunction at this level would be prudent. Table 13.3

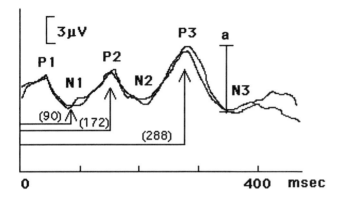

FIGURE 13.3 A normal late auditory evoked potential and auditory cognitive potential response. The tracing depicts a patient's response to infrequent stimuli (a rare tracing), and its replication. Three positive peaks (P1, P2, P3) are noted, as are three negative peaks (N1, N2, N3). Latency measurements are indicated below the tracings for N1, P2, and P3. The line marker below *a* indicates the peak to trough measurement that would be used to derive the amplitude of P3. The actual amplitude is not specified.

provides information regarding the potential sensitivity of a number of tests that fall within the various test categories reviewed thus far.

A second principle to be considered in the selection of a test of central auditory function is the possible influence of peripheral hearing loss. The presence of a peripheral hearing loss can make interpretation of results of tests of central function difficult, if not impossible. The audiologist, however, may be able to minimize the confounding factors associated with peripheral hearing loss if care is taken to select those tests less likely to be affected by end organ involvement. For example, some tests, such as auditory duration patterns and dichotic digits, are less likely to be affected by hearing loss than other tests (eg, frequency patterns or dichotic consonants–vowels). These factors should be taken into consideration in the selection of tests for use with people with peripheral hearing losses.

Finally, the age appropriateness of the tests under consideration should be evaluated. Most of the tests mentioned in this chapter were originally designed to test adults with neurologic involvement. Only later were norms developed for many of these tests for use with children. Unfortunately, many of these norms remain unpublished. It is critical that age-appropriate norms be used whenever assessing children. If published norms are not available, normative data should be established locally before clinical use of any test is implemented.

Serious consideration should be given to the use of tests designed specifically for use with children. Tests such as the Pediatric Speech Intelligibility Test (Jerger

Table 13.3 Predictions for Expected Results for Common Tests for Lesions at Various Sites Along the Central Auditory Nervous System

Test Classification	Low Brainstem	High Brainstem	Auditory Cortex	Interhemispheric Pathways
Monaural low redundancy speech tests	Ipsilateral ear deficit (2)	Contralateral ear deficit (2) Bilateral deficits (2) Ipsilateral ear deficit (1)	Contralateral ear deficit (3)	No deficit (3)
Dichotic speech tests	Ipsilateral ear deficit (2)	Contralateral ear deficit (2) Bilateral deficits (2) Ipsilateral ear deficit (2)	Contralateral ear deficit (3) Bilateral deficits (1)	Contralateral ear deficit (3)
Temporal patterning tasks	Ipsilateral ear deficit (1)	Contralateral ear deficit (1) Bilateral deficits (1) Ipsilateral ear deficit (1)	Bilateral deficits (3)	Bilateral deficits (3)
Binaural interaction tests	Binaural deficit* (2)	Little or no deficit (3)	Little or no deficit (3)	Little or no deficit (3)
Phase tests (eg, MLD)	Binaural deficit* (3)	Little or no deficit (3)	Little or no deficit (3)	Little or no deficit (3)
Auditory brainstem response[†]	Ipsilateral abnormality (3) Bilateral abnormalities (1) Contralateral abnormality (1)	Contralateral abnormality (2) Bilateral abnormalities (1) Ipsilateral abnormality (1)	No deficit (3)	No deficit (3)
Middle latency response[†]	Ipsilateral ear effect (1)	Contralateral ear effect (2) Bilateral ear effects (1) Ipsilateral ear effect (1)	Abnormality at electrode nearest pathology (2) Contralateral ear effect (2)	Little or no deficit (3)
Late response (N1 and P2)[†]	Ipsilateral ear effect (1)	Contralateral ear effect (1) Bilateral ear effects (1) Ipsilateral ear effect (1)	Abnormality at electrode nearest lesion (2) Contralateral ear effect (2)	Little or no deficit (3)
P3 response[†]	Same as late response	Same as late response	Nonlocalizing abnormality (2)	Little or no deficit (3)

Key: 3, high probability of occurrence; 2, moderate probability of occurrence; 1, low probability of occurrence; MLD, masking level difference.

Binaural is used in this context because both ears receive segments of the stimulus and only one score is derived.

[†]Abnormal results may be found for one or more of the indices discussed in the text. Therefore, the use of the singular form in this context does not imply that only one abnormality may exist. It indicates that the abnormal findings may exist.

& Jerger, 1984) and the SCAN: A Screening Test for Auditory Processing Disorders (Keith, 1986) have been specifically developed for, and the norms derived from groups of children. This increases the likelihood that the stimulus items used in the tests will be familiar to young children and within their receptive vocabularies—a situation that may not exist for some of the other tests that were originally designed for use with adults.

MANAGEMENT OF THE CLIENT WITH A CENTRAL AUDITORY PROCESSING DISORDER

Identification of a CAPD is only the first step in the management of a client with such a disorder. As with other hearing disorders, the first action is referral to an appropriate medical specialist if neurologic compromise is suspected. Once any significant neurologic involvement has been managed or ruled out, a variety of intervention strategies may be used. Selection of the strategy (strategies) of choice depends on the nature and extent of the CAPD, the age of the client, and his or her communicative needs. For some people, simply uncovering the deficit and identifying any problems that may be encountered educationally, occupationally, and socially, may be sufficient.

A case of a bright young woman enrolled in a master's degree program immediately comes to mind and provides evidence of the importance of diagnosis and the reassurance that a client receives in simply knowing a CAPD exists. This young woman reportedly struggled with auditory information all her life and was often accused of being "dumb," uncooperative, and lazy throughout most of her elementary and secondary schooling. She struggled to overcome her auditory deficits and managed to succeed in school in spite of her difficulties, although her self-esteem suffered. After a CAPD was diagnosed, compensation strategies were explained to the client, which she could use in processing auditory information as needed. Interestingly, however, the diagnosis itself appeared to be more valuable and helpful to this woman than any of the strategies offered to her. She was openly relieved and appreciative to learn that the cause of her difficulties had been identified. Her self-esteem was restored and she was willing to continue to put effort into her studies and ultimately to obtain her master's degree.

For many people, particularly those whose CAPD is identified later in life, the focus of intervention is likely to be on helping the person identify strategies to overcome any auditory difficulties. Depending on the specific nature of the deficits, these strategies may include preferential seating, the use of speechreading procedures, and many other communication enhancement strategies that are often suggested to people with peripheral hearing impairments. In some cases, specific educational or occupational alternatives are suggested. For example, a modification or waiver of a language requirement may be recommended for a postsecondary student who has difficulty learning a foreign language. Other recommendations for students with a variety of auditory complaints may include use of a note-taking or tutoring service, the tape-recording of lectures for review, enrollment in a specific section of a course when more than one option is available, and the exploration of personal learning styles and time management skills. Use of a personal FM system may be recommended if the client experiences severe difficulty listening in noise.

For children and some young adults, a more aggressive rehabilitative effort is likely to be indicated. Support for an aggressive approach to remediation can be found in recent developments in the field of neuroscience. Key concepts underlying this support are neural plasticity, maturation, stimulation, and long-term memory potentiation. Evidence exists to indicate that the young brain maintains a level of functional plasticity for a certain amount of time (Lenneberg, 1967). Although this time of "potential brain plasticity" has not been established, it does appear that there is a critical period during which functional changes are more likely to occur. Thus, timely and aggressive management is indicated so that the rehabilitative effort may take advantage of the optimal conditions for change. Moreover, the basis for this functional change appears to be stimulation and experience (Akoi & Siekevitz, 1988).

Stimulation activates specific neural pathways that are reinforced on repeated stimulation. Bliss and Lomo (1973) demonstrated that repetitive stimulation increases the strength of neural transmissions at many of the synapses within the central nervous system. Particularly important was the finding that this type of potentiation occurs in two regions of the brain that are important structures in the mediation of memory (ie, the hippocampus and the amygdala) (Gustafsson & Wigstrom, 1988). It therefore appears that early repetitive stimulation may increase the likelihood of positive changes because stimulation enables brain plasticity, and continued stimulation may in fact extend the critical period. If such stimulation does not occur in a timely manner, positive changes are less likely to be realized because neural pathways that are not stimulated may lose their potency with time.

The reception, processing, and comprehension of spoken messages is a complex activity that involves both perceptual and cognitive skills. Understanding requires the coordination of diverse and divergent skills and knowledge. A person needs to be able to process the basic acoustic information on a perceptual level and then to segment the acoustic stream of sounds into smaller constituent units. He or she must have a receptive command of the vocabulary being spoken and have achieved a level of language competence sufficient to process the syntactic and semantic structures represented within the spoken message. In addition, a person must possess adequate general knowledge and appropriate metacognitive skills. To successfully process a spoken message, one must be able to monitor and regulate attention, memory, learning, and language. A breakdown at one or more of these levels can impair language processing in the auditory modality. Efforts should be made to isolate the deficits whenever possible so that therapy can be tailored to the root of the problem. For example, the observation that a client has difficulty understanding speech in noisy environments may imply a deficit in the basic auditory processing of the temporal and spectral features contained within the speech segment. However, it may also represent a deficit in a metacognitive skill (eg, the ability to regulate attention) or a language-based problem (eg, a receptive vocabulary deficit or a syntactic component deficit).

With appropriate testing, it may be possible to determine the level (or levels) of breakdown in a given client. If a client has a problem with the syntactic component, then language therapy is indicated. If on the other hand, no speech and language problems are identified through testing, then more traditional audiologic interventions may be indicated (eg, efforts to modify the acoustic environment or selection and fitting of an FM system, and so forth). In many cases it may not be possible to isolate all of these areas. In these cases, intervention may be directed toward each level of potential breakdown. Often the procedures are complementary and serve to maximize the rehabilitative efforts. For example, an FM system provided to assist a client in processing speech in noisy environments may also serve to help direct and maintain attention to auditory stimuli.

A comprehensive review of management strategies is beyond the scope of this book. However, many traditional speech and language management procedures may be implemented in the remediation of the auditory processing problems of people with CAPD. The key to successful management of a person with a CAPD is the identification of the problem and tailoring of recommendations and management to the individual client's needs and skills. There is no one program that works for everyone. By far the best and most comprehensive program is one that is generated through a collaborative approach among the speech-language pathologist, the educator, the audiologist, and other involved health care professionals working together to design a program tailored to meet the needs of the individual client. Additional resources can be found in Bacon (1992) and Chermak and Musiek (1992).

CASE PRESENTATION

The following case is presented to demonstrate the value of CAPD testing and to elucidate several of the principles and considerations discussed in this chapter.

History

A 71-year-old man awoke one morning with a right-sided headache that he described as the worst in his life. The headache waxed and waned over the next 2 days. On the third morning, the patient awoke feeling well and attended to his woodstove before returning to bed. He later awoke with acute left hemiparesis and some slurring of his speech. He was admitted to the hospital where a working diagnosis of a cerebrovascular accident (CVA) was rendered. An initial computed tomographic (CT) scan on the day of admission was read as normal. However, a

CT scan obtained 5 days after admission confirmed the diagnosis of CVA and revealed a large area of edema in the distribution of the right middle cerebral artery, specifically in the anterior internal capsule. In addition, there was a mass effect associated with the edema with effacement of the anterior horn of the right lateral ventricle. The patient's previous medical history was unremarkable with the exception of a myocardial infarction sustained 2 years before the current medical condition. The patient had been a moderately heavy consumer of cigarettes until about 15 years before the CVA.

Audiologic Findings

The patient underwent audiologic testing during his hospital stay. Results of a routine peripheral auditory assessment revealed a mild to moderate bilaterally symmetric hearing loss (Figure 13.4). Word recognition scores at suprathreshold levels were excellent bilaterally (96 percent for the right ear, 92 percent for the left ear).

A number of behavioral tests* were administered, and the results are shown in Figure 13.5. Bilateral (but asymmetric) deficits were noted on both monaural low redundancy tests (compressed speech and low-pass filtered speech), with left ear scores being more depressed than right ear scores. On two dichotic speech tests (dichotic rhymes and dichotic digits), severe left ear deficits were evident, whereas on two temporal patterning tasks (frequency patterns and duration patterns) bilateral deficits were noted.

Comments

Data from tests of central auditory function of people with peripheral hearing losses must be interpreted with caution. However, the pattern of test results in this case strongly implicates central as well as peripheral involvement. It is important to note in this case that a clinically significant hearing loss is present in both ears. However, the loss is bilaterally symmetric, and word recognition scores are equivalent. Given these findings, the asymmetric results noted on the dichotic speech tests and the monaural low redundancy speech tests are not likely to be explained by peripheral hearing loss. The peripheral hearing loss may be the basis

---

*Except for the dichotic rhyme test, these tests are described earlier in this chapter. In the dichotic rhyme test, two monosyllabic words that are identical with the exception of the first consonants (eg, dig and pig), are presented simultaneously to the two ears and the client is asked to repeat any words perceived. The nature of the task is such that people with normal hearing perceive only one word. Normal performance on the test is approximately 50 percent correct identification for both ears with a slight right ear advantage typically noted. The test, which is still largely experimental, has been shown to be sensitive to compromise of the interhemispheric auditory pathways (Musiek et al, 1989). Investigative efforts are underway to determine the sensitivity of the procedure to cerebral lesions.

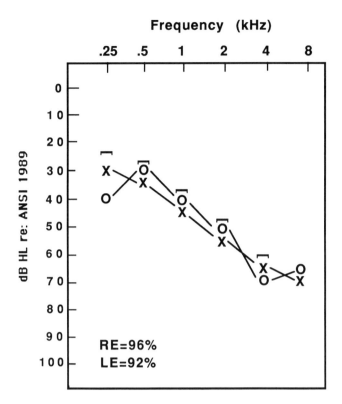

FIGURE 13.4 The audiogram and speech recognition scores of a 71-year-old man who sustained a cerebrovascular accident that resulted in compromise of the right hemisphere.

for some of the deficits noted on the monaural speech tests because the scores for both ears were depressed to some extent. Even these tests, however, may show some evidence of a contralateral ear effect because the left ear scores are lower than the right ear scores for both tests. More striking, however, is the difference in the scores of the two ears on the two dichotic speech tests. In these instances, right ear performance was normal, but clinically significant left ear deficits were noted. Finally, the observation of bilaterally depressed scores on both patterning tests is significant, especially in light of evidence demonstrating that the duration patterns test is largely unaffected by mild to moderate hearing losses (Musiek et al, 1990). Here again, one cannot rule out some contribtion of the peripheral compromise, but the extent of the deficit appears to be inconsistent with the degree of hearing loss. Once one peels away the peripheral deficits, what appears to be left is a classic case of right auditory hemisphere involvement showing contralateral effects on dichotic speech tests and monaural low redundancy speech tests and bilateral deficits on temporal patterning tests.

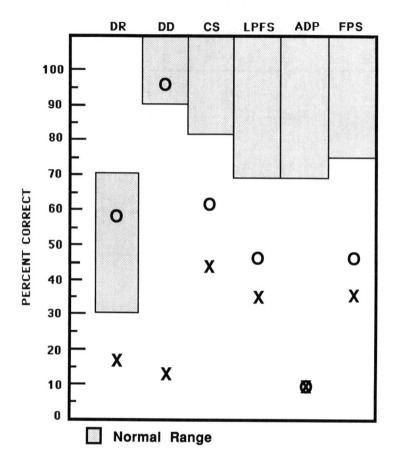

FIGURE 13.5 Behavioral tests of central auditory function of the same patient as in Figure 13.4. Test results are presented for the right (O) and left (X) ears for two dichotic tests (DR, dichotic rhymes; DD, dichotic digits), two monaural low redundancy speech tests (CS, compressed speech; LPFS, low-pass filtered speech), and two temporal patterning tests (ADP, auditory duration patterns; FPS, frequency pattern sequences).

The identification of these deficits has profound implications for the management of this patient. If the patient is to be fit with amplification after medical clearance, as was recommended, consideration needs to be given to the central auditory effects. Given the present results, one must question whether binaural or monaural amplification is preferable. If the patient is to be fit with a monaural device, which often occurs for financial reasons if not for audiologic considerations, the optimal fitting would be for the right ear in this case. If results for the peripheral auditory system alone are considered, however, the advantage of the right ear fitting may not be obvious.

CONCLUSION

The assessment and management of a client with a CAPD is an exciting and challenging area for audiologists. Given the fact that all people with neurologic compromise of the central auditory nervous system, many people with developmental disabilities such as learning disabilities or pervasive language disorders, and virtually all people with hearing losses are at risk for CAPD, central auditory assessment should be undertaken more frequently than currently is the norm. One cannot assume that the auditory system is normal if a client passes a pure-tone hearing test—a practice that is all too common. The implications of CAPD for the design of a management program for people with any of these acquired or developmental disorders are not to be ignored.

Even among audiologists these deficits are often ignored, or at least taken for granted, but their effects on the successful rehabilitation of a client may be staggering. For example, consider the unsuccessful hearing aid user. In many cases, the unsuccessful user is likely to be a client with central as well as peripheral involvement. If the central component is not identified, efforts to remediate this component of the problem may be overlooked. In some cases, little can be done to overcome these deficits, but identification of the deficits allows the audiologist to discuss realistic expectations with the client. Setting realistic expectations often can do much to ensure an honest attempt to use amplification and a successful course of rehabilitation.

REFERENCES

Akoi, C., & Siekevitz, P. (1988). Plasticity in brain development. *Scientific American, 259,* 56-64.

Bacon, S. E. (1992). Speech-language management of central auditory processing disorders. In J. Katz, N. A. Stecker, & D. Henderson (Eds.), *Central auditory processing: A transdisciplinary view* (pp. 199-204). St. Louis: Mosby Year Book.

Baran, J. A., & Musiek, F. E. (1991). Behavioral assessment of the central nervous system. In W. F. Rintelmann (Ed.), *Hearing assessment* (2nd ed.) (pp. 549-602). Boston: Allyn and Bacon.

Beasley, D. S., Forman, B., & Rintelmann, W. F. (1972a). Perception of time-compressed CNC monosyllables by normal listeners. *Journal of Auditory Research, 12,* 71-75.

Beasley, D. S., Schwimmer, S., & Rintelmann, W. F. (1972b). Intelligibility of time--compressed CNC monosyllables by normal listeners. *Journal of Speech and Hearing Research, 15,* 340-350.

Berlin, C. I., Lowe-Bell, S. S, Jannetta, P. J., & Kline, D.G. (1972). Central auditory deficits after temporal lobectomy. *Archives of Otolaryngology, 96,* 4-10.

Bliss, T., & Lomo, T. (1973). Long lasting potentiation of synaptic transmission in the dentate area of the anesthetized rabbit following stimulation of the perforant path. *Journal of Physiology, 232,* 331-356.

Bocca, E., Calearo, C., & Cassinari, V. (1954). A new method for testing hearing in temporal lobe tumors. *Acta Otolaryngologica, 42,* 289-304.

Chermak, G. D., & Musiek, F. E. (1992). Managing central auditory processing disorders in children and youth. *American Journal of Audiology, 1,* 61-65.

Efron, R. (1985). The central auditory system and issues related to hemispheric specialization. In M. L. Pinheiro & F. E. Musiek (Eds.), *Assessment of central auditory dysfunction: Foundations and clinical correlates* (pp. 143-154). Baltimore: Williams & Wilkins.

Fairbanks, G., Everitt, W., & Jaeger, R. (1954). Methods for time or frequency compression-expansion of speech. *Transactions of the IRE-PGA, AU-2,* 7-12.

Fifer, R. C., Jerger, J. F., Berlin, C. I., Tobey, E., & Campbell, J. (1983). Development of a dichotic sentence identification test for hearing impaired adults. *Ear and Hearing, 4,* 300-305.

Galaburda, A. M., & Kemper, T. (1979). Cytoarchitectonic abnormalities in developmental dyslexia: A case study. *Annals of Neurology, 6,* 94-100.

Galaburda, A. M., Sherman, G. F., Rosen, G. D., Aboitiz, F., & Geschwind, N. (1985). Developmental dyslexia: Four consecutive patients with cortical abnormalities. *Annals of Neurology, 18,* 222-233.

Gustafsson, B., & Wigstrom, H. (1988). Physiologic mechanisms underlying long-term potentiation. *Trends in Neuroscience, 11,* 156-162.

Hall, J. W. (1992). *Handbook of auditory evoked responses.* Boston: Allyn and Bacon.

Hynd, G. W., Semrud-Clikeman, M., Lorys, A. R., Novey, E. S., & Eliopulos, D. (1990). Brain morphology in developmental dyslexia and attention deficit disorder/hyperactivity. *Archives of Neurology, 47,* 919-926.

Hynd, G. W., Semrud-Clikeman, M., Lorys, A. R., Novey, E. S., Eliopulos, D., & Lyytinen, H. (1991a). Corpus callosum morphology in attention deficit disorder/hyperactivity disorder: Morphometric analysis of MRI. *Journal of Learning Disabilities, 50,* 275-296.

Hynd, G. W., Semrud-Clikeman, M., & Lyytinen, H. (1991b). Brain imaging in learning disabilities. In J. E. Obrzut & G. W. Hynd (Eds.), *Neuropsychological foundations of learning disabilities: A handbook of issues, methods, and practice* (pp. 475-511). New York: Academic.

Jasper, H. H. (1958). The ten–twenty electrode system of the international federation. *Electroencephalography and Clinical Neurophysiology, 10,* 371-375.

Jerger, J. F., & Jerger, S. W. (1974). Auditory findings in brainstem disorders. *Archives of Otolaryngology, 99,* 342-349.

Jerger, S. W., & Jerger, J. F. (1984). *The pediatric speech intelligibility test.* St. Louis: Auditec.

Katz, J. (1962). The use of staggered spondaic words for assessing the integrity of the central auditory system. *Journal of Auditory Research, 2,* 327-337.

Katz, J., Stecker, N. A., & Henderson, D. (1992). Introduction to central auditory processing. In J. Katz, N. A. Stecker & D. Henderson (Eds.), *Central auditory processing: A trandisciplinary view* (pp. 3-8). St. Louis: Mosby Year Book.

Keith, R. W. (1986). *SCAN: A screening test for auditory processing disorders.* San Antonio: Psychological Corporation.

Kimura, D. (1961a). Cerebral dominance and the perception of verbal stimuli. *Canadian Journal of Psychology, 15,* 166-171.

Kimura, D. (1961b). Some effects of temporal lobe damage on auditory perception. *Canadian Journal of Psychology, 15,* 157-165.

Lasky, E. Z., & Katz, J. (1983). Perspectives on central auditory processing. In E. Z. Lasky & J. Katz (Eds.), *Central auditory processing disorders: Problems of speech, language, and hearing disorders* (pp. 3-10). Baltimore: University Park Press.

Lenneberg, E. H. (1967). *Biological foundations of language.* New York: Wiley.

Morest, D. K., & Bohnes, B. A. (1983). Noise-induced degeneration in the brain and representation of inner and outer hair cells. *Hearing Research, 9,* 145-151.

Musiek, F. E. (1983). Assessment of central auditory dysfunction: The dichotic digit test revisited. *Ear and Hearing, 4,* 79-83.

Musiek, F. E. (1985). Application of central auditory tests: An overview. In J. Katz (Ed.), *Handbook of clinical audiology* (3rd ed.) (pp. 321-336). Baltimore: Williams & Wilkins.

Musiek, F. E., Baran, J. A., & Pinheiro, M. L. (1990). Duration pattern recognition in normal subjects and patients with cerebral and cochlear lesions. *Audiology, 29,* 304-313.

Musiek, F. E., Baran, J. A., & Pinheiro, M. L. (1994). *Neuroaudiology: Case studies.* San Diego: Singular.

Musiek, F. E., Kurdziel-Schwan, S. A., Kibbe, K., Gollegly, K. M., Baran, J. A., & Rintelmann, W. F. (1989). The dichotic rhyme task: Results in split-brain patients. *Ear and Hearing, 10,* 33-39.

Olsen, W. O., Noffsinger, D., & Carhart, R. (1976). Masking level differences encountered in clinical populations. *Audiology, 15,* 287-301.

Pinheiro, M. L., & Ptacek, P. H. (1971). Reversals in the perception of noise and tone patterns. *Journal of the Acoustical Society of America, 49,* 1778-1782.

Reeves, A. G. (1985). Overview of disorders of the central nervous system. In M. L. Pinheiro & F. E. Musiek (Eds.), *Assessment of central auditory dysfunction: Foundations and clinical correlates* (pp. 131-142). Baltimore: Williams & Wilkins.

Saunders, G. H., & Haggard, M. P. (1989). The clinical assessment of obscure auditory dysfunction. *Ear and Hearing, 10,* 200-208.

Schwaber, M., Garraghty, P., & Kaas, J. (1993). Neuroplasticity of the adult primate auditory cortex following cochlear hearing loss. *American Journal of Otology, 14,* 252-258.

Staudt, M., Schropp, C., Staudt, F., Obletter, N., Bise, K., & Breit, A. (1993). Myelination of the brain in MRI: A staging system. *Pediatric Radiology, 23,* 169-176.

Tillman, T. W., & Carhart, R. (1966). An expanded test for speech discrimination utilizing CNC monosyllabic words. Northwestern University Auditory Test No. 6. Technical Report No. SAM-TR-66-55. Brooks Air Force Base: USAF School of Aerospace Medicine.

Willeford, J. (1976). Differential diagnosis of central auditory dysfunction. In L. Bradford (Ed.), *Audiology: An audio journal for continuing education* (Vol. 2). New York: Grune & Stratton.

Willeford, J. A. (1985). Assessment of central auditory disorders in children. In M. L. Pinheiro & F. E. Musiek (Eds.), *Assessment of central auditory dysfunction: Foundations and clinical correlates* (pp. 239-256). Baltimore: Williams & Wilkins.

Yakovlev, P. I., & LeCours, A. R. (1967). The myelogenic cycles of regional maturation in the brain. In A. Minkowski (Ed.), *Regional development of the brain in early life* (pp. 3-70). Oxford: Blackwell Scientific.

SUGGESTED READINGS

Baran J. A. & Musiek, F. E. (1991). Behavioral assessment of the central nervous system. In W. F. Rintelmann (Ed.), *Hearing assessment* (2nd ed.) (pp. 549-602). Boston: Allyn and Bacon.

Hall, J. W. (1992). *Handbook of auditory evoked responses*. Boston: Allyn and Bacon.

Katz, J., Stecker, N. A., & Henderson, D. (Eds.) (1992). *Central auditory processing: A transdisciplinary view*. St. Louis: Mosby Year Book.

Musiek, F. E., & Pinheiro, M. L. (Eds.) (1985). *Assessment of central auditory dysfunction: Foundations and clinical correlates*. Baltimore: Williams & Wilkins.

Musiek, F. E., Baran, J. A., & Pinheiro, M. L. (1994). *Neuroaudiology: Case studies*. San Diego: Singular.

Obrzut, J. E., & Hynd, G. W. (Eds.) (1991). *Neuropsychological foundations of learning disabilities: A handbook of issues, methods, and practice*. New York: Academic.

Index

Abbott, G. D., 318
Abrahamson, I., 381
AB Special Instrument (company), 317
Accommodation, 381-382
  range of, 382
Acoustic admittance, 187
Acoustic environment, communication of,
    and sensory aids, 313
  background acoustic stimulation, 313
  comprehension, 315-316
  detection, 313-314
  discrimination, 314-315
  identification and recognition, 315
  localization, 314
Acoustic impedance, 187
Acoustic neuroma, 79. *See also* Vestibular
    schwannoma
Acoustic reflectometer, 149-150
Acoustic reflex, 192-193, 195-196
Acoustic reflex testing, 112, 187, 192-194
  decay test, 200
Acoustic reflex threshold, 86, 131
Acoustic stimulation, background, and sensory
    aids, 313
Acoustics, and auditory perception, 1-3
Acquired immunodeficiency syndrome (AIDS),
    61, 62
Acute otitis media, 50
Adaptation, 199
Adaptive compression. *See* Noise reduction
    circuits
Adhesive otitis media, 53
Air-bone gap, 40, 174
Air-conduction testing, 171-175, 186
Akoi, C., 432
Alarm clocks. *See* Alerting devices
ALDS. *See* Assistivelisteningdevices
Alerting devices, 266, 298-300
  cuing mechanisms for, 303-304
  signal transmission for, 301-303
  sound pick-up for, 300-301
Alford, B. R., 75
Alpiner, J., 357, 358, 380

Alternate Binaural Loudness Balance (ABLB),
    198-199
Alternate Monaural Loudness Balance (AMLB),
    198-199
American Academy of Audiology, 117
American Academy of Ophthalmology and
    Otolaryngology, 113-114
American Academy of Otolaryngology–Head
    and Neck Surgery, 117, 411
American Academy of Pediatrics, 114, 117
American Association of Retired Persons
    (AARP), 226
American Deaf Society, 359
American National Standards Institute (ANSI),
    151, 171, 175, 221, 223
American Sign Language, 348, 359
American Speech-Language-Hearing Association
    (ASHA), 88, 113, 114, 142, 187, 189
  Ad Hoc Committee on Hearing Screening in
    Adults, 157, 160
  and audiogram, 171
  Committee on Audiometric Evaluation, 148
  Committee on Infant Hearing, 103, 116,
    124, 125
  Guidelines for Acoustic Immittance Screening
    of Middle Ear Function, 151
  Guidelines for Identification Audiometry,
    148, 149, 150, 151, 157
  Guidelines for Screening for Hearing
    Impairment and Middle Ear Disorders,
    148, 149, 151, 159
  Guidelines for the Audiologic Assessment of
    Children from Birth Through 36
    Months of Age, 124-127, 133
  Identification Audiometry, 142
  and Individuals with Disabilities Education
    Act, 121, 123
  and Joint Committee's position statement,
    117
  and speech threshold testing, 179
  and visual reinforcement audiometry, 110
Americans with Disabilities Act (ADA, 1990),
    237, 297

Aminoglycoside antibiotics, 93
Amplifiers
  special, 238
  telephone, 293-295
Anatomy, 1-2
Anderson, M., 347
Anderson, R., 374
Anderson, S. M., 388
Andrews, J., 358, 359, 360, 361
Anotia, 41, 239
Antibiotic prophylaxis, for otitis media, 56, 57
Antibiotic treatment, for otitis media, 56, 57
Antibiotics, aminoglycoside, 93
Apple Tree curriculum, 347
Arenberg, D., 386
Armaly, M., 382
Arnst, D., 289, 379
Asphyxia, 63
Assessment protocol
  for children from birth through 4 months
    of age, 126
  for children 5 to 24 months of age, 126
  for children 25 to 36 months of age, 126-127
  individualized and timely, 125
Assistive listening devices (ALDs), 160, 207,
    220, 221, 254, 265
  coupled with personal hearing aids, 237,
    255-256, 280-285
  definition of, 266-267
  delivering signal from, to listener, 279-285
  and direct audio imput, 237
  frequency modulation systems, 273-276
  hardwired systems, 267-269
  induction loop systems, 269-272
  infrared systems, 276-279
  three categories of, 266
  use of, by elderly, 288-289, 391
  use of, in health care system, 290
  use of, in school system, 285-288
  use of, without personal hearing aid, 280.
    See also Alerting devices; Telecommuni-
    cation devices
Atelectasis, 54
Atherly, G., 380
Atresia, 72
  aural, 41-43
Atrophy, 374, 375
Audiogram, 171-172
  interpreting, and applying speech acoustics,
    337-338
  slope or configuration of, 177, 178
Audiological Engineering, 317, 318
Audiologic assessment report, understanding
    pediatric, 128
  acoustic reflex thresholds, 131
  auditory brainstem response, 129-130
  behavioral testing, 131-133
  tympanometry, 130-131
Audiologic pattern, in cochlear and retro-
    cochlear disorders, 78-79

Audiologic referrals, guidelines for making,
    127-128
Audiologic test results
  fractures, 86-87
  Ménière's disease, 87-89
  multiple sclerosis, 89-90
  noise-induced hearing loss, 90-91
  ototoxicity, 92-95
  presbycusis, 95-97
  sickle cell anemia, 98-99
  sudden hearing loss, 97
Audiologist, school
  contracted basis, 351-352
  full-time, 351
Audiometric evaluation of tumors, 84
Auditory brainstem response (ABR), 81-82, 84,
    86, 202, 425
  audiometry, 107-108
  as electroacoustic measurement, 196-198
  for infants and preschool children, 105,
    129-130
  Joint Committee on, 117
  as objective test of neural abnormalities,
    199-200
Auditory cortex, 32-34
Auditory evoked potentials, 202
Auditory Middle Latency Response (AMLR),
    202, 203
Auditory-oral treatment program, 349-350
Auditory perception, acoustics and, 1-3
Auditory periphery
  cochlear nerve, 24-26
  external auditory meatus, 5, 374
  inner ear, 8-24, 375
  middle ear, 5-8, 374-375
  outer ear, 4-5, 373-374
Auditory skills, role of, in link between hearing
    and speech, 338-339
Auditory Skills Curriculum, 343, 347, 355
Auditory Skills Instructional Planning System,
    343
Auditory trainers, 286
Augustsson, I., 144
Aural atresia, 41-43, 239
Automatic gain control (AGC) instruments. See
    Compression instruments
Automatic signal processing. See Noise
    reduction circuits

Bach, S., 63
Bach-y-Rita, P., 311
Bacon, S. E., 433
Ballenger, J. J., 40, 41, 44, 67
Bankowski, S., 273
Baran, J. A., 415, 418, 419, 422, 423, 424
Barratt, J. J., 90
Barry, J., 239
Basilar membrane traveling wave, 13-16
Batteries, hearing aid, 225-227
  safety precautions regarding, 226-227

Beachler, C. R., 320
Beasley, D. S., 419
Behavioral observation audiometry (BOA), 109-110
Behavioral observation screening, 106, 108
Behavioral test(ing)(s), 131-133
  of abnormalities of outer and middle ear, 194-195
  of central auditory dysfunction, 200-202
  of cochlear function, 198-199
  of neural function, 199
Behind-the-ear (BTE) hearing aids, 227, 228-229, 230
  earmold considerations for, 242
  selecting, 233-235
Behind-the-ear frequency modulation (BTE FM) hearing systems, 284-285
Behrens, T. R., 103, 105, 106, 107, 108, 134
Belal, A., 374
Bender, A., 383
Bendet, R., 252
Benecke, J. E., 84
Berg, F. S., 142
Berger, K., 286
Bergman, M., 267, 356, 376, 379
Bergstrom, L., 43, 44, 92-95, 144
Berliner, K. I., 321
Bernstein, L. E., 320, 321, 327
Berry, S., 343
Bess, F. H., 40, 41, 44, 58, 59, 68, 95, 96, 105, 134, 145, 224, 238-239, 246, 288, 358
BICROS hearing aid, 239
Bilger, R. C., 321
Binaural fusion, 201
Binaural interaction tests, 423-424
Bing test, 194, 195, 205, 207, 208
Binnie, C., 357
Birk-Nielson, H., 380
Birren, J., 386
Birthweight, low, 63
Blamey, P. J., 318, 325, 330
Blazer, D., 389
Bliss, T., 432
Blood, G., 388
Blood, I., 388
Blosser, D., 185
Bluestone, C. D., 46, 47, 48, 49, 50, 51, 52, 53, 54, 55, 56, 57, 143, 144
Bocca, E., 200, 201, 379, 418
Body hearing aids, 227, 228-229, 230, 233
  earmold considerations for, 242
Boettcher, F. A., 90-91, 94
Bohne, B. A., 418
Boies, L. R., 43, 44
Boisen, G., 234
Bone-conduction hearing aids, 239-240
Bone-conduction testing, 171-175, 186
Boothroyd, A., 318
Borg, E., 193
Bowles, N., 386

Brackett, D., 113, 355
Brackman, D. E., 84
Bradley, S., 251-252
Brain abscess, from otitis media, 55-56
Brasel, K., 348
Bratt, G. W., 75, 76
Brimacombe, J. A., 322, 324
Brody, H., 376
Brooks, D. N., 144
Brooks, P. L., 318, 321
Brown, B. H., 322
Brown, M. C., 36
Brown, S. C., 95-96
Brugge, J. F., 314
Bruhn, M., 357
Brummet, R. E., 93
Bührer, K., 149, 150
Bureau of the Census, U.S., 156, 384

Cadman, D., 143, 159, 160
Calearo, C., 379
California Consonant Test, 183-184
Calvert, D., 339
Carhart, R., 181, 183, 245, 419
Carney, A. E., 320
Carter, B. S., 60
Castle, D., 297
Cataracts, 381
Cazals, Y., 88
Central auditory dysfunction, 200-202
  intervention in, 211
  objective measurements of, 202-203
  tests of central auditory function, 210-211
  tests of peripheral auditory function, 210
Central auditory nervous system, 26-27
  age-related changes in, 376-380
  auditory cortex, 32-34
  cochlear nucleus, 27-28
  inferior colliculus, 31-32
  interhemispheric connections, 34
  medial geniculate body of thalamus, 32
  olivo-cochlear bundle, 29-30
  superior olivary complex, 28-29
Central auditory processing disorder (CAPD), 415, 437
  assessment of client with, 418-431
  bases of, 416-418
  case presentation of, 433-436
  definitions and symptoms of, 415-416
  management of client with, 431-433
Central Institute for the Deaf (CID), 342
  Auditory Test W-1, 180
  Everyday Sentence Test, 185
  W-22 word lists, 183
Central nervous system (CNS), 26, 80, 89
Central-peripheral ratio, 379
Cerebrovascular (CVA), 433
Cerumen, 43-44, 72, 374
Ceruminoma, 72-73
Chaiklin, J. B., 142, 180

Chandler, J., 374
Chapman, J., 68
Chapman, R., 349-350
Charcot, J.-M., 89
Chermak, G. D., 433
Chickenpox, 62
Chloroquine, 93
Cholesteatoma, 375
   from otitis media, 53-54
Cholewiak, R. W., 316
Chomsky, N., 104
Chronic otitis media, 51-52
   active, 51
   inactive, 51-52
Chronic suppurative otitis media, 53
Cisplatin, 94
Clark, B. S., 46
Clark, G. M., 318, 321, 322, 329
Clark, J., 175
Clark, S., 342, 343, 346, 347
Clinical assessment techniques and practices,
   109-113
Clinical audiologic assessment of infants and
   young children, 124
   birth through 36 months of age, 124-127
Clinical findings, expected, 203-211
Clinical test battery, routine, 171-186
Closed captioning, 298
Cochlear abnormalities, objective measurements
   of, 195
Cochlear and retrocochlear disorders, 78
   audiologic pattern, 78-79
   audiometric evaluation of tumors, 84
   concussion, 86
   meningiomas, 83
   traumatic factures, 85
   vestibular schwannoma, 79-83
Cochlear Corporation, 321, 322, 326, 327,
   352, 354
Cochlear function, behavioral tests of, 198-199
Cochlear implants, 207, 311
   device, selection, and fitting of, 352-354
   expected benefits of use of, 354-355
   performance of single-channel and multi-
      channel, 324-325
   processing strategies and transducer design
      of, 321-323
   role of speech-language pathologist in,
      355-356.
   See also Sensory aids; Tactile aids
Cochlear mechanics, of inner ear, 13-24
Cochlear nerve, 24-26
Cochlear nucleus, 27-28
Cochlear otoacoustic emissions, 198
Cohn, A. M., 72, 74
Coleman, J. R., 31
Collapsing ear canals, 44-45
Collet, L., 24
Commission on Education of the Deaf, 105

Committee on Hearing, Bioacoustics, and
   Biomechanics (CHABA), 267, 385
Commtram program, 326
Communication modality, two approaches to
   selecting, 349-351
   problems, strategies for solving, in adults
      with acquired hearing losses, 358
   problems, treating, in children with hearing
      impairments, 346-351
Compensated static acoustic immittance, 112
Competing Sentences Test, 201
Comprehension, and sensory aids, 315-316
Compression instruments, 223, 224
Compton, C., 237, 266, 271, 276, 284, 294,
   298, 302
Computed tomography (CT), 81, 82
Concussion, 86-87
Conditioned play audiometry, 111
Conductive auditory impairment
   intervention in, 206
   test results of, 204-206
Conductive hearing loss, 39-40, 173, 374-375
   cerumen in external auditory canal, 43-44
   collapsing ear canals, 44-45
   congenital malformations of outer and
      middle ear, 40-43
   foreign bodies in external auditory canal, 43
   longitudinal temporal bone fractures, 45-46
   and middle ear disease, screening for, 144
   otitis externa, 44
   otitis media, 46-58
   perforations of tympanic membrane, 45
Configuration of hearing loss, 177-178
   cookie-bite, 177
   falling, 177
   flat, 177
   precipitous, 178
   rising, 177
   sharply dropping, 178
   ski-slope, 177
   sloping, 177
   trough-shaped, 177
Congenital, defined, 58
Congenital malformations of outer and middle
   ear, 40-43
Contralateral routing of signals (CROS) hearing
   aid, 230, 233, 238-239, 243
Cooper, H., 313, 315, 327, 329
Coren, S., 158
Cornett, R., 348
Corso, J., 374, 378, 381
Corwin, J. T., 35
Covell, W., 374
Cowan, R. S. C., 321, 330
Cowie, R., 356
Cox, H., 156
Coyne, A., 386
Craig, J. C., 316
Craik, F., 386

Cranford, J. L., 89
Crawford, M. R., 98
Crib-O-Gram, 106-107, 108
CROS hearing aid, 230, 233, 238-239, 243
Cross, A. W., 143
Cross-hearing, 185-186
Cued speech, 372
Cuing mechanisms, for alerting devices,
    303-304
Cytomegalovirus (CMV) infection, 59, 60-61

Dalebout, Susan D., 39, 103
Dallos, P., 22
Darley, F., 142
Davidson, Stephanie A., 219, 265, 282, 289
Davis, H., 184, 185
Davis, J., 338, 340, 341, 345, 349, 356, 357,
    358, 361, 380
Davis, Lynne A., 337
Deafness
    in adults with acquired hearing loss, 361
    assessment of psychological and psychosocial
        skills, 361-362
    different definitions of, 359
    impact on family of diagnosis of, 360
    psychosocial aspects of, 358-362
DeFilippo, C. L., 320
Delk, M. L., 144
Demorest, M. E., 380
Dennis, J. M., 113
Denton, D., 349
Denver Scale of Communication Function for
    Senior Citizens Living in Retirement
    Centers, 280
Derlacki, E. L., 77, 78
Detection, and sensory aids, 313-314
Developmental Approach to Successful
    Listening, 356
Dichotic Digits Test, 201
Dichotic speech tests, 419-422, 434
Dickins, J. R. F., 87
Difference limen for intensity (DLI), 199
Direct audio input (DAI), 237
    and coupling of assistive listening device with
        personal hearing aid, 283
Direct electrical connection, for alerting devices,
    300-301
Directional microphones, 237
Dirks, D. D., 173, 201
Discrimination, and sensory aids, 314-315
Dispenser-adjustable controls, 235
Distortion product otoacoustic emissions
    (DPOAEs), 22, 24
Diuretics, loop-inhibiting, 94
Djourno, A., 321
Donahue, A., 266, 267, 273, 277
Douglas-Cowie, E., 356
Dowdy, L. K., 179
Dowell, R. C., 325

Downs, M. P., 41, 43, 44, 46, 49, 53, 54, 58,
    59, 60, 61, 62, 63, 64, 65-67, 104, 105,
    106, 113, 114, 244
Doyle, W. J., 104
Dunham, M., 240
Durieux-Smith, A., 107, 117
Durrant, J. D., 94

Eagles, E., 145
Ear canal(s)
    collapsing, 44-45
    volume, 190-191
Early intervention, 112-113
Early Intervention Program for Infants and
    Toddlers with Handicaps law, 142
Ear-specific assessment, 125
Easterbrooks, S., 341
Easter Seal Society, 363
Easy Listener, 273-274
Echoic memory, 385-386
Education of the Handicapped Act (1975), 121,
    142
Education of the Handicapped Act Amend-
    ments (1986), 121, 142
Effusion
    otitis media with (OME), 51, 118, 144
    otitis media without, 50
Efron, R., 415
Egan, J. P., 183
Eichwald, J. G., 114
Ekhaml, L., 286
Elderly, 373
    adjustment disorders in, 388
    affective disorders in, 389
    central auditory system, changes in, 376-380
    clinical intervention with, 389-393
    cognitive considerations in, 385-388
    dementia in, 388
    demographic factors and, 384
    financial considerations and, 384
    hearing handicap in, 380-381
    impact of auditory dysfunction on, 380-389
    identification programs for, 156-160
    memory changes in, 385-386
    mobility of, 385
    motivation of, 387-388
    nervous system of, 383
    peripheral physiologic changes of auditory
        system in, 373-375
    pharmacology and, 383
    psychiatric function and disorders in,
        388-389
    psychologic aspects of, 385
    pulmonary function in, 382-383
    sociologic issues and, 383-384
    use of assistive listening devices by, 288-289
    use of linguistic and visual information by,
        387
    visual system in, 381-382

Eldert, M. A., 184
Eldredge, L., 39
Electroacoustic analysis (EAA), 221-222, 225, 247
Electroacoustic measurements, 196-198
Electrocochleography (ECoG), 196
Electroencephalogram (EEG), 203
Electrophysiologic tests, 424-425
Elssman, S., 117
Endres, D., 42
Engen, E., 342
Engen, T., 342
Environmental microphones, 287-288
Environmental Protection Agency (EPA), 402
Equipment, for screening program, 149-150
Erber, N., 358
Etholm, B., 374
Eustachian tube, 374
Evoked otoacoustic emissions, 198
Ewertsen, H., 380
External auditory canal
    cerumen in, 43-44
    foreign bodies in, 43
External auditory meatus, 5
    age-related changes in, 374
External ear. See Outer ear
External redundancy, 379
Eyeglass hearing aids, 227, 229-230, 233
    earmold considerations for, 242
Eyries, C., 321

Facial paralysis, from otitis media, 55
Fairbanks, G., 419
Federal Communications Commission (FCC), 236, 273, 276, 292
Fein, D., 156
Feldman, A. S., 189
Ferre, J., 288
Feth, Lawrence L., 1
Fifer, R. C., 202
Finitzo-Hieber, T., 267
Fire, Kevin M., 171, 373
Fisher, H., 373
Fitzgerald, E., 347
Fitzgerald key, 347
Flexer, C., 267, 286, 288
FM airborne system, for alerting devices, 302-303
FM line carrier, for alerting devices, 301-302
Fodor, W. J., 410
Follow-up, parental and educational, 156
Food and Drug Administration (FDA), U.S., 240, 321, 352
Foreign bodies, in external auditory canal, 43
Forge, A., 35
Forner, L., 339
Fourcin, A. J., 324, 325
Fowler, E. P., 198
Fractures
    audiologic test results, 86-87

follow-up care for, 87
    temporal bone, 45-46, 67
    traumatic, 85
Framingham Heart Survey, 377
Franklin, D. J., 90
Frasier, G. R., 144, 312
Freedman, S., 373
Frequency modulation (FM) ALD systems, 273
    large-area, 273
    personal, 273-275
    strengths and weaknesses of, 275-276
Frequency-specific stimuli, use of, 125
Frerebeau, P., 81
Friedman, H., 240
Friel-Patti, S., 52
Frisina, D., 349
Frolsch, M., 72
Functional Auditory Speech Treatment (FAST), 346-347
Functional Speech Sound Test (FSST), 341-342
Funding, sources of, for people with hearing impairments, 362-364
Furman, J. M. R., 90

Gaeth, J., 252, 378
Gagné, J.-P., 357
Galaburda, A. M., 417
Gallaudet University, 343
Gantz, B. J., 329
Garrard, K. R., 46
Garstecki, D., 148, 392
Gates, G., 95
Gault, R. H., 316
Geers, A. E., 320, 321, 325, 328, 342
Geffner, D., 104
Genetic hearing loss, 58-59
Gerber, S. E., 41, 58, 59, 60, 61, 62, 63, 64
Gerkin, K. P., 113, 114
Gerwin, J. M., 62
Gescheider, G. A., 316
Gillis, L., 389
Giolas, T. G., 286, 357, 358, 380, 392
Glasscock, M. E., 75
Glaucoma, 382
Glomus tumor, 75-76
Glorig, A., 377
Goehl, H., 356
Goetzinger, C., 378
Goff, G. D., 316
Goldberg, B., 103, 109
Goldstein, B. A., 186
Goldstein, M. H., Jr., 320
Goodman, A., 175
Gordon-Salant, S., 388
Gould, H. J., 98
Graham, J., 322
Graham, P., 382
Graham, S. S., 87
Grahl, C., 247

Grammatical Analysis of Elicited Language (GAEL), 342
Grammatico, L., 348
Grant, K. W., 315
Gravel, J. S., 110, 111, 124, 133
Gray, B., 379
Green, D. S., 199
Greenwood, J., 252
Griffiths, J. D., 183
Grimes, A. M., 251
Guilford, F. R., 75
Gustafsson, B., 432

Haggard, M. P., 417
Hair-cell excitation, 16
Hair-cell regeneration, 34-35
Hair cells
    in organ of Corti, 12-13
    role of inner and outer, 18-22
Hakansson, B., 240
Hakkinen, L., 382
Hakstian, A. R., 158
Hall, D. M. B., 144
Hall, J. W., 85, 105, 134, 425, 427, 428
Hamill, T., 240
Hamilton, J. L., 123
Handicaps, state programs for children with medical, 362-363
Hanners, B. A., 252
Hansen, C., 376
Harbert, F., 378
HARC Mercantile, 255
Hardick, E., 338, 340, 341, 345, 349, 356, 357, 358, 361, 380
Hardwired ALD systems, 267-268
    large-area, 268
    personal, 268
    strengths and weaknesses of, 268-269
Hardwired connection, for alerting devices, 301
Harford, E., 239
Harris, J. P., 42
Harris, K., 339
Harvard University, Psychoacoustic Laboratories at, 183
Harvey, J., 121, 122, 123
Haskins, H. A., 184
Hawke, M., 40, 41, 42, 43, 44, 45, 46, 49, 51, 66, 71, 72-74, 75, 76-77, 80, 83, 85, 87, 88, 89, 91, 92-95, 96, 97
Hawkins, D., 221, 237, 241, 247, 267, 282, 283, 284, 287
Hawkins, J., 375, 376
Hayes, D., 193-194, 289, 379
Head, J., 347, 355
Healey, W. C., 252
Health and Human Services, U.S. Department of (DHHS), 105, 134
Health care system, use of assistive listening devices in, 290

Health Examination Survey (1960-1962), 377
Healthy People 2000, 105, 134
Hearing
    and language, link between, 339-341
    and speech, link between, 337-341
Hearing aid(s), 160, 219
    adjustment programs, 254
    batteries, 225-227
    behind-the-ear, 227, 228-229, 230
    body, 227, 228-229
    bone-conduction, 239-240
    candidacy, 220-221
    characteristics, verification of, 246-251
    components of, 256-257
    contralateral routing of signals, 230, 233, 238-239, 243
    coupled with assistive listening devices, 237, 256, 280-285
    direct audio input in, 237
    and directional microphones, 237
    dispenser-adjustable controls in, 235
    earmold considerations of, 242-245
    for elderly, 390-391
    electroacoustic characteristics of, 221-225
    eyeglass, 227, 229-230
    gain and frequency response of, 222-223
    hybrid, 240-241
    in-the-canal, 227, 228, 230, 232-233
    in-the-ear, 227, 228, 230-232
    listening check, 257-258
    monaural vs. binaural amplification in, 241
    noise reduction circuits in, 238
    orientation and follow-up, 251-258
    performance, daily check of, 254-258
    problems, troubleshooting, 255, 258-260
    purpose of, 220
    saturation sound pressure level of, 223-225
    selection and fitting, 245-251
    special amplifiers in, 238
    with special applications, 238-241
    special options available in, 235-238
    style, 227-233
    style, selecting, 233-235
    telecoil in, 235-237
    use of assistive listening device as alternative to, 288-289
Hearing handicap, in elderly, 380-381
Hearing Handicap Inventory for the Elderly (HHIE), 380-381, 392
Hearing Handicap Inventory for the Elderly—Screening Version (HHIE-S), 158, 159, 170
Hearing impairments, children with assessing communication skills of, 341-346
    tests designed for, 342-343
    treating communication problems in, 346-351
    using tests not designed for, 343-346
Hearing Instruments, 240, 241

Hearing loss
  adults with acquired, 356-358, 361
  conductive, 39-58, 173
  configuration of, 177-178
  degree of, 175-176
  genetic, 58-59
  mild, 175
  mixed, 68, 175, 207, 208
  moderate, 176
  moderately severe, 176
  noise-induced, 67-68, 90-91, 401-411
  from otitis media, 52-53
  profound, 176, 311
  sensorineural, 58-68, 175
  severe, 176
  sudden, 97
Hearing screening. *See* Screening Hearing
    Screening Inventory (HSI), 158, 159,
    166
Heffner, H. E., 34
Heffner, R. S., 34
Hemenway, W. G., 113
Herpes simplex virus, 59, 62
Herpes zoster, 62
High, W., 380
High-risk register, 106
Hill, P., 144
Hinchcliffe, R., 374, 376
Hirsh, I. J., 180, 183
Hixon, T., 339
Hnath-Chisholm, T., 318
Hochmair-Desoyer, I. J., 321
Hodgson, W. R., 254, 311
Hohmann, M., 348
Holmes, A., 150
Holtzman, R., 387
Horner, K. C., 88
Horstmeier, D., 347
Hosford-Dunn, H., 117
Hough, J. V. D., 85
Houle, G. R., 123
House, W. F., 321
House Ear Institute, 321
Hudgins, C., 339
Hull, R., 373, 374
Human immunodeficiency virus (HIV), 62
Humes, L. E., 41, 44, 58, 59, 246
Hussung, R., 240
Hutman, L., 382
Hybrid hearing aids, 240-241
Hyde, M. L., 196
Hynd, G. W., 417
Hyperbilirubinemia, 64

Identification, and sensory aids, 315
Identification audiometry, 142. *See also*
    Screening
Immittance, 145, 187, 195
  acoustic, 151, 152, 155, 187
  audiometry, 112

Immittance meter, electroacoustic, 187, 189,
    190
Impedance, 187
Incidence, 143
Individualized Education Plan (IEP), 122
Individualized Family Service Plan (IFSP), 118,
    123
Individuals with Disabilities Education Act
    (IDEA, Public Law 102-119), 118, 120,
    121-123, 124, 127, 134, 142
Induction loop ALD systems, 269-270
  large-area, 270-271
  personal, 271
  strengths and weaknesses of, 271-272
Inductive coupling, of assistive listening device
    with personal hearing aid, 280-282
Inductive pick-up, for alerting devices, 301
Ineraid multichannel cochlear implant,
    329-330
Infants and preschool children, hearing loss in,
    103, 133-134
  clinical assessment techniques and practices,
    109-113
  clinical audiologic assessment of, 124-127
  guidelines for making audiologic referrals,
    127-128
  importance of early identification, 104-105
  Individuals with Disabilities Education Act,
    121-123
  neonatal hearing screening, 113-121
  screening techniques and practices, 106-109
  understanding pediatric audiologic assess-
    ment report, 128-133
Inferior colliculus, 31-32
Influenza, 62
Infrared ALD systems, 276
  large-area, 276-277
  personal, 277-278
  strengths and weaknesses of, 278-279
Inner ear, 8-9
  age-related changes in, 375
  cochlear mechanics of, 13-24
  structure of, 9-13
Inner hair cells
  in organ of Corti, 13
  role of, 20-22
Instruments, hearing screening, for older adults,
    158-159
Insurance
  Medicare, 362
  private, 362
Interagency Coordinating Council, 123
Interaural attenuation, 186
Interhemispheric connections, 34
In-the-canal (ITC) hearing aids, 227, 228, 230,
    232-233, 242
  selecting, 233-235
In-the-ear (ITE) hearing aids, 227, 228,
    230-232, 242
  selecting, 233-235

Intracranial complications, of otitis media, 55-56
Intratemporal complications, of otitis media, 52-55
Intrinsic redundancy, 379
Inventories, hearing handicap, 158. *See also* Hearing Screening Inventory (HSI)
Ivey, R. S., 201

Jacobson, C. A., 147
Jacobson, G. P., 90
Jacobson, J. T., 90, 105, 112, 117, 147, 196
Jahn, A. F., 40, 41, 42, 43, 44, 45, 46, 49, 51, 66, 71, 72-74, 75, 76-77, 80, 83, 85, 87, 88, 89, 91, 92-95, 96, 97
Jensema, C., 298, 349
Jerger, J., 106, 109, 130-131, 184, 185, 197, 199, 201, 289, 375, 378, 379
Jerger, J. F., 144, 145, 193-194, 431
Jerger, S., 184, 194, 197, 375
Jerger, S. W., 429-431
Jesteadt, W., 388
Jewett, D. L., 196
Johnson, J. J., 198
Johnson, J. L., 112
Johnson, M. J., 105, 106
Johnson, R. J., 240, 348
Johnsson, L., 375, 376
Joint Committee on Infant Hearing, 103, 108, 109, 114, 116
    position statement (1994) of, 117-121, 123, 128
Jokinen, K., 379

Kalikow, D. N., 185, 387
Kalmus, H., 382
K-Amp, 238
Kaplan, H., 178
Katz, J., 201, 380, 415, 416
Kaufman, D., 356
Keith, R. W., 431
Kemp, D. T., 22, 198
Kemper, T., 417
Kenworthy, O. T., 288
Kernicterus, 64
Khetarpal, V., 88
Kibbe-Michel, K., 203
Kimura, D., 422
Kirikae, I., 376
Kirkwood, D. H., 227
Klatzky, R. L., 385
Klein, J. O., 46, 47, 48, 49, 50, 51, 52, 53, 54, 55, 56, 57
Konkle, D., 379
Koop, C. E., 133-134
Kopelman, J., 94, 95
Kopra, L. L., 185, 377, 378, 379
Kozak, V., 342
Kretschmer, L., 340, 342
Kretschmer, R., 340, 342

Kretschmer Spontaneous Language Analysis Procedure, 342
Kricos, P., 289
Kristensen, S., 73
Kuhl, P. K., 117

Labor, U.S. Department of, 403, 410, 411
Labyrinthitis, from otitis media, 54-55
Language
    link between hearing and, 339-341
    skills, development of, 347-349
Larose, G., 298-299
Lasky, E. Z., 416
Late auditory evoked response, 427-428
Late auditory potentials, 203
Late evoked responses (LER), 203
Late latency responses (LLR), 203
Lazzaroni, M., 379
Leavitt, R., 266
LeCours, A. R., 417
Lehnhardt, E., 321
Lenneberg, E. H., 104, 432
Lerman, J., 184, 224
Levine, E., 359
Levine, S. C., 39, 46, 58, 62
Levitt, H., 104, 339, 341
Light emitting diodes (LEDs), 276
Linear instruments. *See* Peak-clipping instruments
Ling, D., 257, 338, 339, 342, 346
Lions Club International, 363
Localization, and sensory aids, 314
Lomo, T., 432
Longitudinal temporal bone fractures, 45-46
Loop-inhibiting diuretics, 94
Loudness discomfort levels (LDLs), 224, 250
Lounsbury, E., 252
Low-pass filtered speech, 200
Low-redundancy speech tests, 419
Lucite, 243, 244
Luetke-Stahlman, B., 340, 350
Lybarger, S., 223, 225, 230, 236, 245, 292
Lyles, A. C., 97
Lynch, M. P., 320, 327
Lyxell, B., 357

MacDonald, J., 347
Mackey-Hargadine, J., 85
Magladery, J., 374
Magnetic resonance imaging (MRI), 81-82, 84, 417
Mahoney, T. M., 114
Malloy, P., 251-252
Mangham, C. A., 95, 96
Manley, G. A., 35
Marge, M., 143, 157
Margolis, R. H., 189
Marshall, L., 96, 388
Martin, F. N., 44, 45, 59, 62, 67, 106, 179, 185, 186, 194

Marx, J., 61
Masking, 185-186
Mastoiditis, from otitis media, 53
Mateer, C. A., 85, 86, 87
Matkin, N., 340
Mattox, D. E., 97
Matzger, J., 201
Mauk, G. W., 103, 105, 106, 107, 108, 117, 134
Maurer, J., 373, 374
Maximum power output (MPO). *See* SSPL90
May, A. E., 234
McAfee, M., 340-341
McCandless, G., 379, 380, 392
McFadden, D., 409
McFarland, R., 382
McFarland, W. H., 84
McGarr, N. S., 104, 339
McWilliam, R. A., 122, 127-128
Meadow, K., 348
Measles, 62
Mecklenburg, D., 321
Medial geniculate body of thalamus, 32
Medicaid, 363, 384
Medicare, 362, 384
Melnick, W., 145, 151, 401
Ménière's disease, 24, 87-88, 196
    audiologic test results, 89
Meningiomas, 81, 83
Meningitis
    from otitis media, 55
    from sensorineural hearing loss, 65-66
Meredith, R., 234
Metz, O., 192, 194, 196
Meyerhoff, W. L., 40, 41, 42, 43, 46, 55, 67, 374
Microphone pick-up, for alerting devices, 300
Microphones, environmental, 287-288
Microstructure, of audibility curve, 22
Microtia, 41, 239
Middle ear, 5-7
    age-related changes in, 374-375
    behavioral tests of abnormalities of, 194-195
    congenital malformations of, 40-43
    function of, 7-8
    objective tests for abnormalities of, 187-194
    status, determination of, 126
Middle ear disease, 143-144, 145
    and conductive hearing loss, screening for, 144
Middle ear disorders, 74
    glomus tumor, 75-76
    otic barotrauma, 76-77
    otitis media, 75
    otosclerosis, 77-78
Middle latency response (MLR), 202, 425-427
Middlelweerd, M., 387
Middleton, R., 286
Mild hearing loss, 175

Miller, S., 348
Millin, J., 286
Mills, J. H., 224
Mindel, E. D., 360
Minifonator, 319
Minimum response levels, 132
Minivib, 317, 319
Mitchell, D., 386
Mixed hearing loss, 68, 175, 207
    intervention in, 208
    test results of, 208
Miyamoto, R. T., 80, 81
Moderate hearing loss, 175-176
Moderately severe hearing loss, 176
Modified Rhyme Test, 183-184
Moeller, M. P., 340, 346, 348, 350
Moller, A. R., 196
Monosyllabic stimuli, for speech recognition testing, 183-185
Monsell, E. M., 79, 84
Monsen, R., 339
Moog, J. S., 321, 325, 328, 342
Moore, J. M., 110, 388
Moores, D., 349
Morehouse, R., 117
Morest, D. K., 418
Morrison, R. B., 93
Moscicki, E., 377
Most comfortable loudness level (MCL), 185
Mueller, H. G., 224, 237, 251
Muller, C., 324
Multiple sclerosis (MS), 89-90, 208
    audiologic test results, 90
Mulvihill, J. J., 80, 81
Mumps, 62
Musiek, F. E., 415, 416, 418, 419, 422, 423, 424, 425, 427, 428, 433, 435
Mycins, 66
Myringotomy, for otitis media, 56-57

Naatanen, R., 203
Nabelek, A., 266, 267, 273, 277, 286
Naidoo, Sharmala V., 1
National Association for the Deaf (NAD), 359-360
    Junior NAD, 360
National Battery Hotline, 227
National Captioning Institute (NCI), 298
National Center for Health Statistics, 144
National Health Interview Survey, 96
National Health Survey (1935-1936), 377
National Institute on Aging, 384
National Institutes of Health (NIH), 80, 81, 82, 83, 84, 108
    Consensus Development Conference on Acoustic Neuroma of, 79
    Consensus Development Conference on Early Identification of Hearing Impairment in Infants and Young Children, 109
    and noise-induced hearing loss, 401

National Technical Institute for the Deaf (NTID), 297
Neonatal hearing screening
background of, 113-114
guidelines for audiologic, 116
Joint Committee's position statement (1994) on, 117-121
Neonatal intensive care nursery (NICU), 103, 108
Nerbonne, M. A., 156-157, 158, 251, 289, 357
Neural abnormalities, objective tests of, 199-200
Neural disease
intervention in, 209-210
test results of, 208-209
Neural function, behavioral tests of, 199
Neural redundancy, 379
Neurofibromatosis 1, 80
Neurofibromatosis syndrome, 80-81
Neurofibromatosis 2, 81
Newby, H. A., 240
Newman, C. W., 158, 186, 374
Nicolet Phoenix, 240
Nielsen-Abbring, F. W., 93
Nitchie, E., 357
Noble, W., 380
Noe, C., 267, 273, 277, 282, 286
Noise and hearing loss, 67-68, 90-91, 401-403
anatomic and physiologic pathology, 403-404
audiologic characteristics of, 405-407
audiologic test results of, 91
and hearing conservation, 411
legislation and regulation of, 409
relationship between, 404-405
susceptibility to, 407-409
Noise Control Act (1972), 402
Noise reduction circuits, 238
Normal auditory systems
intervention in, 204
tests results of, 203-204
Northern, J. L., 41, 43, 44, 46, 49, 53, 54, 58, 59, 60, 61, 62, 63, 64, 65-67, 106, 144, 152, 155, 244
Northwestern University
Auditory Test Number 6, 419
Children's Perception of Speech (NU-CHIPS) test, 127, 133
NU-6 word lists, 183
Norton, S. J., 109
Nozza, R. J., 132
Nucleus multichannel implant, 321, 322, 323, 326, 327
Numbers, F., 339
Nursing home, assistive listening devices in, 289

Objective tests (measurements)
for abnormalities of outer and middle ear, 187-194
of central auditory dysfunction, 202-203
of cochlear abnormality, 195
of neural abnormalities, 199-200
Obscure auditory dysfunction, 417
Occlusion effect, 194-195
Occupational Safety and Health Act (1970), 409-410
Ohio Department of Health, 142
Older adults. *See* Elderly
Oleinick, A., 410
Olivo-cochlear bundle, 29-30
Olsen, W., 267
Organ of Corti, hair cells in, 12-13, 25-26
Osberger, M. J., 321, 328, 340, 346
Osguthorpe, J. D., 411
Ossicular discontinuity and fixation, from otitis media, 54
Osteosis, 374
Otic barotrauma, 76-77
Otitis externa, 44, 74
Otitis media, 46, 75, 375
acute, 50
adhesive, 53
chronic, 51-52
chronic suppurative, 53
classification of subtypes, 49-52
complications and sequelae, 52-56
with effusion (OME), 51, 118, 144
without effusion, 50
prevalence and predisposing factors, 46-49
treatment, 56-58
Otoacoustic emissions (OAEs), 108-109
cochlear, 198
Joint Committee on, 117
spontaneous or evoked, 22-24
Otosclerosis, 77-78, 205, 375
Otoscope, 149
Otoscopic inspection, 154-155
Ototoxicity, 66-67, 92
audiologic test results, 94-95
mechanism of toxicity, 92
ototoxic drugs, 92-94
Otte, J., 329
Otto, W., 379, 380, 392
Outer ear, 4-5
age-related changes in, 373-374
behavioral tests of abnormalities of, 194-195
congenital malformations of, 40-43
objective tests for abnormalities of, 187-194
Outer ear disorders, 71
atresia, 72
cerumen occlusion, 72
ceruminoma, 72-73
otitis externa, 74
perforation of tympanic membrane, 73-74
stenosis, 72
tympanosclerosis, 74
Outer hair cells
in organ of Corti, 12-13
role of, 18-19
Owens, E., 183, 325
Oyer, H., 356

PAL PB-50 word lists, 183
Palva, A., 379
Paparella, M. M., 45, 46, 47, 48, 50, 51, 52, 55, 56, 57
Pahor, A. L., 73
Pappas, D. G., 65, 117
Parisier, S. C., 85
Parry, D. M., 80, 81
Parving, A., 234
Pass–fail criteria, of screening tests, 145-146
Pathologic condition, tests for auditory site of, 186-203
PBmax, 184, 185, 379
Peak-clipping instruments, 223-224
Pediatric Speech Intelligibility (PSI) test, 127, 133, 429-431
Peek, B., 68
Pehringer, J., 286
Perforations of tympanic membrane
    in adults, 73-74
    in children, 45
    from otitis media, 53
Performance-intensity (PI) function, 184, 378
Perinatal causes, 58
    of sensorineural hearing loss, 63-64
Peripheral auditory function, tests of, 210
Peripheral auditory system, 9, 175, 210
    physiologic age-related changes of, 373-375
Perkell, J., 325
Perlmutter, M., 386
Permanent threshold shifts (PTS), 403
Perry, E., 374
Personal amplification systems (PASs), 268, 269
Personal FM systems, 286-287, 288
Pestalozza, G., 378
Petros, T., 386
Petrositis, from otitis media, 54
Phillips, A. J., 320
Phillips, D. P., 314
Phonemic balance, 183
Phonetically Balanced Kindergarten (PBK-50) lists, 184
Phonetic balance (PB), 183, 184, 378
Phonetic balance maximum (PBmax), 184, 185
Phonetic Level Speech Evaluation, 342
Phonic Ear, 273
Physiology, 3-4
Pickett, J., 267
Pickles, J. O., 13, 30
Picton, T., 203
Pikus, A., 84
Pinheiro, M. L., 423
Pinna, age-related changes in, 373-374
PI-PB function, 184
Plant, G., 326
Plastic surgery, 41
Plath, P., 234
Plattsmier, H. S., 409
Plomp, R., 357, 387

Pochapin, S. W., 361
Pollack, D., 348
Poon, L., 386
Popelka, G. R., 240
Postnatal causes, 58
    of sensorineural hearing loss, 62, 65-68
Potts, P. L., 252
Power-deFur, L., 121, 122, 123
Prematurity, 63-64
Prenatal causes, 58
    of sensorineural hearing loss, 58-62
Presbycusis, 24, 95-96, 375, 376
    audiologic test results, 96-97
    inner ear conductive, 375
    metabolic, 375
    neural, 375
    sensory, 375
Presbyopia, 381-382
Preschool children. See Infants and preschool children
Preschool Extension, 347
Prevalence, 143
Probe microphone measurement system, 247-250
Probst, R., 36
Proctor, A., 320
Profound hearing loss, 176, 311
Protruding ears, 41
Psychosocial aspects of deafness, 358-359
    adults with acquired hearing loss, 361
    assessment of psychological and psychosocial skills, 361-362
    deaf community, 359-360
    impact on family of diagnosis of deafness, 360
Ptacek, P. H., 423
Public Law 94-142, 121, 142, 350
Public Law 99-457, 121, 142
Public Law 102-119. See Individuals with Disabilities Education Act
Pulec, J. L., 87, 88
Punch, J., 144
Pure-tone audiometry, 145, 149, 155, 171-175
    and configuration of hearing loss, 177-178
    and degree of hearing loss, 175-176
    fail–rescreen, 151
    frequency, 150
    intensity, 150-151
    for older adults, 158, 159
    problems encountered with, 152
Pure-tone average (PTA), 175, 181
Pure-tone average (two frequency, PTA2), 175, 181
Pure-tone sensitivity loss, prevalence of, 377-378

Questionnaires, self-report, 158-159
Quigley, S., 343, 348, 349
Quinine, 93

Ramsdell, S. A., 313
Range of accommodation, 382
Rapin, I., 104
Read, T., 312, 325
Real, R., 62
Real-ear insertion gain (REIG), 248
Real-ear insertion response (REIR), 248
Real-ear measurement system. *See* Probe microphone measurement system
Recklinghausen, F. D. von, 80
Recognition, and sensory aids, 315
Recruitment, 198-199
Reed, C. M., 317
Reeves, A. G., 416
Referrals
  audiologic and otologic, 155
  and recommendations for older adults, 159
Reger, S. N., 198
Reichman, J., 252
Reliability, of screening test, 146
Remein, Q. R., 147
Resource Access Projects (RAP), 118
Retraction pocket, from otitis media, 53, 54
Retrocochlear site of lesion, 378. *See also* Cochlear and retrocochlear disorders
Reynell, J., 342
Reynell Developmental Language Scales, 342
Rhode Island Hearing Assessment Project, 108
Rhode Island Test of Language Structures, 342
Richardson, B. L., 314, 319-320
Rintelmann, W. F., 185, 224
Riske-Nielsen, E., 376
Rivera, V. M., 89-90
Robbins, A. M., 326
Roberts, A., 377
Robinette, M. S., 24
Robinson, D. O., 252
Rock, J. P., 79, 84
Roeser, F. J., 144, 152, 155
Rollover, 184-185, 378
Rönnberg, J., 357
Rosenhall, U., 96
Rosner, B., 46, 49
Ross, M., 184, 224, 241, 258, 273, 286, 392
Rothenberg, M., 316
Roush, J., 122, 127-128, 151
Royster, L. H., 408
Rubel, E. W., 34-35
Rubella, 59, 60
Ruben, R. J., 63, 65, 66, 67, 104
Ruby, R., 375
Rupp, R., 373, 374
Russell, A. F., 319, 320
Rutherford, S. D., 359
Rybak, L. P., 107

Sachs, O., 359
Said, F., 381
Sakai, C. S., 85, 86, 87

Salamy, A., 39
Salicylates, 93
Salthouse, T., 386
Sanders, D., 357
San Diego County Fair Hearing Survey (1948), 377
Saunders, G. H., 417
Savage, H., 288
SCAN (Screening Test for Auditory Processing Disorders), 431
Schein, J. D., 144
Schloss, M. D., 51
School-aged population, hearing disorders in, 143-145
Schools, speech-language pathologists as case managers in, 351-352
School system, use of assistive listening devices in, 285-286
  auditory trainers, 286
  personal FM systems, 286-287, 288
  use of environmental microphones, 287-288
Schow, R. L., 157, 158, 159, 160, 251, 289, 357
Schubert, E. D., 183
Schuknecht, H. F., 88, 375, 376
Schum, D., 282, 283, 287
Schwaber, M., 418
Schwartz, D., 150
Schwartz, R., 150
Schweitzer, V. G., 89, 90
Scott, B. L., 320
Screening
  vs. identification, 142
  procedures, 148-156
  program, prerequisites of, 142-147
  programs for older adults, 156-160
  state laws pertaining to hearing, 141-152
  techniques and practices, in infants and young children, 106-109
  tests, 145-147
  universal, of newborns, 109
Seigel, D., 381
Sekular, R., 382
Self-Assessment for Communication (SAC), 158, 159, 167-169
Selters, N. A., 84
Senescence, 373. *See also* Elderly
Sensitivity, of screening test, 146-147
Sensorineural hearing loss, 58, 78, 175, 184
  perinatal causes of, 58, 63-64
  postnatal causes of, 58, 62, 65-68
  prenatal causes of, 58-62
  screening for, 144-145, 146
Sensory aids, 311, 329-330
  and communication of acoustic environment, 313-316
  successful users of, 328-329
  team approach to, 312-313
  training and rehabilitation for, 325-329
  See also Cochlear implants; Tactile aids

Sensory impairment
  intervention in, 207
  test results of, 206-207
Sentence tests, used to test speech under-
  standing, 185
Sequelae, 52
Sertoma, 363
Service organizations, for funding of people
  with hearing impairments, 363-364
Severe hearing loss, 176
Shadden, B., 157
Shanas, E., 377
Shanks, J. E., 189
Shannon, R. V., 324
Shaw, E., 373
Shea, D. R., 144
Shepard, N., 89, 90
Sherrick, C. E., 316, 326
Shimon, D., 225
Shirinian, M., 289, 379
Shore, I., 246, 378
Short Increment Sensitivity Index (SISI), 199
Sickle cell anemia, 98
  audiologic test results, 98-99
Siekevitz, P., 432
Siemens Hearing Instruments, 2, 319
Sierra-Irizarry, B., 202
Signal-to-noise ratio, assistive listening devices
  to improve, 289
Signal transmission, for alerting devices, 301
  FM airborne system, 302-303
  FM line carrier, 301-302
  hardwired connection, 301
Silverman, S. R., 185
Simmons, F. B., 8, 97, 144, 145, 321
Sitton, A. B., 252
Ski*Hi Language test, 342, 343, 346, 347
Ski*Hi Model, 356
Skinner, M. W., 229, 320
Slager, R., 293, 295
Slataper, F., 382
Slater, S., 103, 106
Slope, sloping, 177
Smith, C., 339
Smith, I. M., 81, 84
Smoke detectors. *See* Alerting devices
Somers, M. N., 329
Sommer, A., 72
Sound pick-up, for alerting devices, 300
  direct electrical connection, 300-301
  inductive pick-up, 301
  microphone pick-up, 300
Speaks, C., 185, 201
Specificity, of screening test, 147
Speech
  and auditory skills, developing, 346-347
  cued, 372
  effect on, of adults with acquired hearing
    losses, 356

link between hearing and, 337-341
low-pass filtered, 200
Speech awareness threshold (SAT), 132
Speech detection threshold (SDT), 132, 179-180
Speech discrimination ability, in elderly, 378
Speech discrimination testing, 182, 183-184
Speech-language pathologists
  as case managers in schools, 351-352
  role of, in cochlear implants, 355-356
  services provided by, to adults with acquired
    hearing losses, 356-357
Speech noise, 186
Speech perception, degraded, in elderly, 378-380
Speech Perception in Noise (SPIN) test, 185, 387
Speechreading, 160, 312, 327-328, 329
  for adults with acquired hearing losses, 357
Speech recognition (identification) testing, 182
  monosyllabic stimuli for, 183-185
Speech recognition threshold (SRT), 132,
  179-181, 419
Speech therapy, 160, 207
Speech understanding, tests of, 178-185
Sperduto, R., 381
Spitzer, J., 374
Spondees, 180-181
Spondee threshold, 181
SSPL90, 224-225, 246, 250-251
Staab, W., 225, 236, 292
Stach, B. A., 90, 145, 267, 274, 288, 379, 391
Staggered Spondaic Word Test (SSW), 201
Staller, S. J., 79, 84, 325
Stapedial reflex testing, 192-194
State programs, for people with hearing
  impairments, 362-364
Static admittance, 187, 189-191, 195
Staudt, M., 417
Stein, D., 347, 355
Stein, L. K., 65, 66
Stenger effect, 194-195
Stenosis, 42, 72
Stephens, S., 234
Sterling, G. R., 252
Sterritt, G. M., 113
Stevens, J. C., 322
Stevenson, E., 348
Stewart, J. M., 58, 144
Sticht, T., 379
Stimulus-frequency otoacoustic emissions
  (SFOAEs), 22
Stout, B., 356
Strauss, K., 297
Studebaker, G., 246
Sudden hearing loss, 97
  audiologic test results, 97
Summit, 317
Superior olivary complex, 28-29
Suprathreshold tests, 178, 182-185
Swimmer's ear, 44
Symbion/Richards, 329

Synthetic Sentence Identification (SSI) test, 185
  with contralateral competing messages (SSI-CCM), 201
  with ipsilateral competing messages (SSI-ICM), 98, 201
Synthetic sentences (SSI), 379
Syphilis, 59-60

Taba, H., 348
Tactaid I, 317
Tactaid II, 317-318, 320, 326
Tactaid VII, 318, 326
Tactile aids, 311, 316
  performance of, 318-321
  processing strategies and transducer design of, 317-318.
  See also Cochlear implants; Sensory aids
TAM, 317
Tangible reinforcement operant conditioning audiometry (TROCA), 111
Tardy, E. M., 41
Taylor, W., 405
Teacher Assessment of Grammatical Structure Test, 342-343
Tectorial membrane, 12
Teele, D. W., 46, 47, 49, 149-150
Teele, J., 149-150
Telecaption 4000, 298
Telecoil, 235-237, 291-292
Telecommunication devices, 266, 290
  for the deaf (TDDs), 266, 295-297
  telephone, 290-297
  telephone amplifiers, 293-295
  television, 298
Telecommunications for the Disabled Act (1982), 236, 273
Tele-Consumer Hotline, 297
Telephone, 290-292
  amplifiers, 293-295
  text, 295-297
  training people with hearing losses to use, 297
Telesensory Systems, Inc., 106
Television, closed captioning on, 298
Television Decoder Act, 298
Temporal bone fractures
  longitudinal, 45-46
  transverse, 45-46, 67
Temporal patterning tasks, 422-423
Temporary threshold shifts (TTS), 403
Teranishi, R., 373
Test of Auditory Comprehension (TAC), 343
Test of Syntactic Abilities (TSA), 343
Text telephones. *See* Telecommunication devices for the deaf (TDD)
Thalamus, medial geniculate body of, 32
Tharpe, A. M., 40, 105
Thibodeau, L., 289

Thielemeir, M., 324
Thomas, M., 62
Thompson, G., 110, 132
Thompson, P. L., 92-95
Thorner, R. M., 147
Thornton, R. D., 320
3M/House single-channel implant, 321, 322, 325
Threshold tests, 178, 179-181
Tillman, T. W., 183, 267, 419
Tinnitus, 402
  subjective, 407
Tobey, E. A., 325
Tone-decay tests, 199
Tonndorf, J., 171
Tonotopic organization, 15-16, 27
TORCH infections, 59-62
Total communication treatment program, 350
Townsend, P., 377
Toxoplasmosis, 59
Training, for screening program, 148-149
  personnel and, 148
  sample, 164-165
Trammel, J., 343
Transient evoked otoacoustic emissions (TEOAEs), 22, 24
Transverse temporal bone fractures, 45-46, 67
Traumatic fractures, 85
Trybus, R., 349
Tsai, H., 373
Tumors, audiometric evaluation of, 84
Turner, J., 382
Turner, R. G., 116
Tye-Murray, N., 325, 339
Tyler, R. S., 324, 325, 356
Tympanic membrane, perforations of
  in adults, 73-74
  in children, 45
  from otitis media, 53
Tympanogram(s), 146, 187-192, 205
  gradient, 191-192
  Type Ad (deep), 190
  Type As (shallow), 189-190
  Type B, 190
  Type C, 190
  width (TW), 191-192
Tympanometry, 112, 130-131, 158, 187, 195
Tympanosclerosis, 74
  from otitis media, 54
Tympanostomy tube insertion, for otitis media, 56-57

Uncomfortable loudness level (UCL), 185
Unilateral sensorineural hearing impairment, 144-145
Unisensory approach, 348
U.S. Public Health Service, 377-378
Universal screening, 109
Upfold, L. J., 234

Validity, of screening test, 146
Vanderbilt/Veterans Administration (VA)
  consensus statement, 221, 241, 246-247, 251
  Hearing Aid Conference, 246
van Rooij, J., 357
Van Tassel, D., 238, 241, 282, 283, 287
Vash, C., 360
Ventry, I., 158, 380, 381, 392
Vernadakis, A., 383
Vernix, 109
Vernon, M., 358, 359, 360, 361
Verrillo, R. T., 316
Vestibular schwannoma, 79, 208
  alternative approaches to, 82
  classification of, 79-80
  detection and treatment of, 81-82
  follow-up care for, 82-83
  with neurofibromatosis syndrome, 80-81
  sporadic, 80
  surgical procedures for, 82
Veterans Administration, 384. See also
      Vanderbilt/Veterans Administration
Villchur, E., 150
Viral infections
  postnatal, 62
  prenatal and perinatal, 59-62
Visual reinforcement audiometry (VRA),
      110-111
Visual reinforcement operant conditioning
      audiometry (VROCA), 111
Vocational rehabilitation, 363

Walden, B. E., 246, 357, 380
Wall, L. G., 71, 141, 148, 149, 150, 151, 289
Walton, W. K., 151
Warchol, M. E., 35
Waters, G. S., 94
Watson, T., 342, 343, 346, 347
Wayner, D., 254
Weaver, M., 79, 84
Weber, B. A., 110
Weber, H., 113
Weber, J., 339
Weber test, 194-195, 205, 207, 208
Webster, D. B., 104
Webster, M., 104
Wedderburn, D., 377

Weikart, D., 348
Weinstein, B., 158, 380, 381, 392
Weinstein, S., 316
Weisenberger, J. M., 311, 313, 314, 316,
      318-319, 320, 321, 327
Weisleder, P., 34-35
Welling, D. B., 79, 81-82, 84
Welsh, L., 376, 379
Welsh, R., 103, 106
Wernick, J., 232, 234
West, J., 339
White, K. R., 105, 106, 108
White, T., 380
Widen, J. E., 110, 111
Wigstrom, H., 432
Wilkening, R. B., 60
Willeford, J. A., 416, 424
Williams, C., 389
Williams Sound PockeTalker, 268
Williams-Steiger Occupational Safety and
      Health Act (1970), 67
Williston, J. S., 196
Wilson, B. S., 322, 329
Wilson, W. R., 132, 151
Windle, J., 356
Wingfield, A., 379, 387
Withrow, F. B., 252
Wolf, E., 382
Word Intelligibility by Picture Identification
      (WIPI) test, 127, 133, 184
World Federation of the Deaf, 360
World's Fair (1939), 377
Wright, L. B., 107
Written Language Syntax Test, 343

Yacullo, W., 237
Yakovlev, P. I., 417
Yantis, P., 171
Yanz, J. L., 388
Yarington, C. T., Jr., 95, 96
Yellin, M. W., 103, 113

Zabrow, A., 389
Zarnoch, J., 380
Zeta Noise Blocker, 241. See also Noise
      reduction circuits
Zikk, D., 375
Zrull, M. C., 31

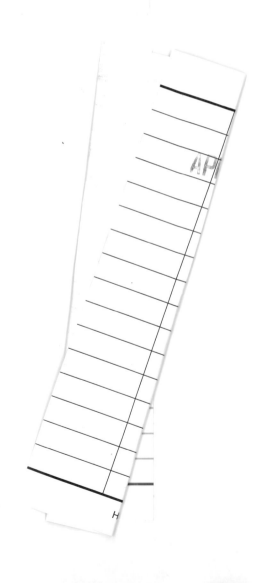